HUMAN DEVELOPMENT IN INDIA

HUMAN DEVELOPMENT IN INDIA

Volume–1

Cross-National Perspective and Profiles

Edited by

B. Suresh Lal

SERIALS PUBLICATIONS

NEW DELHI (INDIA)

First Published – 2009

ISBN: 978-81-8387-244-7

Published by

SERIALS PUBLICATIONS
4830/24, Prahlad Street, Ansari Road
Darya Ganj, New Delhi-110002 (India)
Phone : 23245225 Fax : 91-11-23272135
E-mail: serials@satyam.net.in

CONTENTS

EDITOR'S NOTE

The two volume study on "Human Development in India" is mainly based on empirical studies by researchers, who have zeal to present the issues from a new angle.

The first volume contains perspectives collected from different states in India as well as cross-national perspectives. The first study on capacity approach to human development emphasizes Amartya Sen's concept of development as freedom and some of the cross-country studies are also based on this theme. In line with the above theme, some of the studies deal with the emerging issues in social sector, especially in the educational field and health care. Another theme that had been often debated is the role of information technology in the era of globalization and this aspect had been covered by some of the studies in this volume. Another stand of studies encompasses the experiences of African countries in lieu of their uneven development such as poverty, drought and often human development concerns.

Studies on Gender and Subaltern Dimensions have been intermingled together in the second volume on human development. These studies are primarily intended to throw more light on the alteration of the livelihood patterns of tribals due to the development paradigm adopted in the country. A significant number of studies reveal the deficiencies of the present delivery systems in improving capabilities of poor and disadvantaged groups either in the attainment of education or receiving good health care. The role of self-help groups in enhancing entrepreneurial ability among women is another theme, besides other aspects like NGO's activities is fostering rural development and joint forest management. Research contributions from hitherto less researched areas like North-Eastern states figure in this volume.

Volume-1
Cross-national Perspectives and Profiles

Gopala Krishna Studies capability approach to human development. According to him, human development refers to a long and healthy life, to acquire knowledge and have a decent standard of living, the author opined that human development is as old as Aristotle. Amartya Sen's human capability approach focuses on the ability of human beings to lead lives they have reason to value and enhance their substantive choice. It has direct relevance to the well being and freedom of people, influences economic production and social change. He argues that absence of human capabilities represents poverty. Human development approach of Sen categorically states that development is not merely confined to the acquisition of wealth but is also about the enhancement of freedoms or choices. It primarily focuses on health, food and education.

Rattan Chand analyzed intra-state, inter-state and rural-urban disparities in house hold consumption expenditure during the period of 1973-2000 in his article "Inequality in Household Consumption Expenditure" using Gini-Coefficient, monthly per capita consumption expenditure (MPCE) of bottom, 30 percent and top 30 percent people in rural and urban areas, coefficient of variation (C.V), ratio of rural expenditure in total MPCE based on the NSS data. An attempt was also made to elicit changes that took place in the composition of expenditure on food and non-food items and among food items the trends in MPCE. It was shown that inequalities in MPCE declined in rural areas of 15 states during the period and no such decline was noticed in the urban areas in all the 15 states: In two states- Assam and Tamil Nadu, inequalities increased. Inter-state disparities shown a decline during 1973-94 but increased in 2000. MPCE has increased in all states. Though Rural-Urban disparities remained same at national level, they increased in seven states and declined in eight states. It is observed in the study that the proportion of expenditure on food items decreased and that on Non-food items increased in rural as well urban areas. It is also observed that there is a change in the expenditure on food items. The share of cereals in the food basket declined and the share of milk, vegetables, meat, fish increased in all the states except in the rural areas of Assam, Bihar, Orissa and West Bengal.

It may be concluded that Rattan Chand succeeded in successfully using NSS data in analyzing the disparities in MPCE. The study would have been strengthened if an attempt was made to analyze changes in rural-urban disparities in MPCE and changes in composition in expenditure on food and non-food items in relation to economic development.

In the study on Demographic Transition and Food Security in South Asia: Some Policy Options. The author **Faladra K. Sudan** analyzed the status of food security in South Asian Countries-India, Pakistan, Bangladesh, Nepal and Sri Lanka. In the beginning an attempt was made to explain how balance between population and food is achieved by using Malthusian, Anti Malthusian and Neo-Malthusian views of "Demographic Transition Theory". In the latter part of the article, trends in population growth and increase in the food production were analyzed to show that these countries are moving towards food crisis and going to get into population-environment-food trap by heavy population growth. The study rightly suggested that, to over ride this problem, focus should be on population control and increasing food production on one hand and even distribution of food supplies and protecting the efficiency and quality of environment on the other. There is scope for detailed study of the adverse impact of over population and over exploitation of natural resources by rich people on the environment and resultant impact on food production.

V. Vijayalakshmi analyzed the green consumerism and corporate sector responsibility in the current globalised scenario. She explained the nexus between consumer sovereignty and corporate social responsibility to facilitate sustainable development. She discussed the role of citizen consumers in providing food security to the poor. She insists that in the context of potentials and pitfalls of globalization it is necessary to build alternative identities arising from conscientious consumption. Responsible consumption and empowerment of the rural poor is needed to achieve optional and sustainable production. She concluded that global economic integration is neither a panacea nor a curse. It can't be halted but definitely altered to advance prosperity and values.

T. Pathinathan and others examine the various reasons for school dropouts through a mathematical approach with the help of fuzzy models (FRM). They foresee the people of the country as its real wealth and the basic purpose of development is primarily meant to enlarge the human freedoms. The people in the process become the beneficiaries of such development and also the agents of the progress and change that it brings about. Underlying the importance of literacy helps them to become knowledgeable which helps them to realize their full potential. They correlate the relations between the parent and children of dropouts using fuzzy relational maps. Authors identify the gap between the rich and poor widens day by day and the earning capacity of the poor decreases tremendously. Because of competitive market forces, the cost of living goes up along with the cost of good education, resulting in an increase in inequality, exploitation, unethical things in society and causing negative impact on income, as well as employment opportunities and freedom.

Naresh Singh examines the teledoc project for health care in India. Human health is an important indicator of the development of the nation. Further it is very important for the attainment of the twin developmental goals of poverty reduction and economic growth. He feels that the project is delivering low-cost immediate health care to rural people at affordable rates with service motto.

Madhan Mohan Upadhyay studies the participative model of organizational development in government. The author focuses on the importance of organization development (OD) strategies to help the development of government agencies in a systematic way. There are three popular OD models.

Participative model is a help to common and gross root people to have transparency and accountability on various schemes and programs sponsored by central and state government to uplift the needy and poor people.

Anil Kumar and Geeta Khurana analyzed the trends in productivity of labor and capital in dairy industry in India during pre and post reform periods. They used Measurement of productivity Growth Model for their study. They revealed in their study that the Indian dairy sector at aggregate and disaggregate levels i.e. state levels registered increasing growth in labour productivity during post-liberalisation period in comparison with pre-liberalisation period. They concluded that growth of capital productivity at both aggregate and disaggregate level did not respond well during liberal environment. They suggested adopting human resource management practices, modern technology, productivity linked reward system and encouragement to rural youth to improve the labour productivity.

Ezhil Jasmine examines the performance of tea industry in the country. In India no house is an exception in taking tea. The study shows that there is a strong correlation between tea drinkers and producers and it is part and parcel life of Indians. The author feels that growth of tea production is appreciable, Assam and Tamilnadu are the two states dominating in tea production. Though India got first place in the world in tea production, compound annual growth rate of exports is negative in India. High cost of production is a fundamental problem of tea industry. If the industry can cutout it's cost of production, it would lead to earning of foreign exchange by way of exports and providing employment opportunities to local people.

To achieve inclusive growth objectives of 11th five year plan, the author **Alpana Vats** emphasized the importance of financial inclusion of a large section of people in the article on Promoting Financial Inclusion. An analysis of the role of Banks, using 55th round NSSO data, the author proved that the delivery systems of formal financial sector has not reached poor and down trodden people despite several schemes being launched for the betterment of the poor and down trodden and they have been made to depend on informal sector. Analyzing the data of banks in this regard, the author proved the failure of the banks even to adhere to the norms fixed by RBI to maintain CDR. The analysis presented the experiences and measures taken by various countries, especially of the Bangladesh, to achieve the aim of financial inclusion. The author stressed the importance of micro finance and suggested banks to think out side the box in reaching that section of the people who constitute the Bottom of Pyramid. Banking with low income people is also commercially profitable.

In the lengthy article "Impact of Information and Communication Technology (ICT) on E-Governance" **M. Chakraborthy** has explained the use of information and communication Technology (ICT) and its impact on E-Governance by defining Governance as a process of collecting, using, supplying information so as to achieve desired goals. The importance of information, the role of technology in collecting processing, using and supplying information and the multiple benefits that can be derived by using various forms of ICT, different steps involved in employing ICT have been explained vividly. No doubt ICT has crept into all aspects of individual and social activities and things are getting done speedily with ICT. But the matter of concern of an average citizen is irregularities and ill activities, they have also increased with the same speed with the use of ICT. Negative aspects of the use of IT need to be analyzed so as to enable application of ICT in all needy fields without the fear of negative consequences of using ICT.

Pradeep Nair emphasizes that community economic development depends. on electronic communication technologies it has become a potent force in transforming social, economic and political life globally. E-commerce is a dominating business system in information age. It reduces cost, inventory process and delivers on time. Electronic commence has given way to businesses like e-money(ATM), on line demand, entertainment, music and movies , medical care, to name a few among the various uses to which it is being utilized.

T. Karthikeyan & others studied impact of globalization on branding self help group products the role of women in a developing society like India has been tremendous in recent times and it is the status of women that guides the destiny of a nation. In this paper authors examine the impact of branding on SHG's products. In India lot of production and marketing activities are taking place in rural areas by SHG's. If SHG products are branded it becomes easy for identification and differentiation. The same we could find in NGO SEWA where the branding of products avoids duplication, and creates markets in rural areas. It also results providing in employment opportunities and improving standard of living and curb poverty.

B. Sripirabaa & Krishnaveni emphasized a comparative study of the capacity assessment of organization capacity building is one of the methodologies available for managers to assess and build the capabilities of organizations. This concept has been used by non-profit organizations. Authors considered POET to assess and enhance organizational capacity, so that all the organizations work in a meaningful way and assess their on time achievements of goals in development process. Authors try to compare various tools that are available for measuring and building the capacity of organizations.

Yogesh Ranjit studies in detail the various forest policies and legislations in India & Nepal. He has given a historical account from Pre-British government i.e. before 1757 to joint forest management guidelines formulated in 2002 in India and from Pre-Unification of Nepal i.e. before 1768 to community forestry in Nepal. In a both countries the author covered ancient time policies as well as modern time policies and guidelines in a detailed manner. The author further examines that as the demand for food, forest products and land for settlement increases, the productivity function of forest dominates its protective function, so that both sides of the people and government started over exploitation of forest and forest resources. As a result environmental degradation and ecological imbalance pervades at local, regional and national levels. He suggested that people's participation and favorable policies lead to better forest protection management, its optimal use and sustainable development in both the countries.

Shaista Alam & others studied openness, stock market development fostering factor productivity growth in Pakistan. The study provides that openness to trade and stock market development have a long run equilibrium relationship with total factor productivity growth. They examined the empirical findings that lend support to the above hypothesis. For the openness and stock market development are among the key determinants of total factor productivity growth. Further this study suggests that stock market development facilitates productivity growth by reducing the incremental cost of external capital.

Shankar Chatterjee & Jayasree studied development of African countries would depends on the control measures of various societal issues like militants' problems, illiteracy, civil war, corruption, women problem, aids, sexual violence etc. Many countries in Africa are facing the above problems inspite of its rich resources and labour intensive technology.

Ravinder Rena studies challenges for research development in Eritrea. Research is a scientific investigation for new facts of knowledge. The paper is broadly divided into five sections. The paper reveals that Eritrea is a developing country in Africa and its main occupation is agriculture and allied activities. But its contribution to GDP is very low because of lack of technologies and innovations, lack of high yielding varieties, traditional cultivation, no encouragement to research and development and lack of resources. As a whole the country is lacking young researchers. Thus it could be said that there is an urgent need to have a policy that takes into account priority for research and other basic needs of research of the society so that development could take place rapidly

In his study "Poverty Alleviation Measures In Eritrea: A country Located In North East Africa" **Shankar Chatterjee** tried to establish the effectiveness of the SMCP (Savings and Micro Credit Programme), a programme in the direction of eradicating poverty in Eritrea-an infant independent country in Africa, with empirical evidences.

D.V. Madhusudhan Rao and Shankar Chatterjee explained the industrial development in Eritrea during post liberation era. This study reveals that after liberation of Eritrea, the more medium and large scale manufacturing establishments are being established every year. This provides more employment opportunities and eradication of poverty which is 66 percent in the country.

The authors **Arshad and Rahaman** in their study 'Drought in Saharan Eritrea! Socio economic consequences attempted to study the impact of drought on Eritrea. In the first part of the study the meaning of drought and its magnitude were explained and the consequences of drought with empirical evidences were analyzed. It was established that drought is a recurring phenomena, due to its climatic condition in Eritrea. The livelihoods of Eritreans remain vulnerable due to severe crop failure, loss of livestock and asset depletion as eighty percent of populations depend on agriculture. Drought results in a vicious cycle of socio-economic impacts. In view of recurrence phenomena and devastating effects of drought, the development of non agriculture sector as an alternative sources of employment was suggested on one hand and conservation of water by micro dams, digging water wells etc., encouraging allied activities, particularly poultry and dairy on the other along with institutional and policy frame work.

In the article Eritrean trade with Italy in post independence period–analytical study, its author **Ravinder Rena** explained the importance of and factors responsible for trade between Eritrea and Italy and trends in the trade. Instead of looking for foreign assistance, recognizing the importance of the foreign trade and investment for country's economic development, Eritrea attempted to develop trade relations with it neighboring countries especially with Italy. Colonial historic background of Eritrea, existing conditions of its economy, its geo-economic strategic location to make possible entry to other part of the world etc., are the main factors influencing trade between these two countries. Italy made an imperialist entry into Eritrea and made Eritrean its colony. To continue imperialist exploitation in new form, to continue its hold on Eritrean resources it is necessary for Italy to trade with Eritrea. In view of this observation, it is desirable to analyze the positive impact of trade with Italy on Eritrean economy, in the post independence period.

Shankar Chatterjee's probe that a majority of women in Eritrea do not have independent house hold activities and they are in poverty is the basis for his article. In contrast government has initiated saving and micro credit programme (SMCP) that has brought a change in the quality of life of the beneficiaries, not only benefiting them economically but they are now socially and culturally advanced. They have self–confidence to mange an enterprise, where the mind is without fear and head is held high.

Hakeem Ijaiya has studied discrimination against female children, such as female genital mutilation, born out of wedlock, early marriages, child abuses and exploitation are common practices in many parts of Nigeria. Female Genital Mutilation (FGM) is a most inhuman practice in the country. The age of mutilation varies from 3 months to 17 years. As a result many female children are facing serious health risks including HIV infection due to unhygienic problems. The author feels that the government should create awareness on the rights of the female children in Nigeria. There should be a modality for the protection of the rights and help to meet their basic needs, expand their opportunities to reach potentials.

Volume-2
Gender and Subaltern Dimensions

R. Venkata Ravi & V. Narayana Reddy emphasis women's participation in development, which bring their concerns for developmental activities and decision-making regarding societal issues. Women elected in PRIs are playing a pivotal role in the implementation of various programmes and schemes to various sections of people. On the other hand downtrodden women have not been involved in any decision making process and women from upper caste have not shown interest to work under leadership of lower caste women. This study suggests that elected women in PRIs need support of their family members, prior political experience and capacity to convince others.

Nirmala & Dhulasi Birinda in their study "Welfare of Indian Women and Children: Responsibility of Politicians" explained that for improving the welfare of the society, focus needs to be on the welfare of the women and children who are integral part of the society and the economy. It was stated that due to lack of political will and irresponsibility of political parties and politicians, several programmes intended for the welfare of women and children have been jeopardized in implementation. It is suggested that for the betterment of women and children and better functioning of our democratic system, political parties and politicians are to be made accountable to people and their presence should be restricted in all fields whenever it is found that their role is not necessary.

Avishek Hazara & others examine domestic environment and women's health in a study of northeast India. Any undesirable change in the physical, chemical or biological component of the environment can cause harmful effects on various forms of life while indoor pollution affects the health of women. In rural area a majority people used wood, crop residues, dung cakes, coal lignite, charcoal and kerosene as means of cooking and lighting. As a result it affects the women's health in causing respiratory diseases, eye irritation and headache. Further it affects the neural systems of women.

Lal Suresh & Priyamvada have studied health conditions of tribal women. Generally tribal people are living in remote and geologically diverse climate areas and modern medicine has not been accepted as essential to their functioning by most of tribes. This paper examines the relationship between education and health care; more the education levels less the ill health. A majority of women are facing the problem of anemia. Biological and socio-economic factors are highly responsible for high fertility in tribes, infant and maternal mortality rates per 1000 population being 103 and 5 to 8 respectively in India and AP. Authors feel that tribal women are facing different health problems due to lack of health facilities and lack of awareness.

Women's entrepreneurship has a significant role in achieving employment of women, there by achieving the objective of economic development with social justice. Women in India were degraded to lower position in social political and economic spheres from a higher position which they enjoyed earlier. By implementing the various programmes to promote women entrepreneurship and thereby achieve economic self reliance of women, a little progress was made. A concrete and comprehensive set of action is needed to make the desired progress. This is the analysis of **Niraj Kumar** in his Article "Woman Entrepreneurship in Rural Areas".

Soumitra Sarkar examines the issue of mushroom cultivation by women having microfinance as a tool of socio-economic development and poverty alleviation in most of rural areas in general in India and West Bengal in particular. The author feels that rural women who are in below poverty line have joined in self help groups (SHGs) starting different economic activities earning money. This helps them to take independent decisions at their work place and it leads to a better position for them at home. It also represents hopes and dreams of the deprived women enterprising for the creation of a social environment which is free of inequalities and provides them economic space to participate actively in the development process. The study covers women entrepreneurs chosen from six districts in West Bengal where SHG & SGSY group women actively are engaged in mushroom cultivation. These women needed more training for scientific cultivation and they also require financial marketing support from Government.

In the article on Self-Help Groups and Non-Convention products: A study of Micro Enterprises in North Bengal" **Sumithra Sarkar** has demonstrated that Micro enterprises taken up by women Self Help Groups in Non-Conventional economic activities are profitably moving ahead in North Bengal, showing a positive impact on rural women. He suggested extension of support from Governments, NGOs and people for a better future of micro enterprises in the field of Non-Conventional Products, run by SHGs

Sritharan & Rajkumar's analysis on the brand of commodities and consumers preferences or commitment to particular brand in the article "a study on the Brand Loyalty among women" explained what brand loyalty is and what factors influence the consumers to be loyal to the brand of a commodity. The study revealed that young age group, lower income group consumers are more loyal to a brand. An increase in the prices beyond a certain limit would lead to a decline in the demand for a brand. Direct relationship with consumers, assurance; of quality are key aspects in maintaining the brand loyalty in the long run.

M. Arun Kumar traces tribal women participation in local bodies, women in tribal society play a vital role in their social, cultural, economic and religious ways of life and are considered as an economic asset in their society. But still they are lagging far behind in the different walks of life like education, employment, good health. Tribal women's participation in panchayat raj institutions will help to foster a new image of women who can come into politics themselves and perform independently. In contrast there are many hurdles in the process of empowering women. In order to overcome the hurdles women need education, awareness and boldness.

D. C. Nanjunda & M. Annapurna In their article on "Combating Child Labour Listen What Employers Say" attempted to establish that inspite of various constitutional provisions, laws and prohibitions preventing employers from employing child labour in work, the problem of child labour is increasing day by day. The problem of child labour was analyzed with a new angle from employers' point of view. They suggested proper understanding of the nexus between poverty child labour's families and educational programmes and linking of poverty eradicating programmes with educational programmes to curb the child labour system. There is scope for some more analysis in the light of 93rd constitutional amendment which made primary education a fundamental right of children. This has a link with child labour problems. The problem of child labour is likely to increase if the right to primary education is not safeguarded. The question of debate here is who has to take the responsibility of safeguarding this right, the state or parents of children living in poverty?

K. M. Naidu & others discussed the social sector growth in India and allocation among states focusing on Andhra Pradesh. The status of expenditure on education, enrolment and dropouts and expenditure on health has been analyzed. They gave suggestions for judicious growth, like allot by more resources for education and health, decreasing the dropout rates particularly among girls, free coaching, imparting skill oriented education strengthening the base of primary education, improving rural health services, more involvement of Panchayat Raj institutions in health and education and coordination of public sector and private sector in the proper implementation of health programmes in Andhra Pradesh.

In the study "Impact of Joint Forest Management on Ecological Sustainability and Related Issues: A comparative study of Jahubug and Mandla Districts of Madya Pradesh" the investigators **R. Singh and S P. Singh** attempted to assess the impact of Joint Forest Management (JFM) system on the sustainability of eco-system of regional level where JFM system is being practiced in two ways; one, by analyzing changes in the habitat in terms of forest coverage to show the sustainability of the habitat and two, by analyzing variations in the population of domestic animals for sustainability of Biological life cycle. With empirical evidences, the study concluded that the JFM programmes have short-run impact in terms of enhanced access to resources. Doubts have been raised about long-run positive impact of JFM on regional eco-system. The study suggested alternative policy in view of population pressure on resources and nitration of forest protection programmes with development programmes in tribal villages.

In the study "Intensive Forest Protection and Expected Benefits. A Case of Western Ghats of Tamilnadu". The authors **Subramanian & Others** analyzed Topography, Geology and Soil, Climate and Rainfall conditions in Gudalur Range and Meghamalai Range of Theni Forest Division in Tamil Nadu. The study showed that there is a decline in the study area Meghamalai Wildlife Sanctuary is created to protect wild life and diverse fauna and flora of the area but it is being disturbed by local tribal people for their livelihood.

Ram Krishna Mandal, studies herbs in Arunachal Pradesh, economic viability and sustainability. A majority of the word's medicinal flora is found in Himalayan ranges of India, Arunachal Pradesh comes under Himalayan belt. It is covered with more geographical area as forest. Many rare herbs are being grown in this state. All types of herbs are not in records and more studies are to be conducted to find these medicinal plants and necessary steps are to be taken to make viability and sustainability of herbs to protect biodiversity. AP state is developing day by day and needs of people are increasing and its impact on urbanization, area of cultivation, shifting cultivation, population growth, transportation, and industrialization are responsible for the deforestation of the herbal flora/wealth in Arunachal pradesh.

M. Romesh Singh studied the relevance and implications of Tribal development policy in Manipur. He reviewed the development schemes implemented in tribal areas of Manipur, role of development institutions in tribal areas and tribal unrest and tribal development. He revealed that most of the various development schemes implemented through different agencies for socio economic development of tribals have failed to serve the real purpose due to many constraints. There are no separate planning and development strategies for tribals in hill areas and plain areas though there are differences in socio-economic growth between them. The tribals in plain areas are well advanced than tribals in hill areas. So, he advised separate allocation of funds and development strategies for the tribals living in plain and hill areas for a justified distribution of development benefits and to protect the due share of the poor tribals living in hill areas.

Prasant Kumar Acharya has studied the development of Primitive Tribal Group (PTG) project established in Orissa in the article "Monitoring and Education of Micro projects Established for Tribal Development in Orissa". This study stressed the importance of Monitoring and Evaluation of the projects for effectiveness and achievement of desired results.

The study concluded that the existing system of Monitoring and Evaluation of Micro project is not planned with regard to the time aspects, indicators, methods and process of data collection and lacked mechanism for operationlizing participatory monitoring. Hence it suggests the integration of appraisal, the monitoring and evaluation activities by setting up only one state level cell.

T. Prabhakar Reddy and V. Ramesh have studied the legal issues of tribal land alienations where, tribes are being exploited for centuries by forest people and non-tribes of their area. They state that there were many commissions set up to look into the grass root level issues but they have not been able to perform the job as was expected and instead they were servicing the interests of non-tribes which has also contributed to the skewed land alienations in tribal areas. Authors also argue that various laws and regulations are passed to safeguard the tribal's interest but the situation still remains same. It shows that there are gaps in existing laws i.e., from 1839 (British Administration) to 1 of 1970 and LTR / Acts. They suggested that changes made in LTR should be implemented immediately. All the pending land disputes should be settled at the earliest.

Y. Nilachandra Singh examines the poverty as a determinant of the of living standard in Mizoram with reference to Maimit district. He has taken into account two parameters i.e. sum total house hold expenditure (STHE) and per capita house hold expenditure (PCHE).for that he has selected 400 Mizo respondents and 200 each from Chakmas and Tuikuks belonging of various age groups, socio-economic conditions and other demographi aspects. Mizos are urban and rural staying while chakmas and tuikuks are more rural oriented. Their main occupation is shifting cultivation. He also examines that mizos are very advanced socio-economically than the chakmas and tuikuks. STHE and PCHE are more in mizos than in chakmas and tukiks. Because of low literacy lack of exposure to external world and rural chakmas and tuikuks have low STHG &PCHE in mamit district of Mizoram State.

The paper of **Mousumi Roy** studies agrarian development and employment scenario in post-reform era in West Bengal.

Reforms helped to improve the growth of GDP, but there is a negative impact on employment of labour. In agricultural sector, the negative impact is more on rural households, where employment opportunities have not been concentrated. This condition is prevailing in entire West Bengal's rural packets. Government should take initiation to provide different employment programs to utilize rural people potentiality for economic development of state and country.

Patil Vijay R. studies the farmer's suicides in Maharastra, agriculture is a biological industry and still a way of life of the people in India. In globalization era farmers are committing suicides because of various reasons such as debt, mono-cropping systems, spurious seeds, high cost of pest and fertilizers, apart from cost of production increasing. As per author's investigation in Maharastra, moneylender, mortgage, decline in yield, lack of irrigation, drought, lack of credit facilities from banks are the main causative factors for formers' suicides.

D. Rajasenan analysed the Kerala Model of Fisheries Development and indigenous fishermen's responses. He discussed the crises in the fishing industry, impact of modernization and changing paradigms of marine fishery conservation. He concluded that the modernization process of the fishery through technology resulted in overcapitalization and the concomitant fishery resources related problem. The traditional fishermen's response in the form of new technology not only accorded economic gains but also created an environment challenging the unwanted modern technological intrusion and regaining the lost control of the production process. He suggested for a small change in the policy paradigm favouring the traditional fishery and conservation.

Sitakanta Sethi & others discussed in their study NGOs as the third sector in development. They also discussed the need for the motivation of the students towards development actions and growing relevance of rural development management and research. They argued out case for a change in attitude and bahaviour towards the poorest of the poor both from the development administrators as well as young generation. By going to the rural areas, visiting the slums and sometimes interacting with the people belonging to these sections of society the development administration well on youth can change their attitude to a great extent. The scene of the paid and unpaid staff is not very much encouraging either to count NGO's work as a profession. In the line with globalization and liberalization, the third sector in development needs to be reformed in a number of areas in a professional manner with strong motivation. Missionary approach needs to be welcomed in this sector.

In view of failures and lags in effectively implementing various programmes in the various poverty alleviating and employment generating schemes which aimed at benefiting rural poor people, by government, government agencies and NGOs, the idea of participatory research, planning and action which aims at actively involving people, who are actual beneficiaries, in taking up various poverty eradicating programmes for effective results was analyzed in the article "Can Participatory Research, Planning and Action by Panchayat and NGOs Assure Rural people's Livelihood" by **Sitakant Sethi**. The author suggested that issues to be taken into account while adopting this approach, for better results. However it is desirable to assess the role played by NGOs with a truism that when Government itself is a voluntary organization and trustee of people what is the need to have NGOs.

Human development is a process of enlarging people's choices. The most critical ones are to lead a long and healthy life, to be educated and enjoy a decent standard of living. Additional choices include political freedom, guaranteed human rights and self-respect what Adam Smith called the ability to mix with others without being "ashamed to appear in publick". The inference drawn from the perusal of the papers presented in the two volumes clearly show that human development is a multidimensional concept and its level is influenced to a large extent by the performance of its various facets such as measures, initiatives and efforts by government and its agencies to promote human development under different social heads, such as the education, literacy, health, sanitation, housing, nutrition and other basic social services.

It is in this background that the present volume attempts to analyze and uncover various dimensions of human development such as the process, content, behaviour, gender, ethnic and other related dimensions. The contributors being from diverse disciplines, it is hoped that the volumes contribute to the scantly explored area of study of human development in India.

FOREWORD

The concept of human development is a process of enlarging people's choices. In principle, these choices can be infinite and can change over time. But at all levels of development, the three essential ones are for people to lead a long and healthy life, to acquire knowledge and to have access to the resources needed for a decent standard of living. Additional choices include political freedom, guaranteed human rights and personal self-respect. If these essential choices are not available, many other opportunities remain inaccessible. It is age old concept as civilization. Earlier economist observed that economic development measured in term of gross domestic product (GDP). More the volume of GDP per capita, higher the state of development, it means more the GDP, more the country's progress and prosperity. The concept of GDP completely ignores the well-being of the people.

Human development is the primary purpose of UNDP. The publication of annual Human Development Report, under the stewardship of Mahbub hl Haq, has stimulated many countries, including India, to launch Human Development Initiatives. The eighth Five Year Plan's ultimate goal was human development. There was a moment in 90s in India's history when major change of course in some basic economic policies was under way. That was a moment of hope and anxiety. It was a time when old certainties and dogmas have given way to an open-minded quest for policies that can work to improve the human condition of the people who live in this country. It is indeed a time for new ideas and bold innovations. The present edited volumes of Dr. B. Suresh Lal on "Human Development in India,

Volume-I: Cross-National Perspectives and Profiles & Volume-II: Gender and Subaltern Dimensions" is useful to critical understanding of dynamics of human development particularly women and tribes in a very unequal world social setting.

Dr. Lal, worked for these books, all the papers contained in this volumes, will be a valuable addition to the growing literature on this subject, by a variety of scholars on very wide ranging issues. That there are forty seven papers is both a challenging task but also a limitation as it is difficult to put all of them in a running theme. It has a rainbow character. What is common to all the papers is the concerns of the scholars on the unfolding social reality more so the women and tribal development experience.

The issues covered relate to human development This includes capability approach to human development, inequality in household consumption, food security, green consumerism, sustainable health care in rural India, trends in productivity of labour and capital in dairy industry, information & communication impact on e-governance, e-commerce and community economic development.

Forest policies and legislations, development of African countries, challenges for research development, poverty alleviation measure, industrial development, drought, trade and impact of micro credit among women in Eritrea, all these papers reveal maximum coverage of Eritrean issues in the country and each paper has a different emphasis. Other paper on human rights and gender discrimination is also focus on women problems in Nigeria.

The scholars who have touched gender and subaltern issues and its impact point out some of the concerns as to how the world is under the control of globalization and its affect on economies of transitional societies. These papers cover participation of women in development, welfare of Indian women and children, domestic environment and women's health, tribal women's health conditions, women entrepreneurs, women self help groups, brand loyalty among women, tribal women in local governance and combating child labour these are papers on women and health issues where privatization and coporatization of health is taking place very rapidly. Few papers cover the important areas like social sector infrastructure, joint forest management impact on ecological sustainability, intensive forest protection and expected benefits, herbals sustainability and economic viability, tribal development policy, monitoring and evaluation of micro project in tribal areas, issues of tribal land alienation, poverty determinants, agrarian development, factors affecting farmer's suicides, Kerala fisheries model, participatory research, planning and action by panchayath and non-governmental developmental initiatives. In nutshell all the papers compiled in this great little book discuss the societal issues and these papers put together are multi-dimensional and raise certain questions about core-issues of our society. The content and concerns are very relevant. That such a range of issues could be brought under a volume i.e, Human Development in India by Dr. Suresh Lal, young scholar is an accomplishment by itself. This is a new and refreshing experience.

PROF. SHAIK AHMED HUSSAIN
Keller Graduate School of Management
DeVry University, New York, USA

ACKNOWLEDGEMENTS

This book would not have been possible without the encouragement and support of many individuals and institutions. I along, with the contributors to the volume, owe a debt of gratitude to Serials publishers, New Delhi for giving me the task of editing. I am glad to thank Prof. Shaik Ahmed Hussain, DeVry University, New York, USA for foreword. Our special thanks to Prof. C. Siva Rama Krishna Rao and Prof. G. Srineevas Reddy, Kakatiya University. They offered continuous encouragement and extremely valuable inputs on these volumes. I am thankful to my friends and scholars Dr. M. Ravinder and AV Ramana for their encouragement, inspiration, at every stage. My family members also deserve my heartfelt thanks for working tirelessly round the clock providing all the logistic support to finish the job of editing.

1

CAPABILITY APPROACH TO HUMAN DEVELOPMENT: SOME REFLECTIONS

Gopalakrishna B. V.

Introduction

Till the sixties, economic growth was considered the principal objective of a government and per capita income is the most appropriate yardstick to measure human well-being. The experience of industrial economies in the postwar period indicates however that the benefits of rapid economic growth may not reach all segments of a country's population, under such circumstances, per capita income may not be a satisfactory indicator of the well-being of a country. The persistence of mass poverty even when income was rising was proof that the benefits of growth do not reach poor families without active state intervention. As a result there was a distinct change in the approach to development in the seventies and eighties[1].

Socio-economic development replaced economic growth as the focus of attention and fresh emphasis was placed on the concept of income distribution and equity. Several new measures of welfare and development were tried out and discarded–the Level of Living Index, The State of Welfare Index, The Quality of Life Index, the Physical Quality of Life Index etc. However since 90s, Human Development Index (HDI) has emerged as a universally accepted index of development.

Objectives of the Paper

The following are the objectives of the study:

1. To understand the conceptual clarification of human development, its growing importance and its foundation.
2. To focus on the Capability Approach to Human Development.
3. To perceive some reflections on the contours of Capability Approach to Human Development.

Concept of Human Development

Human development is a process of enlarging people's choices. In principle, these choices can be infinite and can change over time. But at all levels of development, the three essential ones are for people to lead a long and healthy life, to acquire knowledge and to have access to the resources needed for a decent standard of living. If these essential choices are not available, many other opportunities remain inaccessible.[2]

But human development does not end there. Additional choices, highly valued by many people, range from political, economic and social freedom to opportunities for being creative and productive and enjoying personal self-respect and guaranteed human rights.

Human development thus has two sides. One is the formation of human capabilities, such as improved health, knowledge and skills. The other is the use people make of their acquired capabilities–for productive purposes, for leisure or for being active in cultural, social and political affairs. If the scales of human development do not finely balance the two sides, much human frustration can result. Accordingly the concept of human development, income clearly is only one option that people would like to have, though certainly an important one. But it is not the sum-total of their lives. The purpose of development is to enlarge all human choices, not just income.

The concept of human development is much broader than the conventional theories of economic development. Economic growth models deal with expanding GNP rather than enhancing quality of human lives. Human resource development treats human beings primarily as a input in the production process–a means rather than an end Welfare approaches look at human beings as beneficiaries and not as agents of change in the development process. The basic needs approach focuses on providing material goods and services to deprived population groups rather than on enlarging human choices in all fields.

Human development also encompasses elements that constitute the critical issues of gender and development. There are four major elements–productivity, equity, sustainability and empowerment (HDR, 1995). Through enhanced capabilities, the creativity and productivity of people must be increased so that they become effective agents of growth. Economic growth must be combined with equitable distribution of its benefits. Equitable opportunities must be available to present and to future generation.

Human development goes beyond economic growth, but it is not anti-growth, from a human development perspective, economic growth is not an end in itself. Rather is a means to an end-enlarging people's choices. There is, however, no automatic link between income growth and human progress. In the short run, even in the absence of satisfactory economic growth, countries can achieve significant improvements in human development through well-structured public expenditure[3]. However, it is wrong to suggest that economic growth is unnecessary for human development. In the long run no sustained improvement is possible without growth (HDR 1990 & 1996).

Amartya Kumar Sen has defined Development in term of an expansion in capabilities and 'entitlement' capabilities refers to what a person can (not) do or can (not) be. Freedom from hunger, being free to participate in the political process, being adequately sheltered, access to health and education etc., can be quoted different manifestations of capabilities. His capability approach to human development would be discussed in the following pages.

Measuring of Human Development

It is easier to measure national income than human development. And many economists would argue that national income is a good indicator of human well being while there is evidently a strong relationship, since economic growth is an important means to human development, human outcomes do not depend on economic growth & levels of national income alone. They also depend on how these resources are used–whether for developing weapons or producing food, building palaces or providing clean water and human outcomes such as democratic participation in decision-making or equal rights for men & women do not depend on incomes.

The important human outcomes achieved in countries around the world, such as life expectancy at birth or under-five mortality rates, which reflect the capability to survive, or literacy rates, which reflect the capability to learn. They also include indicators on important means for achieving these capabilities, such as access to clean water and on equity in achievement, such as the gaps between men and women in schooling or political participation.

The traditional concept of planning focused on the expansion of production of goods and services and consequent growth in per capita income has been transformed to enhancement of human well-being. Well-being as an indicator of prosperity is measured on now the planned efforts have succeeded in providing better opportunities for people especially the deprived and those who are living below the normative minimal poverty line, to enjoy a productive and socially meaningful life. As the economic prosperity measured in terms of per capita income does not always ensure enrichment in quality of life reflected in broader dimensions of well being, it has to be measured using indicators such as Human Development Index (HDI), Gender Related Development Index (GDI), Human Poverty Index (HPI) and Technology Achievement Index (TAI) etc.

Human Development Index (Hdi)

The human development index constructed by the UNDP Human Development Report 1990 under the leadership of Mahabub ul Haq (of Pakistan) has derived roots from the writings of Amartya Sen as well as his personal advice to the UNDP. The publication of the human development report by the UNDP since 1990 vastly improved the empirical work related to the measurement of human development by constructing a number of development indices. Given the data constraints and the complexity involved in including many indicative variables, UNDP's approach has been to measure human development by focusing on three essential elements of human life–longevity, knowledge and decent living standards. Human development is defined as the process of enlarging people's choices, in order to enable them to lead a long and healthy life, to be educated and to enjoy a decent standard of living (UNDP, 1990). Since 1990, the HDR has published a composite index of human development called the Human Development Index (HDI) for several countries. The HDI is based on average achievements in the three basic dimensions namely longevity, knowledge and income of human development. Data pertaining to HDI components is collected from estimates reported by the United Nations and its agencies and by other internationally recognised organisations. HDI measures the average achievement in three basic dimensions of human development. Before calculating HDI, an index for each of the three dimensions is created. For this purpose, maximum & Minimum values are chosen for each indicator.

Foundations of Human Development

The human development is not a new invention. It is as old as the subject of Economics itself is. The idea that social arrangements must be judged by the extent to which they promote "human good" dates at least to Aristotle.

Aristotle (384–322 B.C.) argued "Wealth is evidently not the good we are seeking, for it is merely useful and for the sake of something else". He also distinguished between a good political arrangement from a bad one by its successes and failures in enabling people to lead "flourishing lives".

The tradition of treating human development as the real end of all activities was continued in *Kant* (1724–1804) who observed that "So act as to treat humanity. Whether in their own person or in that of any other, in every case an end without, never as a means only".

Adam Smith (1723–90) stated that economic development should enable a person to mix freely with others without being "ashamed to appear in public", while he was expressing a concept of poverty which went beyond counting calories and integrated the poor into the mainstream of the community. A similar strain was reflected in the writings of the other proponents of modern economic thought such as Robert Malthus, Karl Marx, and John Stuart Mill.

McCulloch (1967)–Asserted that human beings are the most important of all machines and every investment in their training and education is an "acquisition of the utmost consequence".

Schultz T.W.–has given three ratios in relation to education and economic growth.[4]

- Education–Labour Ratio- to show the amount of human effort going into education relative to the total labour force.
- Education–Income Ratio – which relates the resources entering into to consumer income.
- Education–Investment Ratio to show the relation between the resources entering into education and the resources going into reproducible physical capital.

The recent theories of human capital are focusing attention on endogenous growth, the origins of which are attributed to *Paul Romer* and *Robert Lucas* among other. Romer is of the view that technological progress is not an exogenous factor influencing development but the result of deliberate action taken in response to market incentives or a sociologists would hold that innovative approaches are adopted as a sequence to the process of education. One can note in this stand of thinking an approach to inter-disciplinarily will concern for change and innovation and its relationship with education.

Romer (1986), in the Endogenous Growth Theory highlights the fact that technological progress in not an exogenous factor influencing development but is the result of 'intentional actions' taken by people who respond to market incentives. Technology is considered to consist of a non-rival component, which being separate from individuals, can grow without bound and, therefore, leads to increasing returns to scale. Thus, private investment in Research and Development (R & D) raises the level of technology so that it acquires the nature of a public good.

Lucas (1988), another endogenous growth theorist who emphasise investment in human capital more directly and links it to long-term rates of economic growth. These human capital theories indicate how investment in education enables the entire production process to benefit from positive externalities. Educated people not only use technology more efficiently, they are also likely to innovate and spread the benefits of such innovation to co-workers thereby increasing the efficiency of all factors of production. The human capital theories attribute the lack of convergence between the growth rates in developed and developing countries to the fact that the poorer countries do not make adequate investments in human capital, which results in their recording low growth rates.

Nancy Stokey (1991) in her paper devises a model aimed at explaining growth phenomena such as that experienced by some successful new industrialized countries in East Asia, where rapid economic growth has been accompanied by higher volume of exports, rapid growth in education and rapid changes in the composition of output[5].

Growing importance of Human Development

Human Development is defined as the process of enlarging people's range of choices. The most critical of these wide ranging choices are to live a long and healthy life, to be educated and to have access to resources needed for a decent standard of living. Additional choices include political freedom, guaranteed human rights and personal self-respect (UNDP 1990).

Human development firstly focuses exclusively on the expansion of only one choice income, while the second embraces the enlargement of all human choices-whether economic, social, cultural or political. It might well be argued that the expansion of income can enlarge all other choices as of income can enlarge all other choices as well.[6]

According to Paul Streeten, human development is necessary on account of the following reasons[7].

1. It is the end while economic growth is only a means to this end
2. It is a means to higher productivity
3. It helps in lowering the family size by slowing human reproduction
4. Human development is good for physical environment. Deforestation, desertification and soil erosion decline when poverty declines.
5. Reduced poverty contributes to a wealthy civil society, increased democracy and greater social stability
6. Human development can help in reducing civil disturbances in a society and in increasing political stability.

The first human development report published in 1990 focussed on how growth failed to translate into improved human lives in many developing countries. The most critical human development indicators are–People to live a long and healthy life, to be educated and to have access to resources needed for a decent standard of living. If these essential needs are not met, people are deprived of many other opportunities that are supposed to be available in a well-functioned democratic society. The Human Development Index (HDI), is constructed as a measure of human development, consists of these three components–Longevity, Knowledge and Decent Standard of Living. For longevity–Life Expectancy at Birth is used as a proxy similarly for–Knowledge, Literacy Rate and a

Combination of Primary, Secondary and Tertiary Enrolment are used as a proxy; and to measure a decent standard of living, GDP per capita, measured in terms of real purchasing power (PPP US $), is used.

Education is always apt to make reasonable choices within a well-designed human development strategy. More over they are the most likely to translate the human development policies into effective and sustainable action, creating upward achievement in all areas of human life. Well- educated people are more productive, healthier, more creative and ultimately richer in all dimensions of the word. Indeed, education stands at the top of those factors determining the human development level. As such, education is both an input and an output, of the human development process. As input, education is indispensable for progress in all spheres of human development. As output, education is the axiom for building up human capabilities, a focal interest of human development, given its primary role in enabling people to fully participate in socio-economic and political development.

The growth of Western European countries and the U.S.A. has been based more on Investment in Physical Capital than in human capital in their earlier phases of development. But in the case of underdeveloped countries, the need for human capital in the form of educated persons in different vocations is greater to provide the missing components in the initial stages of their development. The major problems in human capital formation in developing countries are:

- Rapidly growing population.
- Mounting Unemployment as well as widespread of Under employment especially in agricultural sector.
- Shortages of skills and knowledgeable personnel.
- Inadequate or under developed organisations and institutions for Mobilising human effort.

The implication therefore is, all developing countries need to focus on human development in which case capability approach as a strategy, would acquire lot of significance.

Amartya Sen's Capability Approach to Human Development

Amartya Kumar Sen has defined Development in term of an expansion in capabilities and 'entitlement'. Capabilities refer to what a person can (not) do or can (not) be. Freedom from hunger, being free to participate in the political process, being adequately sheltered, access to health and education etc., can be quoted different manifestations of capabilities. In this context, it will be essential to remember that capabilities are generated by 'entitlements' of an individual (within a society), which is measured not simply as income, but rather as the bundle of rights and opportunities available to an individual. These two together, thus imply, both the available choice set and also the capacity to exercise their right over the choice set. Needless to add, the greater is the capability and entitlements of individuals in a society, the higher is the level of development of that society. (Sen. 1989).

He opines, that human being is a subject, rather than object, of development. According to Sen, human development is a process that expands the capabilities of human being and allows them an opportunity to use them productively. sThat is human development is a process of expansion of opportunities for human beings. Sen also emphasize that at the core of human well-being is freedom of choice. The expansion of human capabilities implies greater freedom of choice. So that people can explore a wider range of option that they find worthwhile.

Development according to Sen is the quality of life in terms of capability expansion. That is the expansion of valuable capabilities–broadening of the set of valuable beings and doings an individual can achieve. Development is the freedom to achieve valuable doings and beings (Functionings). Functionings are ends of human life and they can also be means to human life. Functionings are parts of a person's state of being or doing in leading a good life. Capability gives the combinations of functionings achievable by an individual. It is a set of functioning that reflects the freedom of an individual to make choices of possible livings desired by the individual. Capabilities include endowment, individual capacity and social opportunity that in turn impact on capability and are capable of being developed.

Sen's capabilities approach explains development as freedom and 'capability to function'. That is "what we can do with what we have". From Sen's approach there are three core values of development, which are sustenance the ability to keep individual alive, self-esteem and freedom from servitude and poverty. According to Sen, freedom is the matter but there is implication that the means of having the freedom may not matter. Sen's notion of development as capability expansion has been criticised Dizilbash (1996), for example, argues that capability expansion may include impoverishment of some lives and can be achieved through vicious means. The ways in which expansion of capabilities are achieved may be objected to partly because the means may be anti-social. That is, the means of achieving objectives are important and should be considered, just as well as the ends. Sen does not seem to take this into consideration. Sen neglects incorporating negative freedom into his analysis.

Sen's list of functioning's and capabilities is ill defined. Some items included as valuable functionings could be ability to steal, ability to destroy self or others, which should not be included. So how to achieve a good life is not well explained. Enlarging the number of capabilities may not be what the concept of development should be. More capabilities may not mean a better quality of well-being.

Different cultures within different contexts may provide different conditions for functioning and developing capabilities. What is regarded as correct functioning may not be the same in some cultures; since functioning may differ from culture to culture. Values cannot be measured and so cannot be compared. In discussing development in terms of expansion of capability it is not possible to say anything about development when expansion or contraction in capability occurs in a given situation. This is partly because one's capability cannot be compared with that of another person's. Interpersonal comparison of capability is not possible. We cannot also compare one's loss with that of gain of capability, since capability is not measurable.

Some Reflections of Capability Approach on Human Development

- When the first HDR was published Mr. K.C. Das Gupta regarded HDI as incomplete without considering human freedom. Accordingly Human Freedom Index was devised, which became an essential ingredient of human development. It is in this context, that the capability approach received lot of significance.
- Capability achievement will enable people to enjoy the freedom to those the type of life they want to lead. Hence human freedom also became a dimension of human development.
- A given quality of combination of education and health promote well-being through developing their capabilities.
- The development of capabilities in turn enables people to have entitlement which provides a command over goods and services. This further strengthens human freedom as well as capabilities.
- Human capability approach focuses on the ability of human beings to lead lives they have reason to value and to enhance the substantive choice they have.
- Human Capital and Human Development cannot but be related since both are concerned with the role of human beings and in particular with the actual abilities they achieve and acquire.
- If a person becomes more productive in making commodities through better education, better health and so on, the person can directly achieve more and have freedom to achieve more.
- Capability approach to human development takes us back to an integrated approach to economic and social development championed particularly by Adam Smith in his 'Wealth of Nations' as well as 'The Theory of Moral Sentiments'.
- Human capabilities have their direct relevance to the well being and freedom of people, influence economic production and social change.

- The emphasis of Amartya Sen on the development of social infrastructure is an important determinant of capability development. This in turn becomes the base for human development, entitlement and human freedom.
- Public action is an important means to achieve human capabilities. And hence, government's role is still vital in social infrastructure development.
- Poverty represents the absence of some basic capabilities to function.

Conclusion

The term "Human Development" has come to be accepted in the Development Economic literature as an expansion of human capabilities, a widening of choices, an enhancement of freedom and a fulfillment of human rights. Therefore Human Development intends to keep human beings at the center of development and not at the periphery. Longevity, Literacy and Level of income measure human development, and also determine the capabilities and functioning's of people. Although expansion of income is regarded as a 'Means' to human development and not an 'End' in itself, the policy significance of income expansion is clarified. Therefore, a carefully articulated combination of both income generating and human development strategies have become crucial. But these may not be the domains of private sector and hence public/state participation is inevitable. Human development calls for not only the availability of certain socio-economic amenities, but also their quality, availability as well as the entitlement of people over them. Several studies have rightly confirmed that the neglect of social capital has led to underdevelopment of human capabilities as a result of which both human development and human capital were adversely affected. Therefore, human development through capability Approach deserves a prominent place in development strategy.

Notes

1. Planning Commission (1999) Karnataka Human Development Report, Government of Karnataka.

2. UNDP, HDR 1990, 1991, 1993, 1995 & 1997.
3. Streeten Paul (1994) "Human Development: *Means and Ends*", Vol. 84, No. 2, "AEA Paper & Proceedings."
4. Schultz, T.W. (1971), Education and Economic Growth, Bowman, M.J., *et. al.* (Eds.).
5. Nancy Stokey (1991) A Product Quality Approach.
6. Haq Mahabub Ul (1995) "Reflection on Human Development" Chapter 3 & UNDP First Human Development Report 1990.
7. Paul Streeten (1985), Basic Needs Approach.

References

Harbison F. & Myers C.(1970), "Education, Manpower and Economic Growth", *Oxford and IBH Publishing House Company,* Calcutta.

Kothari, V.N. (1966), "Investment in Human Resources", Rapporteur's Report, *Indian Economic Journal.*

Kiker, B.F. (1967), "The Concept of Human Capital in the History of Economic Thought", *The Indian Economic Journal,* Vol. X, Jan–March.

Kumar, A.K.S. (1991) "UNDP's Human Development Index: A Computation for Indian States", *Economic and Political Weekly,* October 12, pp. 2343–45.

Mahbub Ul Haq (1996), "Reflections of Human Development", *Oxford University Press,* United Kingdom.

MHDC (2003), "Human Development in South Asia 2002", *Oxford University Press,* New York.

Planning Commission (1999), "Human Development in Karnataka", Government of Karnataka_*UBS Publishers Distributors Limited,* Bangalore.

Pratima Trivedi (2000), "Economic Progress and Social Justice: Towards Social Sector Development", *Deep & Deep Publications Private Limited,* New Delhi.

Planning Commissions (2001), "National Human Development Report", *Government of India.* New Delhi.

Ruddar Datt (2002), "Human Development and Economic Development", *Deep & Deep Publications Private Limited,* New Delhi.

Sakiko Fukuda–Parr & A.K. Shivakumar (2003), "Readings in Human Development", HDR Office UNDP, *Oxford University Press*, New Delhi.

UNDP Various Issues of Human Development Reports from 1990 to 2004, *Oxford University Press*, New York.

2

INEQUALITY IN HOUSEHOLD CONSUMPTION EXPENDITURE IN INDIAN STATES 1973- 2000

Rattan Chand

Introduction

The Indian National Sample Survey (NSS) has been conducting Household Consumption Expenditure surveys regularly since its inception in 1950. It used to be an annual feature till the NSS 26th round (1971-72). From the NSS 27th round (1972-73), it became a quinquennial survey integrated with employment and unemployment surveys. The results of the quinquennial surveys with large sample sizes are used for the estimation of poverty and for evolving various policy interventions. Six quinquennial surveys on household consumption expenditure have been conducted so far during 27th, 32nd, 38th, 43rd, 50th and 55th rounds of NSS in the years 1972-73, 1977-78, 1983, 1987 88, 1993 94 and 1999-2000 respectively. Seventh quinquennial survey was conducted during the NSS 61st round (July 2004-June 2005) and the results for this are not available yet.

Of late, there has been a lot of discussion about the relative performance of states in India. It is well known that regional disparities are large in India, and there is widespread perception that these have increased in the recent past (Nirvikar Singh *et al.* 2002). In these studies of inter-state disparities, growth rate of per capita income or state domestic product has been used. However, for a population with low per capita income levels, monthly per capita consumption expenditure (MPCE) is perhaps a better indicator of the economic well being of people than per capita income estimates (Planning Commission, 2002). The MPCE is considered to be a fair indicator of human living standards, since it aggregates the monetary value of all goods and services actually consumed during a particular reference period. This includes consumption out of purchase, home produce, free collection, gifts etc.

The objective of this paper is to study intra-state and inter-state consumption expenditure inequality, rural-urban disparity in consumption expenditure and relationship between consumption expenditure and inequality, using NSS data from the six quinquennial rounds of survey. The analysis has been restricted to 15 major states where sample sizes are large enough to provide reliable estimates of parameters.

Data and Methods

The use of the Lorenz curve is an effective way of showing inequality of income or consumption within and between regions. The cumulative percentage of population is plotted

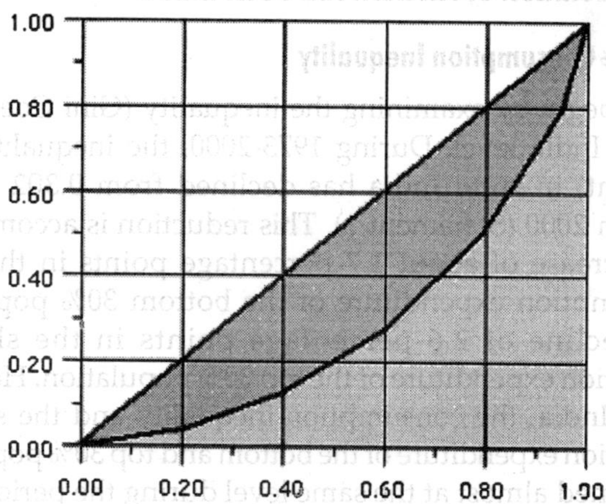

Figure 1 : **Lorenz Curve**

along the horizontal axis while the cumulative percentage of income (consumption in our case) is plotted along the vertical axis (Figure 1). The curve shows the actual relationship between the percentage of income (consumption) recipients and the percentage of income they in fact actually receive. For most people, however, a curve may be less descriptive than a score or value. Therefore, for better understanding, economists have popularised a measure known as the 'Gini Coefficient' named after Corrado Gini, an Italian statistician and demographer. Gini Coefficient is obtained by dividing the area between the Lorenz Curve and the 45-degree equality line by the entire area below the 45-degree line. A Gini coefficient of '0' indicates perfect consumption or income equality, while a '1' would imply that a single person incurs all consumption expenditure or possesses all income.

For studying the intra-state inequality, Monthly Per Capita Consumption Expenditure (MPCE) data by household expenditure classes and the distribution of population in each MPCE class has been used for calculation of Gini Coefficients. Inter-state inequality and rural-urban disparity in household consumption have been studied using state-wise MPCE data at constant prices from the six quinquennial rounds of NSS. To study the relationship between consumption and inequality, use of correlation coefficient has been made.

Intra-State Consumption Inequality

One can begin by examining the inequality (Gini Coefficient) at the all India level. During 1973-2000, the inequality (Gini Coefficient) in rural India has declined from 0.302 in 1973 to 0.260 in 2000 (Statement 1). This reduction is accompanied by an increase of about 1.7 percentage points in the share of consumption expenditure of the bottom 30% population and a decline of 2.6 percentage points in the share of consumption expenditure of the top 30% population. However, in urban India, the consumption inequality and the share of consumption expenditure of the bottom and top 30% population has remained almost at the same level during the period 1973-2000.

Statement 1
Household Consumption Inequality Trends in India

Year	*rural*			*urban*		
	Gini Coefficient	*share in consumption expenditure (%)*		*Gini Coefficient*	*share in consumption expenditure (%)*	
		Bottom 30% population	*Top 30% population*		*Bottom 30% population*	*Top 30% population*
1972-73	0.302	15.0	50.9	0.341	13.9	54.3
1977-78	0.337	14.3	53.9	0.345	13.5	54.9
1983	0.298	15.2	50.9	0.330	13.9	53.7
1987-88	0.291	15.8	50.4	0.352	13.4	55.3
1993-94	0.281	16.0	49.9	0.340	13.6	54.7
1999-00	0.260	16.7	48.3	0.343	13.4	54.7

A close examination of the values of the Gini Coefficients of MPCE for all the six quinquennial NSS rounds (1973-2000) for the rural and urban sectors of the 15 major states (Tables 1R and 1U) reveals as follows. In the rural areas, the inequality has declined in 13 states during 1973-2000 whereas it has marginally increased in two states. These two states are Assam and Tamil Nadu. Maximum decline in the value of Gini coefficient has been observed for the state of Rajasthan. The decline in Bihar, West Bengal, Gujarat, Orissa, Punjab, Madhya Pradesh and Maharashtra is higher than the decline at the national level whereas in Andhra Pradesh, Kerala, Haryana, Karnataka, and Uttar Pradesh, the decline is lower than the decline at the national level. Interestingly, the share in consumption expenditure of the bottom 30% population has gone up in the rural areas of all the states except Assam and Tamil Nadu, where it has declined or remained at the same level (Table 2R). The percentage share of the top 30% population has declined in all the states except Andhra Pradesh, Assam and Tamil Nadu (Table 3R).

In the urban areas, the Gini Coefficient has declined in 7 states, increased in six states and remained at the same level in 2 states during 1973-2000. The states where the Gini Coefficient has declined (in the order of maximum to minimum decline) are Kerala, Orissa, Rajasthan, Madhya Pradesh, Haryana, Punjab and Maharashtra. The share in consumer expenditure of bottom 30% population (Table 2R) also increased in these states (except Kerala) and the share of top 30% (Table 3R) declined except in (Kerala and Maharashtra).

The states where the urban Gini coefficient increased during 1973-2000 (in the order of increase in the Gini Coefficient) are Tamil Nadu, Gujarat, Assam, Uttar Pradesh, Andhra Pradesh and West Bengal. In Karnataka and Bihar there has been no change in the value of Gini Coefficient. Further, in all these eight states, (except Bihar and West Bengal) the share in consumption expenditure of the bottom 30% population has declined (Table 2U) whereas the share in consumption expenditure of the top 30% population has gone up (Table 3U).

Table 1R
Gini Coefficient for Monthly Per Capita Consumer Expenditure (MPCE)-Rural

	State	*1972-73*	*1977-78*	*1983*	*1987-88*	*1993-94*	*1999-00*	*Col. (7) -col. (2)*
	(1)	(2)	(3)	(4)	(5)	(6)	(7)	(8)
1.	Andhra Pradesh	0.273	0.298	0.294	0.301	0.284	0.233	-0.040
2.	Assam	0.180	0.179	0.192	0.222	0.176	0.200	0.020
3.	Bihar	0.288	0.259	0.256	0.264	0.223	0.206	-0.082
4.	Gujarat	0.302	0.285	0.257	0.233	0.236	0.234	-0.068
5.	Haryana	0.277	0.288	0.272	0.281	0.301	0.238	-0.039
6.	Karnataka	0.273	0.321	0.303	0.292	0.265	0.241	-0.032
7.	Kerala	0.310	0.353	0.330	0.323	0.287	0.270	-0.040
8.	Madhya Pradesh	0.306	0.331	0.295	0.290	0.277	0.243	-0.063
9.	Maharashtra	0.310	0.462	0.285	0.331	0.303	0.258	-0.052
10.	Orissa	0.312	0.301	0.267	0.267	0.243	0.244	-0.068
11.	Punjab	0.307	0.303	0.279	0.295	0.265	0.239	-0.068
12.	Rajasthan	0.316	0.464	0.343	0.303	0.260	0.208	-0.108
13.	Tamil Nadu	0.272	0.319	0.325	0.323	0.306	0.279	0.007
14.	Uttar Pradesh	0.277	0.299	0.290	0.279	0.278	0.245	-0.032
15.	West Bengal	0.305	0.292	0.286	0.252	0.252	0.225	-0.080
	All India	0.302	0.337	0.298	0.291	0.281	0.260	-0.042

Table 1U
Gini Coefficient for Monthly Per Capita Consumer Expenditure (MPCE) -Urban

	State	*1972-73*	*1977-78*	*1983*	*1987-88*	*1993-94*	*1999-00*	*Col. (7) -col. (2)*
	(1)	(2)	(3)	(4)	(5)	(6)	(7)	(8)
1.	Andhra Pradesh	0.297	0.319	0.327	0.361	0.320	0.313	0.016
2.	Assam	0.267	0.324	0.276	0.337	0.287	0.310	0.043
3.	Bihar	0.323	0.304	0.301	0.297	0.306	0.323	0.000
4.	Gujarat	0.242	0.308	0.264	0.285	0.287	0.287	0.045
5.	Haryana	0.315	0.317	0.313	0.297	0.280	0.287	-0.028
6.	Karnataka	0.323	0.342	0.334	0.334	0.315	0.323	0.000
7.	Kerala	0.390	0.395	0.374	0.387	0.337	0.321	-0.069
8.	Madhya Pradesh	0.348	0.377	0.306	0.331	0.327	0.315	-0.033
9.	Maharashtra	0.367	0.362	0.337	0.352	0.352	0.348	-0.019
10.	Orissa	0.347	0.323	0.296	0.324	0.304	0.292	-0.055
11.	Punjab	0.313	0.380	0.319	0.278	0.276	0.290	-0.023
12.	Rajasthan	0.333	0.301	0.304	0.346	0.290	0.280	-0.053
13.	Tamil Nadu	0.315	0.333	0.348	0.348	0.344	0.381	0.066
14.	Uttar Pradesh	0.312	0.327	0.319	0.329	0.322	0.329	0.017
15.	West Bengal	0.338	0.317	0.327	0.353	0.333	0.342	0.004
	All India	0.341	0.345	0.330	0.352	0.340	0.343	0.002

Table 2R

Percentage Share of the bottom 30% population in Total Monthly Per Capita Consumer Expenditure (MPCE)-Rural

State	*1972-73*	*1977-78*	*1983*	*1987-88*	*1993-94*	*1999-00*
(1)	*(2)*	*(3)*	*(4)*	*(5)*	*(6)*	*(7)*
1. Andhra Pradesh	15.9	15.3	15.6	15.5	16.1	18.0
2. Assam	19.8	21.6	19.9	18.9	20.4	18.9
3. Bihar	15.1	16.6	16.7	17.1	18.2	19.2
4. Gujarat	15.2	15.8	17.2	18.3	17.6	17.6
5. Haryana	15.7	15.4	16.3	15.9	14.8	17.0
6. Karnataka	15.9	14.1	14.8	15.5	16.5	17.7
7. Kerala	14.7	13.2	14.4	14.6	14.6	16.0
8. Madhya Pradesh	15.1	14.8	15.5	15.7	16.3	17.7
9. Maharashtra	15.0	11.6	15.9	14.9	15.3	16.7
10. Orissa	14.5	14.9	17.4	16.7	17.3	17.4
11. Punjab	14.7	14.6	18.9	15.3	16.6	17.1
12. Rajasthan	14.3	10.8	16.7	14.2	16.7	18.7
13. Tamil Nadu	16.1	14.6	16.2	14.4	15.2	16.1
14. Uttar Pradesh	16.5	16.9	15.4	16.2	16.0	17.6
15. West Bengal	15.0	15.2	15.3	17.4	17.9	18.2
All India	15.0	14.3	15.2	15.8	16.0	16.7

Table 2U

Percentage Share of the bottom 30% population in Total Monthly Per Capita Consumer Expenditure (MPCE)-Urban

State	*1972-73*	*1977-78*	*1983*	*1987-88*	*1993-94*	*1999-00*
(1)	*(2)*	*(3)*	*(4)*	*(5)*	*(6)*	*(7)*
1. Andhra Pradesh	16.8	14.5	14.8	13.2	14.5	14.6
2. Assam	16.8	15.0	18.0	14.9	15.8	14.5
3. Bihar	14.3	15.1	15.2	16.2	15.1	14.9
4. Gujarat	17.6	15.4	17.2	15.8	15.6	15.6
5. Haryana	14.3	14.9	15.0	15.6	15.6	15.1
6. Karnataka	15.0	13.6	13.3	13.8	14.0	13.9
7. Kerala	17.0	11.5	12.6	12.4	14.1	13.8
8. Madhya Pradesh	14.5	13.1	15.7	14.0	14.6	14.6
9. Maharashtra	12.2	12.2	13.2	12.7	12.5	13.0
10. Orissa	13.5	13.9	19.3	14.0	14.5	15.5
11. Punjab	15.0	12.8	14.9	15.9	15.8	15.6
12. Rajasthan	14.9	15.2	14.8	14.4	15.3	16.1
13. Tamil Nadu	14.7	13.9	13.4	15.3	13.8	12.7
14. Uttar Pradesh	14.9	14.4	14.7	14.1	14.1	14.3
15. West Bengal	13.3	14.0	13.9	14.4	13.6	13.9
All India	13.9	13.5	13.9	13.4	13.6	13.4

Table 3R
Percentage Share of top 30% population in Total Monthly Per Capita Consumer Expenditure (MPCE) - Rural

	State	*1972-73*	*1977-78*	*1983*	*1987-88*	*1993-94*	*1999-00*
	(1)	*(2)*	*(3)*	*(4)*	*(5)*	*(6)*	*(7)*
1.	Andhra Pradesh	48.9	50.9	50.9	51.6	50.6	53.6
2.	Assam	42.3	42.0	43.2	45.6	41.8	43.6
3.	Bihar	49.8	47.3	47.5	48.6	45.7	44.3
4.	Gujarat	51.6	49.1	47.6	46.6	46.1	46.1
5.	Haryana	49.3	50.4	49.0	49.6	51.6	47.1
6.	Karnataka	48.5	52.8	50.9	50.6	48.8	46.7
7.	Kerala	52.0	55.4	53.8	53.6	50.6	50.0
8.	Madhya Pradesh	51.9	51.8	50.5	50.2	49.6	46.7
9.	Maharashtra	51.4	62.7	50.0	53.7	51.2	48.1
10.	Orissa	51.7	51.0	48.0	48.7	48.3	46.9
11.	Punjab	51.5	50.7	50.7	51.0	49.6	47.3
12.	Rajasthan	52.5	63.4	54.4	51.6	48.2	44.4
13.	Tamil Nadu	48.9	52.6	52.8	53.1	52.1	49.7
14.	Uttar Pradesh	49.3	48.0	50.1	49.8	49.7	47.3
15.	West Bengal	49.8	50.4	49.5	47.6	47.8	45.2
	All India	50.9	53.9	50.9	50.4	49.9	48.3

Table 3U
Percentage Share of top 30% population in Total Monthly Per Capita Consumer Expenditure (MPCE) - Urban

	State	*1972-73*	*1977-78*	*1983*	*1987-88*	*1993-94*	*1999-00*
	(1)	*(2)*	*(3)*	*(4)*	*(5)*	*(6)*	*(7)*
1.	Andhra Pradesh	47.9	53.0	53.3	56.0	53.1	52.4
2.	Assam	48.5	52.8	48.5	54.2	55.8	52.1
3.	Bihar	52.7	51.4	51.8	51.3	52.3	53.3
4.	Gujarat	41.9	52.1	48.6	50.2	50.4	50.4
5.	Haryana	52.9	52.5	53.5	51.0	49.6	49.6
6.	Karnataka	50.8	54.5	54.0	53.7	52.4	52.9
7.	Kerala	51.1	58.5	57.6	59.0	54.4	53.0
8.	Madhya Pradesh	54.8	57.2	52.1	53.9	53.3	52.4
9.	Maharashtra	53.6	55.0	54.8	55.0	55.3	54.9
10.	Orissa	54.3	52.8	51.9	53.0	51.6	50.9
11.	Punjab	52.2	56.2	53.7	49.8	49.4	50.6
12.	Rajasthan	53.8	51.4	51.3	54.8	50.5	50.0
13.	Tamil Nadu	52.5	53.8	55.0	49.1	54.6	57.3
14.	Uttar Pradesh	52.4	53.6	53.1	53.3	53.4	53.7
15.	West Bengal	54.4	52.0	53.5	53.7	54.3	54.8
	All India	54.3	54.9	53.7	55.3	54.7	54.7

Assam and Tamil Nadu are the only two states where inequality for consumption expenditure has increased both in rural and urban areas.

Monthly Per Capita Consumption Expenditure

State-wise MPCE (Rs) figures at current prices for the six quinquennial NSS rounds conducted during 1973-2000 have been converted to constant prices (Tables 4R and 4U). The conversion has been done using deflators derived from state specific poverty lines for each of the years. The MPCE has increased in real terms in all the states during the period 1973–2000. In the year 2000, the state of Orissa had the lowest MPCE both in rural and urban areas. In the rural areas, Orissa had the lowest MPCE in all the six quinquennial rounds whereas in the urban areas, its position was relatively better before 2000. The state of Punjab, which had the highest MPCE in 1972-73, has moved to number-two position in 2000. The top position has now been occupied by the state of Kerala. During the period 1973-2000, the state of Kerala has registered the highest growth in MPCE both in rural and urban areas (Tables 4R & 4U). In the rural areas, the states which have registered more than 80% growth in MPCE during 1973-2000 are Andhra Pradesh, Kerala, Maharashtra, Tamil Nadu and West Bengal. In the urban areas, such states are Assam, Gujarat, Karnataka (79%), Kerala and Tamil Nadu. All these states have improved their relative ranking with respect to the MPCE of remaining states. A look at the coefficient of variation (CV) calculated from state-wise rural MPCE (last line in Table 4R) indicates that the inter-state disparity among states showed a declining trend during 1973-1994 but it again increased in 2000. However, in the urban areas the inter-state disparity did not show any trend though it is approximately 1 point higher in 2000 as compared to 1973.

The composition of consumption expenditure between food and non-food items also reflects the economic well being of the population. Generally, poor households are expected to spend substantially more on food items as against the non-food. One expects the proportion of expenditure on food to decline with

Table 4R
Monthly Per Capita Consumer Expenditure (MPCE) (Rs.) at constant* prices Rural

	State	1972-73	1977-78	1983	1987-88	1993-94	1999-00	% Growth 1973-2000
	(1)	(2)	(3)	(4)	(5)	(6)	(7)	(8)
1.	Andhra Pradesh	39.79	57.11	66.24	72.65	73.87	71.96	80.8
2.	Assam	41.67	48.71	57.27	60.05	55.41	58.10	39.4
3.	Bihar	41.20	56.23	55.48	65.45	59.35	66.69	61.9
4.	Gujarat	51.70	60.53	69.40	66.02	70.68	81.42	57.5
5.	Haryana	70.07	77.77	85.60	87.24	82.26	98.35	40.4
6.	Karnataka	44.53	59.05	66.25	67.44	68.19	76.26	71.3
7.	Kerala	42.19	65.14	75.53	83.67	82.74	105.58	150.2
8.	Madhya Pradesh	40.72	53.47	60.37	66.61	65.51	64.74	59.0
9.	Maharashtra	41.55	66.81	63.17	70.18	70.60	78.69	89.4
10.	Orissa	34.96	41.76	43.55	49.22	53.10	54.00	54.5
11.	Punjab	74.62	96.24	96.05	99.25	92.51	102.30	37.1
12.	Rajasthan	51.98	96.31	80.66	77.12	76.10	81.30	56.4
13.	Tamil Nadu	37.70	50.43	52.63	58.84	67.36	75.35	99.9
14.	Uttar Pradesh	42.12	60.77	60.82	63.48	62.88	67.76	60.9
15.	West Bengal	38.45	50.99	53.99	64.05	68.82	70.77	84.1
	All India	44.17	60.15	62.28	68.11	67.85	73.66	66.8
	CV	25.03	25.57	21.04	17.83	15.12	19.82	

Table 4U
Monthly Per Capita Consumer
Expenditure (MPCE) (Rs) at constant* prices Urban

	State	1972-73	1977-78	1983	1987-88	1993-94	1999-00	% Growth 1973-2000
	(1)	(2)	(3)	(4)	(5)	(6)	(7)	(8)
1.	Andhra Pradesh	56.32	72.85	77.81	81.81	79.27	91.25	62.0
2.	Assam	60.75	77.32	79.38	107.17	108.51	118.95	95.8
3.	Bihar	59.91	75.72	75.92	76.04	90.69	97.10	62.1
4.	Gujarat	57.58	86.67	82.55	86.39	95.01	116.85	102.9
5.	Haryana	69.88	78.59	94.66	92.15	96.20	113.78	62.8
6.	Karnataka	57.89	77.44	80.57	75.77	81.33	103.70	79.1
7.	Kerala	58.27	77.46	90.28	102.35	110.50	122.73	110.6
8.	Madhya Pradesh	61.88	77.00	74.33	83.38	81.09	90.75	46.7
9.	Maharashtra	74.84	88.69	86.70	87.89	95.91	107.27	43.3
10.	Orissa	62.35	71.29	71.99	80.79	80.09	77.57	24.4
11.	Punjab	77.88	96.16	94.68	96.69	104.57	120.25	54.4
12.	Rajasthan	63.87	79.72	84.49	86.29	90.72	102.47	60.4
13.	Tamil Nadu	54.02	66.24	70.15	77.33	76.16	105.29	94.9
14.	Uttar Pradesh	53.55	67.94	70.51	80.66	86.28	95.14	77.7
15.	West Bengal	68.23	78.87	87.95	90.81	105.22	116.07	70.1
	All India	63.33	77.60	81.37	87.48	92.40	106.86	68.7
	CV	11.65	9.92	10.08	10.80	12.36	12.43	

* adjusted for inflation using deflators derived from state specific poverty lines for each of the years.

development and economic prosperity. The percentage of expenditure on food to total consumption expenditure has declined in rural and urban areas of all the states during 1973 – 2000 (Tables 5R & 5U). At the national level, the share of expenditure on food declined from 72.9% in 1973 to 59.4% in 2000 (in rural areas) implying a corresponding increase in the expenditure on the non-food items. The share of expenditure on food items has also declined in the rural areas of all the states during 1973-2000. In 1973, the state with lowest share of expenditure on food items was Punjab with 63% share. In 2000, eleven states have share of expenditure on food lower than 63% and only four states have more than 63% share of expenditure on food items. These four states are Assam, Bihar, Orissa and West Bengal.

In 1973, the share of expenditure on food items in the urban areas was the lowest in Maharashtra and Punjab, each having 61% share. In 2000, all states have share of expenditure on food lower than 61%. In 1978, the lowest share of expenditure on food was for Punjab (55%) whereas in 2000, only Assam, Bihar and Orissa have share on food expenditure more than 55% (Table 5U).

In rural and urban areas of all the states, the share of expenditure on cereals has declined (Tables 6R and 6U) during 1973-2000 implying switch over to better quality food such as milk, vegetables, meat, fish, eggs etc. However, in the rural areas of Assam, Bihar, Orissa and West Bengal it still continues to be over 45% as against the share of about 20% in Punjab and Haryana. In the urban areas, Assam, Bihar and Orissa and West Bengal have 30% or more share as against 18-19% in Gujarat, Haryana and Punjab.

Rural-Urban Disparity in Consumption Expenditure

The rural-urban disparity in consumption can be studied by using the ratio of rural to urban MPCE (Table 7). An increasing ratio (towards 100) indicates a reduction in rural-urban disparity whereas a declining ratio (away from 100) indicates an increase in rural-urban disparity. At the national level, the ratio of rural to urban MPCE increased from 70% in 1973 to 78% in 1988 but

Table 5R

Percentage Expenditure on Food to Total Consumption Expenditure

	State	*1972-73*	*1977-78*	*1983*	*1987-88*	*1993-94*	*Rural 1999-00*
	(1)	*(2)*	*(3)*	*(4)*	*(5)*	*(6)*	*(7)*
1.	Andhra Pradesh	73.4	64.6	60.3	59.3	59.6	60.5
2.	Assam	77.5	75.0	73.4	70.2	72.3	67.6
3.	Bihar	78.1	75.5	73.6	69.7	71.0	66.5
4.	Gujarat	73.4	68.6	66.1	69.1	67.1	59.8
5.	Haryana	67.3	62.3	63.6	60.8	60.1	55.5
6.	Karnataka	73.5	63.3	63.5	63.6	62.0	59.1
7.	Kerala	70.4	61.2	61.7	59.9	60.5	53.7
8.	Madhya Pradesh	72.2	65.7	66.5	64.3	61.2	58.1
9.	Maharashtra	67.6	49.8	61.5	58.2	59.5	54.7
10.	Orissa	75.1	71.4	73.6	68.9	68.1	64.1
11.	Punjab	62.6	59.7	58.7	57.6	57.9	52.3
12.	Rajasthan	73.9	48.9	60.7	62.0	62.3	59.5
13.	Tamil Nadu	72.0	65.7	65.1	64.1	62.8	58.7
14.	Uttar Pradesh	70.1	65.8	63.3	62.2	61.5	57.4
15.	West Bengal	77.4	72.7	74.0	71.0	66.8	65.9
	All India	72.9	64.3	65.6	64.0	63.2	59.4

Table 5U

Percentage Expenditure on Food to Total Consumption Expenditure- Urban

	State	*1972-73*	*1977-78*	*1983*	*1987-88*	*1993-94*	*1999-00*
	(1)	*(2)*	*(3)*	*(4)*	*(5)*	*(6)*	*(7)*
1.	Andhra Pradesh	67.7	59.2	79.2	52.8	53.8	47.4
2.	Assam	68.4	62.0	66.4	57.6	59.7	55.3
3.	Bihar	70.4	69.4	66.5	63.9	62.9	57.2
4.	Gujarat	72.9	59.4	61.7	60.3	58.4	49.6
5.	Haryana	63.2	59.7	57.7	57.9	53.9	45.9
6.	Karnataka	67.2	61.5	58.1	56.8	55.7	46.3
7.	Kerala	64.8	61.6	59.4	57.1	53.9	49.0
8.	Madhya Pradesh	62.6	58.3	60.4	56.6	52.9	47.6
9.	Maharashtra	61.1	56.1	58.2	55.9	53.0	45.3
10.	Orissa	65.4	66.0	65.3	60.7	57.8	57.0
11.	Punjab	60.6	54.5	55.8	55.2	53.0	47.1
12.	Rajasthan	66.1	60.9	57.6	56.8	56.7	50.8
13.	Tamil Nadu	64.1	60.8	58.4	54.8	54.6	45.6
14.	Uttar Pradesh	66.2	62.3	59.7	57.2	56.0	50.5
15.	West Bengal	64.2	63.4	60.8	57.6	55.9	52.3
	All India	64.5	60.0	59.1	56.4	54.7	48.1

Table 6R

Percentage Expenditure on Cereals to Total expenditure on Food-Rural

State (1)	*1972-73* (2)	*1977-78* (3)	*1983* (4)	*1987-88* (5)	*1993-94* (6)	*1999-00* (7)
1. Andhra Pradesh	62.8	55.9	49.8	41.8	41.2	40.7
2. Assam	58.2	55.8	56.0	48.9	48.6	47.8
3. Bihar	65.7	62.8	64.8	54.8	52.0	48.9
4. Gujarat	45.6	39.4	33.7	28.1	24.9	24.5
5. Haryana	36.8	34.2	28.6	25.5	21.2	19.9
6. Karnataka	63.1	52.8	47.9	38.3	36.8	34.8
7. Kerala	45.4	38.7	38.9	29.8	29.0	26.9
8. Madhya Pradesh	60.7	57.0	53.4	43.9	42.9	43.0
9. Maharashtra	57.6	46.5	41.5	32.6	30.0	32.3
10. Orissa	69.7	69.3	68.0	60.1	57.3	56.2
11. Punjab	26.8	26.7	25.2	19.1	18.2	19.0
12. Rajasthan	50.3	41.5	39.8	35.0	28.9	30.1
13. Tamil Nadu	57.8	54.8	53.8	43.8	39.3	30.7
14. Uttar Pradesh	57.6	47.7	46.5	38.9	35.2	36.6
15. West Bengal	65.3	58.2	60.7	52.5	50.7	47.7
All India	55.7	51.0	49.2	41.0	38.3	37.3

Table 6U

Percentage Expenditure on Cereals to Total expenditure on Food-Urban

State (1)	*1972-73* (2)	*1977-78* (3)	*1983* (4)	*1987-88* (5)	*1993-94* (6)	*1999-00* (7)
1. Andhra Pradesh	47.4	42.7	26.3	44.4	33.3	32.8
2. Assam	41.8	42.3	45.3	33.3	33.7	34.1
3. Bihar	48.2	45.2	48.2	40.7	36.4	37.2
4. Gujarat	36.3	28.9	25.1	20.6	19.4	18.7
5. Haryana	29.0	27.1	23.4	20.4	19.2	18.7
6. Karnataka	44.8	39.7	34.9	28.8	29.4	28.0
7. Kerala	37.5	32.8	33.6	22.5	24.1	23.1
8. Madhya Pradesh	39.0	38.2	35.1	26.0	27.8	29.4
9. Maharashtra	26.6	26.6	25.9	21.1	21.4	22.8
10. Orissa	44.7	44.1	48.5	36.3	34.4	39.9
11. Punjab	22.4	23.4	21.3	17.5	17.0	17.3
12. Rajasthan	35.6	31.7	29.7	24.7	22.4	22.9
13. Tamil Nadu	40.9	40.6	40.5	31.1	29.9	23.8
14. Uttar Pradesh	39.1	35.1	33.1	26.4	25.3	26.4
15. West Bengal	34.2	35.6	36.3	31.2	30.5	30.0
All India	36.2	34.1	33.0	26.5	25.7	25.7

Table 7
Rural to Urban MPCE Ratio (%)-Constant prices

	State	*1972-73*	*1977-78*	*1983*	*1987-88*	*1993-94*	*1999-00*	*Change 1973-2000*
	(1)	(2)	(3)	(4)	(5)	(6)	(7)	(8)
1.	Andhra Pradesh	70.65	78.39	85.13	88.79	93.18	78.85	8.20
2.	Assam	68.59	63.00	72.15	56.03	51.07	48.84	-19.75
3.	Bihar	68.77	74.26	73.08	86.07	65.44	68.68	-0.09
4.	Gujarat	89.79	69.84	84.07	76.42	74.40	69.68	-20.11
5.	Haryana	100.27	98.96	90.43	94.68	85.51	86.44	-13.83
6.	Karnataka	76.92	76.25	82.23	89.01	83.85	73.54	-3.38
7.	Kerala	72.40	84.10	83.66	81.75	74.88	86.03	13.62
8.	Madhya Pradesh	65.80	69.44	81.21	79.89	80.79	71.34	5.53
9.	Maharashtra	55.52	75.33	72.86	79.85	73.61	73.36	17.84
10.	Orissa	56.07	58.58	60.49	60.92	66.29	69.61	13.54
11.	Punjab	95.81	100.08	101.45	102.64	88.47	85.08	-10.74
12.	Rajasthan	81.38	120.80	95.47	89.37	83.89	79.35	-2.04
13.	Tamil Nadu	69.79	76.13	75.03	76.09	88.45	71.56	1.77
14.	Uttar Pradesh	78.66	89.44	86.26	78.70	72.88	71.23	-7.43
15.	West Bengal	56.35	64.65	61.39	70.53	65.41	60.97	4.62
	All India	69.75	77.52	76.53	77.86	73.43	68.93	-0.81

thereafter it again declined to 69% in 2000. The ratio has increased in seven states during 1973-2000 indicating reduction in rural-urban disparity. Maximum increase in the ratio is observed in the state of Maharashtra (17.8 points) followed by Kerala (13.6 points), Orissa (13.5 points), Andhra Pradesh (8.2 points), Madhya Pradesh (5.5 points), West Bengal (4.6 points) and Tamil Nadu (1.8 points). On the other hand, the ratio has declined in seven states during 1973-2000. It declined by over 10 percentage points in Assam, Gujarat, Haryana and Punjab and by less than 10 points in Rajasthan, Karnataka and Uttar Pradesh. In Bihar it has remained almost at the same level.

In 2000, the states with the lowest to the highest rural-urban disparity (in that order) were Haryana, Kerala, Punjab, Rajasthan, Andhra Pradesh, Karnataka, Maharashtra, Tamil Nadu, Madhya Pradesh, Uttar Pradesh, Gujarat, Orissa, Bihar, West Bengal and Assam.

Relationship between Gini Coefficient and MPCE

The relationship between inequality and MPCE has been studied with the help of correlation coefficient between the values of these variables for the six quinquennial rounds. As there are only six pairs of values, the correlation coefficients presented here are purely indicative. A negative correlation indicates that the inequality decreases with increase in MPCE and vice versa. On the other hand a positive correlation indicates increase in inequality with increase in MPCE and vice versa.

In the rural areas, negative correlation is observed between Gini Coefficient and MPCE in 12 states as well as for all India level (Statement 2). The correlation is only positive in Assam, Rajasthan and Tamil Nadu. The correlation is, however, *statistically significant* (at 5% level of significance) only for the states of Gujarat (-0.85), Orissa (-0.95) and West Bengal (-0.95). In the urban areas, the correlation coefficient is negative in eight states and positive in seven states as well as for all India. However, the correlation is *statistically significant* only for Kerala (-0.82) and Tamil Nadu (0.98).

Statement 2
Correlation Coefficient between Gini Coefficient and MPCE

	State	Rural	Urban
1.	Andhra Pradesh	-0.04	0.48
2.	Assam	0.66	0.51
3.	Bihar	-0.72	0.04
4.	Gujarat	-0.85	0.66
5.	Haryana	-0.66	-0.73
6.	Karnataka	-0.33	-0.11
7.	Kerala	-0.54	-0.82
8.	Madhya Pradesh	-0.59	-0.36
9.	Maharashtra	-0.07	-0.46
10.	Orissa	-0.95	-0.61
11.	Punjab	-0.56	-0.31
12.	Rajasthan	0.41	-0.63
13.	Tamil Nadu	0.02	0.98
14.	Uttar Pradesh	-0.25	0.74
15.	West Bengal	-0.95	0.29
	All India	-0.55	0.14

Conclusion

The analysis covering 15 major states based on data from the NSSO's six quinquennial surveys conducted during the period 1973-2000 revealed that the inequality for consumption expenditure has declined in the rural areas of all the major states except Assam and Tamil Nadu. This decline is generally accompanied by an increase in the consumption share of the bottom 30% population and a decline in the consumption share of the top 30% population. In the urban areas, the situation is mixed as the inequality in consumption expenditure has increased or remained at the same level almost in half of the states and declined in the remaining half. Assam and Tamil Nadu are the only states where the inequality has increased in rural as well as urban areas. The MPCE has increased in real terms in rural as well as in urban areas of all the states. The state of Orissa continued to have the lowest MPCE during 1973-2000. The highest MPCE position has now been achieved by Kerala moving Punjab to the second slot. In the rural areas, the interstate disparity in consumption expenditure has declined during 1973–1994 but has increased in 2000. In the case of urban areas, the inter-state disparity has not shown any trend and it is almost at the 1973 level. Rural to urban disparity has remained almost same at the national level. The rural-urban disparity has increased in seven states and declined in eight states. In 2000, the rural-urban disparity was the lowest in Haryana and the highest in Assam. During 1973-2000, the rural-urban disparity has worsened most in Gujarat followed by Assam, Haryana, Punjab, Uttar Pradesh Karnataka, Rajasthan and Bihar while it has improved most in Maharashtra followed by Kerala, Orissa, Andhra Pradesh, Madhya Pradesh, West Bengal and Tamil Nadu. The correlation between MPCE and Gini coefficient has been found to be negative in 12 states in rural areas and in eight states in urban areas. In rural areas of Gujarat, Orissa and West Bengal, the correlation is negative and statistically significant. In the urban areas, the correlation is negative and statistically significant only in Kerala and positive and statistically significant in Tamil Nadu.

References

Sarvekshana Issue No. 7: First Quinquennial Survey on Consumer Expenditure: 27th Round, 1972-73.

Sarvekshana Issue No. 26: Second Quinquennial Survey on Consumer Expenditure: 27th Round, 1977-78.

NSS Report No. 332: Pattern of Consumer Expenditure of Schedule Caste and Schedule Tribe Households, 1983.

Sarvekshana Issue No. 48: The Fourth Quinquennial Survey on Consumer Expenditure: 43rd Round, 1987-88.

NSS Report No. 402: Level and Pattern of Consumer Expenditure in India, 1993-94.

NSS Report No. 457: Level and Pattern of Consumer Expenditure in India, 1999-2000.

National Human Development Report, 2001, Planning Commission, March 2002, New Delhi.

Nirvikar Singh, Laveesh Bhandari, Aoyu Chen and Arti Khare, 'Regional Inequality in India: A Fresh look' Santa Cruz Centre for International Economics, University of California, Santa Cruz, December, 2002.

P.D.Joshi, Sarvekshana, Analytical Report No. 2: Changing Pattern of Consumption Expenditure in India and Some Selected States, National Sample Survey Organisation Department of Statistics, Ministry of Planning and Programme Implementation, Government of India, New Delhi, 1998.

3

DEMOGRAPHIC TRANSITION AND FOOD SECURITY IN SOUTH ASIA: SOME POLICY OPTIONS

Falendra K. Sudan

Introduction

Demographers refer to changes from stable population with high fertility and mortality to a new stability in population due to low fertility and mortality patterns as demographic transition. Different countries in the world have entered the demographic transition at different periods of time. There are also substantial differences in the rate of demographic transition and time taken to achieve population stabilization. Population growth and its relation to economic growth has been a matter of debate for over a century. The early Malthusian view was that population growth is likely to impede economic growth because it will put pressure on the available resources, result in reduction in per capita income and resources; this, in turn, will result in deterioration in quality of life and level of food security. Contrary to the Malthusian predictions, several of the East Asian countries have been able to achieve economic prosperity and improved quality of life and food security in spite of population growth.

South Asian nations are moving through the demographic transition at more gentle speeds. The deep-rooted sentiments against cultural change in Pakistan, and widespread poverty in Bangladesh, delay the process. Sri Lanka underwent demographic transition at the same time as South East Asian countries but has not achieved the economic transition and improved food security. It is now realized that population growth or demographic transition can have favourable impact on economic growth only when there are optimal interventions aimed appropriate utilization of available resources. For India the current phase of demographic transition with low dependency ratio and high working age group population, represents both a challenge and an opportunity. The challenge is to ensure human development and optimum utilization of human resources. The opportunity is to utilize available human resources to achieve rapid economic development and improved food security.

Experts are divided on whether future increases in agriculture outputs will be sufficient to meet the growing demand resulting from population growth. However, most analysts-including (Alexandratos, 1995; Bongaarts, 1994, 1996; Dyson, 1996, 2003; FAO, 1996a, 2003a, 2003b; Smil, 2000) - while acknowledging that the world food situation has many problems, are cautiously optimistic and predict progress in reducing undernourishment in many regions. The demographic growth is likely to complicate efforts to improve food security in South Asia where recent trends in food demand and food production, coupled with the likelihood of considerable future population increases, do not augur well for a major reduction in the proportion of hungry people (Brown, 1993; Myres, 1991: Postel, 1992).

South Asian region is still in a mid-low position as regards per capita food supplies. Nevertheless, considering India alone we see tremendous advances over the last 50 years-food grain production has increased four fold (50 to 200 Mt), while population has increased three fold (from 330 million to over 1000 million). These successes of the Green Revolution should be widely acknowledged but the shortcomings also need to be recognized. The resource-poor farmers and landless and especially those in marginal areas have not benefited significantly. The inability of such groups to improve their food security, in spite of substantial food production gains, is now recognized as a general failure to alleviate poverty within the context of enhancing agricultural resources so that employment and incomes may increase.

Despite remarkable performance in food production scenario, food insecurity remains a chronic problem (Brklacich, 2000). Population density in relation to arable land increased considerably since 1950 and is expected to increase further. The population density is less than 100 in South Asia. This, however, does not reveal the whole picture. The density varies from peak above 700 in Bangladesh to the low depths of below 140 in Pakistan (United Nations, 1994). Since 1950, area of cultivated land per capita has declined significantly. In India, for example, it has dropped from 1.11 acres in 1921 to 0.62 acres in 1971 and a further decline has also been observed in recent past too. In order to counter the decrease in cultivated land per capita and meet the increasing demand for agricultural goods, including food, it is necessary to raise agricultural productivity. From 1900 to 1945, the increase in overall agricultural output was over taken by population increase. In India (then comprising present-day India, Pakistan and Bangladesh), population increased by 18.4 per cent and overall agricultural output increased by 13 per cent (Bhattacharjee, 1958). In other words, despite the increase in total area under cultivation the agricultural sector did not show any growth. Since mid-1965, growth of food production has been observed to be higher than population growth in all but two. In Bangladesh, these growth rates have been almost the same, but in Nepal, the population growth rate has been significantly higher than growth in food production (Sudan, 2001).

If the nutritional level of a given population judges the adequacy of the food supply, South Asia is still a long away from providing the minimum daily requirement of nutritional food. The bulk of South Asian population suffers from general debilitation and lower physical energy and productivity (World

Bank, 2001). The position is worse in respect of nutrient types of food, which are generally outside the reach of the mass of population. Apart from the low level of income, the inability of the people to have sufficient food and a balanced diet is also related to overpopulation. In South Asia, productivity of food grains till recently did not keep pace with the increased demand resulting from population growth and rise in per capita income and, consequently, the prices of food grains rose and the consumption levels of the poorer sections of the society has been depressed. Thus, rapid population growth in South Asia not only affects food production and consumption, but also will profoundly affect the distribution of overall income and assets in the present century. The land tenure patterns, distribution of agrarian incomes and farm holding by size and rates of rural-urban migration is likely to be significantly modified. The rapid population growth seems certain to increase the number of landless, subsistence or disadvantaged peasantry and raise the administrative burdens and social costs of absorbing urban arrivals as well as managing the food aid and assistance. Conversely, the slower population growth could lessen the severity of these effects, once its cumulative influence on numbers began to take effect.

Objectives

The main objective of the paper is to examine the interrelationship between population and food security in South Asian perspective and to suggest some policy options for ensuring food security.

Materials and Methods

The study is based on secondary data sources such as publications of United Nations, Food and Agricultural Organization, World Bank and Governments of India, Nepal, Bangladesh, Pakistan and Sri Lanka, and published and unpublished studies of individual researchers. Five South Asian Countries have been selected for comparative study of population situation and food security scenario in the post World War Second period with an object of drawing some policy options to make the sub-continent free of hunger. The study has utilized potentially rich secondary data sources, which has been analyzed to draw meaning inferences.

Findings

Population and Food: Theoretical Perspective

(a) Malthusian Principle of Population: Malthus was not the first person to suggest that population growth might outstrip the capacity to produce food (Malthus, 1798). Nor was he the first to suggest that this might limit population size by raising death rates (see Blaxter, 1986; Saether, 1993). But he was certainly most influential and impressive; and modern demographers still frequently acknowledge their debt to him. The basic argument of Malthus' *An Essay on the Principle of Population,* can be sketched with the help of a few famous quotations: "Population, when unchecked, increases in a geometrical [i.e. compound] ratio. Subsistence [i.e. food production] increases only in an arithmetical ratio .... By that law of our nature, which makes food necessary to the life of the man, the effects of these two unequal powers (of population and food) must be kept equal. This implies a strong and constantly operating check on population from the difficulty of subsistence. This difficulty (of providing sufficient food) must fall somewhere and must necessarily be severely felt by a large portion of mankind" (Malthus, 1798, p. 14). Malthus then proceeded to argue that the balance between population and food is chiefly maintained by upward pressure on the death rate–and that this 'absolutely necessary consequence' was primarily brought about by hunger, starvation and disease. But, should these factors still be insufficient to restore equilibrium, then: "gigantic inevitable famine stalks in the rear, and with one mighty blow levels the population with the food of the world (Malthus, 1798, p.140).

Malthus significantly revised the simple argument on the relationship between population and food of the *First Essay* in his so-called *Second Essay*. He gave increasing importance to changes in the birth rate as an alternative way of maintaining the balance between 'population' and 'food'. Essentially he argued that when food was scarce and times were hard, prices rose and men and women were forced to delay their marriages. In turn, this reduced the birth rate and helped to restore the equilibrium between population and resources (including food supplies) (Wrigley and Schofield, 1981). Also, he realized that trade-off could occur. For example, a decline in the birth rate would reduce the risk of a rise in the death rate. Malthus' description of the rate of increase of food production as arithmetic (i.e. linear) was a reasonable generalization given the evidence that was available to him (Flew, 1970). He was discussing the increase of food on the implicit assumption that the supply of cropland was fixed. In modern parlance, he was describing the form of growth of agricultural yields – e.g. food output per hectare. During recent decades, the aggregate yields have indeed increased in a fairly linear (Dyson, 1996). So, especially the later writings of the Malthus on the adaptabilities, flexibilities and general complexities of the relationship between population and food contain many valuable insights, which are still valid today.

(b) Views of Anti-Malthusian: Since Malthus' time there have been periodic 'waves' of people who doubted the capacity of the world to produce enough food for its growing population (Kellman, 1987). However, so-called 'anti-Malthusian' presented a more optimistic outlook. Instead of seeing a large and growing population as a problem for systems of food production, the opposing perspective sees these characteristics as both a sign and, indeed, a cause of prosperity. According to anti-Malthusian views, the flexibility and adaptability provided by efficient markets through trade can help solve any problems posed by population growth. Indeed, since population growth increases the volume of demand for food, if scarcity occurs then prices will rise and eventually farmers will be stimulated into producing more food. This leads to the view that, over the long run, population growth actually causes food to be both more plentiful and cheaper (Simon, 1981). Besides markets, scientific research has led to increase in agricultural productivity. Major advances here include the development of

mass production techniques for nitrogen fertilizers around 1913, and the development of so-called 'green revolution' high yielding varieties (HYVs) of wheat and rice during the 1960s (Flew, 1970).

The second main way by which farm productivity may be increased is through the stimulation of agricultural innovation induced by population growth itself. Drawing upon African and Asian data Boserup (1965) noted the positive correlation, which existed between population density and the intensity of land use. Societies living at low population densities tended to practise 'extensive' agriculture; farmers would cultivate a plot of land with a few simple tools and then move on to work another patch, letting the original plot lie fallow for perhaps 20-25 years during which time its productivity would recover. Then the rejuvenated plot would be cultivated again. However, societies living at comparatively high population densities were much more likely to cultivate the same plot of land each year (i.e. practise annual cropping). These communities tended to have more sophisticated agricultural systems and farm tools. Moreover, levels of food production per person were sometimes higher under such more 'intensive' farming regimes, particularly if greater inputs of agricultural labour per person were required (i.e. in terms of time spent in cultivation).

From this essentially cross-sectional observation, Boserup argued that through the challenges to society, which it posed, population growth often actually worked as the major dynamic engine of agricultural change–stimulating, in particular, the adoption of improvements in land use and technology. Moreover, this basically anti-Malthusian perspective can be further developed to argue that–other things being equal–the larger a population is, the larger will be the number of farmers, and therefore the greater will be the chance that someone will discover a new and more productive way of cultivating the available supply of land (Boserup, 1965; Simon, 1992). There is no doubt that historically such Boserupian processes have been very significant in societies all round the world. Indeed demographic increase may well have been the single most important cause of agricultural intensification. Furthermore, potentially there are many ways in which food production can be increased to keep up with population growth (Bilsborrow, 1987). No doubt, increased population density may eventually lead to greater intensification, it is not obvious that this will be necessarily be accompanied by increased levels of food production per head. There is widespread agreement among agricultural economists that the innovations which poor farmers in much of the developing world are likely to be able to generate by themselves will be quite incapable of keeping up with such very high rates of population growth (Hayami and Ruttan, 1987; Pingali and Binswanger, 1991). Indeed, it will be essential to incorporate the benefits of agricultural innovations into the overall processes of adaptive response.

(c) Views of Neo-Malthusian: The world's population is certainly both larger and better-fed now than it was two hundred years ago. In spite of repeated expressions of anxiety, world food production has generally kept ahead of population growth. In large measure this has been due to the more expansion of the area of land in cultivation, plus the continual development of agricultural practices by farmers and, more recently, the application of modern scientific and industrial approaches to the tasks of raising crop yields and transporting and storing food (see Boserup, 1990; Grigg, 1993). Modern neo-Malthusian writers do not deny that these long-term improvements in per capita food production have taken place. But they argue that in the 1980s and 1990s the world has at last reached a critical turning point. They maintain that in certain crucial respects the situation which humanity now faces is different from that it has confronted in the past. In particular, the neo-Malthusian case highlights the extra ordinary scale of contemporary world population growth and the related–and increasingly serious– environmental problems to which growth contributes. The argument acknowledges that issue of distribution–especially the existence of widespread poverty in much of the developing world, coexistent with over-consumption and waste of resources by rich nations–is very important. But it retains at its core grave anxiety about whether food production can possibly keep up with population growth

(see Brown, 1993; Brown and Kane, 1995; Ehrlich and Ehrlich, 1990; Ehrlich *et. al.*, 1993; Myres, 1991).

The basic demographic facts underlying the modern neo-Malthusian case are not in dispute. If it took about 130 years for the human population to grow from 1 billion to 2 billion, the next billion were added in just 30 years, i.e. by about 1960. The rate of demographic growth has been declining since 1960s because the world's birth rate has been falling faster than the death rate. But even so, during the 1980s alone the world's population grew by an estimated 841 million people. Moreover, most population projections broadly agree that in the next three decades up to the year 2020, the absolute increment will be about 870 million people in each decade (United Nations, 1994). The phenomenon of demographic momentum makes most of this growth virtually certain (see McNicoll, 1992). This unprecedented demographic increase is overwhelmingly located in the developing world where birth rates are the highest and population age structures are youngest. In fact, over 95 per cent of the 2.603 billion increment which the United Nations projects for the period 1990-2020 is expected to occur in the developing countries. This increase in population will be the main cause of a tremendous expansion in the demand for food, and therefore of greatly increased exploitation of land for agricultural production.

At this point environmental considerations and judgments enter the argument and things suddenly become much more complicated. Part of the modern neo-Malthusian case is that food production all over the world is increasingly coming up against various constraints, of which perhaps the two most important relate to land and water. The total amount of cropland is shrinking because of population growth. The greater and greater demands, which are being made upon the land, which is in cultivation, are leading to widespread land degradation– in such forms as soil erosion, compaction and desertification. It is claimed that throughout much of the developing world mounting population pressures are directly threatening the inherent productivity of the soil (Brown, 1988; Brown and Kane, 1995). Fast-growing cities are gobbling-up prime agricultural land, and the dwindling supplies of new land which might be brought into cultivation are generally of much poor quality. In case of water, the problems seem to be severe. More than one-third of current world agricultural production is said to come from the approximately 16 per cent of agricultural land that is irrigated. But "Worldwide the prospects for major gains in irrigated area are not good" (Brown, 1988). So the amount of irrigated cropland per person is also declining because of population growth. Again, there are many difficulties relating to irrigation water than just of falling per capita supplies, which includes rising levels of pollution, increased salinization of irrigated croplands, falling water tables and increased competition of water–for example between farmers and city-dwellers, and between nation states. Furthermore, as is often the case apropos environmental problems, these processes frequently combine and interact in synergistic ways. Fast growing cities threaten supplies of both agricultural land and water. Deforestation of upland areas–often fuelled in part by the migration of poor farmers in search of cultivable land–may cause increased flooding and agricultural destruction downstream. Thus, humanity is confronted with a serious dilemma: a population-environment-food 'trap' (Ehrlich *et. al.,* 1993).

The world's population having grown by about 841 million people during the 1980s, the neo-Malthusian case proceeds to argue that these various constraints and threats are already having extremely serious and detectable effects on food production. The 'green revolution', which kept food output ahead of world population growth during the 1960s and 1970s, is portrayed as running out of stream. The best locations for planting the high yielding varieties of major cereal crops like rice and wheat have largely been used up. It is contended that many countries have reached the point where higher and higher doses of fertilizer to each hectare of cropland produce very little increase in yields. In lots of places the yields of major food crops are said to be falling, or only increasing slowly (Myers, 1991). According to neo-Malthusian, the 1970s saw increasingly frequent setbacks in the race between population and food. But in the 1980s, there occurred a critical turning point. Since about 1984 the world's population has been growing faster than its production of cereal grains (which form the principal basis of the human food supply). Put differently, since the mid-1980s, the global output of grain per person has been falling (Brown, 1993; Brown and Kane, 1995; Ehrlich *et. al.,* 1993; Harrison, 1992; Myres, 1991; Population Action International, 1992; Postel, 1992). Furthermore, this negative trend seems to be established in every world region Brown, 1991). These trends mean that the world's reserve stocks of grain have also been falling.

Therefore, a couple of exceptionally bad global harvests–arguably more likely under conditions of rapid climate change–could easily cause a repeat of the food prices rises and 'world food crisis' which occurred in the early 1970s (Brown, 1988, 1991; Brown and Kane, 1995). Beyond this, it is predicted that during the 1990s global agricultural production may grow at an average annual rate of only 0.9 per cent, while population continues growing at around 1.6 per cent. This implies that per capita food production could fall by 7 per cent in the coming decade and raises the prospect of 'an absolute global shortage of food' leading to widespread starvation and famine in developing countries (Brown, 1988; Enrlich. *el al.,* 1993). Thus, the neo-Malthusian view is that in the decades ahead, food shortages will in both frequency and severity. The next ten years could see a major crisis involving 'mounting grain deficits, surging grain prices and spreading hunger among ever larger numbers of people' (Brown and Kane, 1995; Ehrlich and Ehrlich, 1990; Ehrlich *et. al.,* 1993; Myers, 1991). It is seriously proposed that by 2020 there could be several million excess deaths stemming from hunger and famine (Daily and Ehrlich, 1990).

Some features of the neo-Malthusian argument must be taken more seriously. It would be absurd not to acknowledge that population growth may lead to reduced per capita supplies of cropland and renewable water in the years ahead. It is clear that in many parts of the world rapid demographic growth is contributing to damage the environment, and that this often has adverse consequences for local food production. Furthermore, no one doubts that there will be major growth in global food demand in the next few decades–largely because of population growth. This will certainly present humanity with a considerable challenge. Moreover, certain elements of the neo-Malthusian case can be evaluated comparatively precisely. For example, since the mid-1980s either South Asian population has been growing faster than its cereal production, or it has not. Similarly, either population growth has been outstripping growth of cereal production in all South Asian countries, or it has not. Likewise, either there are signs that famine or food crises are becoming more frequent and severe, or there are not. It is true that these issues are not entirely devoid of judgement. But it is also true that they involve relatively 'hard' and objective sets of data. Moreover, demographic studies can provide us with some comparatively firm indicators as to the likelihood that starvation and famine will curtail South Asian population in the next few decades. By evaluating these rather more specific neo-Malthusian claims, we can get a better idea as to whether the more extreme forecasts deserve any consideration at all.

Population and Food Situation in South Asia

The South Asian countries, i.e. Bangladesh, India, Nepal, Pakistan and Sri Lanka cover 85 per cent of the total area of the region, 96 per cent of the irrigated area, 98 per cent of the population and 99 per cent of the gross domestic product. India is by for the largest country in the region with 72 per cent of land area and 76 per cent of the population. On an average, about 55 per cent of the land area is used for agriculture (including pastures). In Nepal and Sri Lanka, this figure is lower (about 35 per cent), probably due to the occurrence of mountains. In Pakistan, the low percentage of agricultural land is due to arid conditions. Due to land pressure and flat topography, in Bangladesh almost 80 per cent of the land area is used for agriculture (Roest, 2000). The arid conditions of Pakistan are reflected in the high per centage of irrigation: almost 80 per cent against 20 to 30 per cent in the other countries of the region. Population growth is highest in Nepal (2.5 per cent), the country with the lowest gross domestic product (together with Bangladesh). Sri Lanka, the most prosperous country, has the lowest population growth of 1.1 per cent (CIA, 1998). Agriculture as a sector produces about 30 per cent of the gross domestic product in the region, but employs about 65 per cent of the labour force. Remarkably, in all countries the income per capita in agriculture is about 50 per cent of the national average.

Between 1970 and 1990, food supplies in the developing world increased by about 16 per cent and have out placed population growth in most regions. However, food insecurity remains a chronic problem and yield increases are also falling, lessening our ability to meet the growing food needs (Brklacich, 2000). As recently as the 1970s, South Asia was sub-continent known for its famines and recurrent food crisis. However, during the last two decades, the situation has changed remarkably and increases in food supply remain ahead of population growth in South Asia. At the end of 1998, Pakistan produced its largest ever harvest of wheat at 18.7 million tons. Bangladesh also recorded good cereal harvests, reinforcing its confidence that it might soon attain food self-sufficiency. In 1999, India enjoyed a bumper harvest so large that its warehouses over flowed and food grains were stored under the open sky for lack of space in the go-downs. However, natural disasters worked in opposite direction and jeopardize the food security scenario in most parts of the region. In 2000, drought devastated agriculture and industry in India and Pakistan. A super-cyclone ravaged India's state of Orissa and saturated more than 1 million ha of cropland (WFP, 2001).

The Indian sub-continent is two thirds larger in population than the entire continent of Africa. The population densities in the region are high: one out of five people live in the region (World Bank, 2001). With about 294 million classified by the FAO as undernourished (over 200 million people in India alone), the region has significant problems related to food security (FAO, 2000). Cereals represent a high share of dietary intake, ranging from 57 per cent in Pakistan to 83 per cent in Bangladesh. In 1997, South Asia produced 29 per cent of the world's rice, 15 per cent of the world's wheat and 11 per cent of the world's oil crop (FAOSTAT, 2000). Most South Asian countries are net importers of wheat and about 6.4 million tons of wheat is imported annually (6.6 per cent of the world wheat trade during 1996-98). During the recent past, India and Pakistan have emerged as net exporters of rice: India exported 3.1 million tons, while Pakistan exported 1.8 million tons during 1996-98. All other countries in the region are importers of rice the largest being Bangladesh at 1.3 million tons. With the exception of Nepal, each of the countries imports pulses to meet national requirements. During 1996-98, the annual average imports amounts to 8.1 per cent of the pulses production in the region (FAO, 2000).

Based on FAO food balance sheets, dietary energy supply per capita is generally higher than it was in 1970. However, in Bangladesh, it has dropped by 4.5 per cent. In Sri Lanka, a decline in dietary energy supply per capita, at the beginning of the 1980s coincides with the resurgence of violence in that country. It is important to note that despite relative prosperity in the country, Sri Lanka's dietary energy supply per capita is the lowest in the region, followed by Bangladesh. Taking 1995 as a benchmark the average dietary energy supply per capita was 73 per cent of the developed world's dietary energy supply (2329) kcal versus 3207 kcal). Normally, standards of adequacy can be achieved only at national calorie supply levels of about 2800 kcal per capita per day (2700 kcal per person per day, is estimated by FAO (1996b), and only if the national food distribution is relatively egalitarian and public health services work satisfactory (Fogel, 1997). All the countries in the region are classified as low income, food deficit country, which suggests a priority status for development assistance under WFP food resource allocation decisions. Gross national product (GNP) per capita in the region ranges from US$ 210 in Nepal, US $ 350 in Bangladesh, over US $ 400 in India and Pakistan, to over US $ 800 in Sri Lanka. Economic growth rates also vary enormously, from a low of 2 per cent in Nepal to a robust 6 per cent per annum in India (World Bank, 2001). In the following paragraphs, a separate account has been given for the individual countries of the region with regard to the food production and availability.

In Bangladesh, all governmental plans have consistently emphasized the achievement of food self-sufficiency. Although the country has not experienced a famine since 1974, food, and the fear of not having enough, plays a crucial role in the agriculture-led political economy of Bangladesh (Ahmed *et. al.*, 2000). Green revolution technologies introduced after in dependence in the 1970s as well as far-reaching market-oriented agricultural reforms undertaken during the late 1980s and early 1990s, led to sustained growth in rice production. Much of the expansion came from a shift from traditional varieties to modern high yielding ones, increased application of fertilizer, and through an expansion of cropped area during the dry season by irrigation. The accompanying reforms comprised considerable deregulation of agricultural markets and prices, such as fertilizers, seeds, and irrigation; and gradual cutbacks of the subsidized food rationing system and public procurement of grains. The growth in grain production stagnated in the early 1990s registering less than one per cent annual growth rate during 1990-97, compared to 2.8 per cent in the 1970s and about 4 per cent in the 1980s. During this period, there were growing doubts about Bangladesh's ability to increase food production to 31 million tons, its projected requirement by 2010. However, several successive bumper harvests (in the late 1990s) have reinforced its confidence that food self-sufficiency is possible in the near future (WFP, 2001).

Overall, the strategy of cereal self-sufficiency has been quite successful, from producing only 11 million tons in 1970, cereal production nearly doubled to over 21 million tons in 1999 (FAOSTAT, 2000). Parallel to the increase in food production, food imports dropped from 26 to 30 per cent of total import volume and 50 to 70 per cent of export earnings in the 1980s, to 18 per cent of all imports and 34 per cent of Bangladesh's total export earnings in recent years. In the 1990s, Bangladesh's annual food-grain imports have been in the range of 1-2.5 million tons. However, hikes tend to occur in response to 'disaster year', such as in 1988,1991, or 1998. When cereal imports increased due to the relief measures that were implemented following widespread floods or major cyclones

(WFP, 2000). Rice imports, for example, reached up to 2.6 million tons in the disaster year of 1998. Despite the impressive increase in domestic production, Bangladesh has still the lowest dietary energy supply per capita in the region. Making the situation worse, the prevalent consumption pattern indicates that the national diet is nutritionally extremely unbalanced, with cereals making up an astonishingly high 82 per cent (FAOSTAT, 2000). Bangladesh's proneness to disaster is a key risk factor for the national food economy and for household food security. As has happened recurrently in the past, disasters wipe out crops and cause immense damage to the physical and social infrastructure. Incorporating disaster mitigation into development policies and programmes is an absolute imperative, more than in any other country of the region. Another impending food insecurity factor is urbanization like other countries in South Asia, Bangladesh's rapidly growing urban population will not to be fed, and pressures on the government to control food prices may have a major effect on reforms in its agricultural and food assistance policies.

Over the last 50 years, India has made significant strides in its food grain production. Its output has increased from about 55 million tons to over 200 million tons, an increase of 263 per cent. During the same period, the population grew from 360 million to above 1000 million (188 per cent increase). This success is attributed in part to the Green Revolution that started in the late 1960s and was characterized by huge public investments in irrigation infrastructure and research, land reforms, introduction of high-yielding varieties of seeds and the expanded use of fertilizer and pesticides. The new agricultural technologies pushed up productivity of wheat and rice. However, the benefits of the "green revolution" were unequally distributed among the farmers. The 'winners' were primarily wheat producers with large and medium landholding under irrigation in the north-west namely in Punjab and Haryana. In the 1980s, India became self-sufficient in food grains and a marginal net-exporter, during that period the average production growth rate was 3.5 per cent per annum (Haller, 1999). Like Bangladesh, India could not maintain this pace. Food grain output grew at a rate only 1.8 per cent per annum, a slightly higher than the growth rate of population (1.7 per cent). Moreover, the huge growth in food grain output since the 1960s was based on just two crops: wheat and rice. The annual growth of production of pulses remained more of less stagnant during last 30 years, and coarse cereal production actually declined (FAOSTAT, 2000).

Currently, India's macro availability dimension of food security is premised on self-sufficiency in wheat and rice, and on net imports of pulses and vegetable oil. Imports of cereals no longer play a significant role given the sheer size of India's domestic production. Since 1990s, India has been twice a net importer of food grain. The trade liberalization had a significant impact in certain agricultural sub-sectors. For instance, domestic production of pulses and vegetable oil has been either stagnant or declining, the trade liberalization in the 1990s has resulted in considerable gain in imports market share, between 20 and 30 per cent of domestic production (FAOSTAT, 2000). This has increased the availability of oil and lower prices in the local market. The large --scale dependence on imports could be dangerous to India, given the food grain supply and demand compared to the international cereal market. The current level of consumption is 175 million MT, whereas the country produces 190 million MT cereals, and the size of world cereal market is about 250 million MT. The dependence on imports would make the country vulnerable to the international price fluctuations and price hikes. In the extreme, situations could arise where the world market supply of food grains cannot meet the domestic demand. Over the period, considerable gains in food availability have been made, this has not resulted in an equitable distribution of food in all parts of the country due to infrastructural constraints, market imperfections, and governmental regulations, resulting in regional food scarcities. The increase in population and changing consumption pattern due to rising incomes and progressive urbanization will influence the future food demand. The total demand for food grains will range from 250 to 360 million tons to feed a population of 1.2 billion by 2010 (Bhalla *et. al.,* 1999). The future challenges for India includes both raising food output and ensuring sustainable, stable, and widely shared growth in food supplies. The larger food supplies must also came from rising biological yields and the replacement of chemical fertilizers with bio-fertilizers, besides area expansion and more irrigation which calls for heavy investment in research, bio-technology development and its dissemination. Keeping the rising income levels, India will be facing a Herculean task if it wants to meet the rising demand from domestic production.

Nepal is an overwhelmingly agrarian economy, with agriculture contributing more than 40 per cent to the GDP, the highest share of all South Asian countries (Mahbub UL Haq Human Development Centre, 2000). Nepal has shifted from a position of national food grain surpluses to chronic food deficits. In the early 1980s, Nepal still has net trade surplus in rice, but since the early 1990s, food imports have increased substantially. Today, 45 out of 75 districts are considered food deficit. During the recent past, the overall agricultural growth rate of 2.2 per cent has not kept pace with population growth (2.4 per cent), which can be attributed to land degradation due to extremes in precipitation, marginal soil and serious erosion of agricultural top-soil, dwindling forest resources, and irrigation constraints (WFP, 2001). One of the most crucial factors affecting food accessibility and availability is the lack of communication and transport infrastructure (Mathema, 1999). An escalating domestic insurgency in many remote mid-hill and mountain districts has had and impact on the food security of the regions. The intensification of agriculture in the *Tarai,* and the diversification of its agriculture in the hills and mountains will be the key to Nepal's food security in the coming decades. There is urgent need for making heavy investment in the road infrastructure in order to open up remote areas, i.e., the areas of acute food insecurity. Alongside the roads, much can be done for food insecure household to help them transform their agricultural practices from unsustainable subsistence pattern to more profitable approaches such as community forestry, agro-forestry, and cash cropping. In Nepal, the future food security is linked to how well it meets this redistribution challenge.

In Pakistan, the breakthrough in agriculture came with the green revolution in the 1960s, with the subsidized supply of new seeds and fertilizers and the increase in water availability, both through canal and tube well irrigation. As a result, agriculture grew by more than 4 per cent per annum in the 1960s, fell to 2.6 per cent in the 1970s, but again picked up in the 1980s. This partly offset the discrimination against agriculture. However, as in other South Asian countries, the impact and benefits of the green revolution were confined mainly to regions with extensive irrigated areas (Punjab, Sindh and parts of NWFP), and the dissemination of the technology package was biased in favour of the large farmers (Islam, 1996). Today, Pakistan's agricultural economy is characterized by self-sufficiency in cereal production and exports of high quality rice and cotton. More than two-thirds of the overall cereal production of 23 million MT is wheat. Despite sustained growth in production, Pakistan has to import 2 to 2.5 million tons wheat per annum to feed its population, which is growing at a persistently high rate of 2.8 per cent (the highest in South Asia). Oilseed production in Pakistan represents another notable setback, from a position of self-sufficiency, the country has now become a net-importer. Efforts to expand the production of non-traditional oilseeds have failed as domestic price policies and wide scale imports of cheap foreign cooking oils have effectively curbed production incentives (WFP, 2001).

A strong focus on sustainable increase in domestic food production might be necessary considering the country's increasing difficulties in financing food imports. Since the mid-1990s, Pakistan faced slow economic growth, rapid inflation, declining foreign exchange reserves, and large fiscal deficits. High and increasing imports of wheat and oil have worsened Pakistan's chronic balance of payments deficits and foreign exchange shortages. All this has led to increases in prices of food. Like India, the agriculture sector in Pakistan has a large potential for growth, and for most crops, the yield gap between current and potential yields is significant. To what extent this gap can be closed depends upon the ability of the country to address the challenges in the agriculture sector. Less optimistic food production projection based on the past trends suggests serious shortfalls in food grains, which will increase from over four million tons in 2000 to over ten million tons by 2025. The future food security in Pakistan will depend on both its natural resource endowments and its policy framework. While Pakistan has sufficient land resources to produce enough food to meet the entire domestic demand, its key constraint is water. Once considered a water-rich country, today Pakistan is in the midst of a growing water crisis. This affects primarily the irrigation system, which currently uses 97 per cent of the water. Cropping patterns have been based on the false premise of abundant water. Pakistan's canal irrigation network was designed in the midst of the green revolution to support cropping intensities of only 70 to 80 per cent annually, with thinly spread supplies for a thinly spread population. Population growth and consequent land fragmentation, combined with low crop yields, have forced the farmers to double their cropping intensity well beyond the design assumptions of the infrastructure. Another determinant of Pakistan's future food security will be closely connected to political and economic developments. In the past, food insecurity has been less an issue due to good marketing network and generalized wheat subsidies. However, latest data suggests that these subsidies still required over US $ 200 million of government funds (Pasha *et. al.,* 2000), have now been terminated. From the perspective of the local food producers, this is a positive step because sustainable increases in food production will require non-distorted food markets. But poor households would suffer, if the macro food security instruments of the past were dropped without any substitute. The newly planned 'National Food Programme' that targets poor families, would be a step in the right direction.

Sri Lanka has a comparatively high degree of food security compared to its other South Asia neighbours. However, in certain areas, its food economy is precarious. Sri Lanka's biggest food security concern is the on-going civil conflict and its impact on vulnerable population. As many as one million people have been displaced by the war, with more than 680,000 fed by the government in 'welfare camps', waiting for the fighting to stop so that they can return home and resume their lives (WFP, 1999). In addition, to the massive economic and property damage caused by the war, food production has also suffered. The north and east of Sri Lanka were major producers of both crops and fish, and production of these has been greatly affected. The second national food security concern is the country's so-called 'dry-zone'. This zone is less densely populated than other parts of Sri Lanka and is rainfed or under minor irrigation; and agriculturally much less diversified than the wetter region of the country. The main crop produced in the dry zone is paddy. But production costs are high and cheaper imports, for example, from India, are increasing the pressure for major structural changes. Sri Lanka has been a net importer of food, and the major proportion of the Sri Lankan diet is imported. The government has taken steps to promote local food production, especially rice. Numerous irrigation projects have increased the amount of land under cultivation (from 340,000 ha in 1948 to 750,000 ha in 1998), which along with the introduction of green revolution technologies have increased yields from 1.4 to 3.5 tons per hectare. Nevertheless, compared to its neighbour, India, Sri Lanka is a high cost producer of rice. As the economy continues its structural transformation, the emphasis on rice production is likely to diminish, especially if regional free trade opens agricultural markets to more competition.

Recommendations and Conclusion

Overall, the application of green revolution technologies in South Asian countries have resulted into greater food security and made food economies more resilient to famine. However, projections suggest that South Asia could face increasing food insecurity during the current decade, as the amount of food needed to maintain consumption at current levels could increase steeply depending on factors such as population growth, a slowdown in the growth in grain cultivation area, and the influence of rising incomes on dietary composition. Pakistan is projected to have the highest status quo food gap. India still has potential for food grain production increases, especially in the North-Eastern states. To a lesser extent, also Bangladesh can squeeze more output from its land with improved agro-technology. Although Bangladesh will continue to import wheat, the country is perched on the edge of rice self-sufficiency. By contrast, Pakistan faces a resource crunch. Its limits to growth relate to water supplies, despite of broad irrigation coverage. The Himalayan Kingdom of Nepal do not has vast potential for irrigation that India, Pakistan, and Bangladesh do. Nepal's comparative advantage lies in exploiting upland-lowland interaction and trade. Given the extreme biodiversity, country has greater potential for growing high value cash crops; and rural accessibility, in terms of both communication and market integration, is a key issue. Sri Lanka has very different food economy than the rest of the region. Sri Lanka's plantation sector with its high degree of export-orientation is an important element of the food economy. With its large earnings from trade, it has been able to import sufficient supplies of basic commodities. Thus, the country-wise food security scenario in South Asia varies greatly. The answer to expected future food insecurity problem lies in strengthening existing food based interventions that have long been instrumental in mitigating the worst effects of access and utilization failure among the poorest household. South Asia has been the recipient of vast quantities of international food aid over the past five decades. It has also been implementing some of the largest and most ambitious national food assistance programmes in the world. There is no doubt that such intervention since 1950s saved millions of people from starvation.

United Nations (2003) assessment of population prospects indicates that a radical slowdown in South Asian demographic growth is likely. However, despite the considerable fall in the growth rate, the annual increments will continue to be large because of population momentum-the tendency for population growth to continue beyond the time that low fertility has been achieved due to the relatively high concentration of people in the childbearing ages. Technological improvements in agriculture over the past century have allowed most countries of the region to increase food production well ahead of population growth at a steady falling economic cost, and without an environmental catastrophe. The crucial question is: can this progress be sustained in the future? Overall, there is no doubt that the demographic transition which is now underway in most South Asian countries-and is fairly advanced in Sri Lanka-helps to slow down the growth in demand for agricultural commodities, and thus facilitates the process of achieving food security. On the other hand, the economic and environmental costs of augmenting per capita food production may well prove too great for countries like Bangladesh and Nepal whose populations grow faster, resulting in greater poverty and fewer resources to fight it. In such countries, much will depend on their governments' ability to develop effective policy responses to the challenges posed by growing human numbers, poverty, and environmental degradation. In order to strengthen food security and address disparities in nutritional levels, a massive increase in food production is needed in these poorer countries, combined with growth in per capita incomes and improvements in international trade. But whatever the policy context, the goal of achieving food security will be made more difficult if population growth rates cannot be reduced.

How can a country reduce its population growth? The evidence on the matter suggests that much can be achieved through policies, which reduce unwanted births, enhance women's education, increase life expectancy, and reduce the demand of households for child labour. In this context it is worth mentioning that the average total fertility rate (TFR) is significantly high in Nepal and Bangladesh indicating that the demographic transition has not started. Reducing fertility levels in these countries would certainly create better conditions for achieving progress in food security in the region. For example, the improvement of household food security and nutritional levels is associated with women's access to gainful employment and education, and with their role in decisions on household expenditure and production matters (FAO, 1997; World Bank, 2003). Therefore, efforts to promote gender equality and empower women are a key component of the fight against poverty and hunger.

Among the major forces expected to influence food production in coming years are investment in agriculture, considerations related to the environment and natural resource base, and government policy. Agricultural growth and development must be vigorously pursued to meet growing food needs, alleviate poverty through employment creation and income generation in rural areas, and stimulate overall economic growth. Agricultural growth is the most efficient and effective means of promoting general economic growth and, hence, of improving food security of the poorest people in low-income South Asian developing countries. Various investments are needed to facilitate agricultural and rural growth, such as agricultural research and technology to generate yield-increasing production technology and improved crop varieties, improved rural infrastructure to facilitate access to markets, modern inputs, credit, and technical assistance.

Natural resource management and environmental considerations are also expected to influence food production. Much of the degradation in the South Asian region - overgrazing, deforestation, and over-exploitation for fuel-wood - results from poverty and from lack of opportunities to intensify agriculture. As population, poverty, and food demands continue to grow, failure to develop and implement appropriate technology in production and marketing could lead to either more food insecurity and hunger, for which the current generation of poor people will pay, or to further degradation of natural resource base, for which future generations will pay. Trade-offs between meeting future food demands and maintaining production capacity can be avoided and sustainability in food production can be assured only if investment in appropriate research and technology is accelerated, relevant externalities are internalized into production and consumption decisions or effectively dealt with by government policy, and poverty is significantly reduced or eradicated.

Net imports are a reflection of the gap between production and demand. The gap between production and need will be even wider, as many of the poor are priced out of the market and are unable to exercise their demand for needed food. The poorer countries in the region will lack sufficient foreign exchange to import food in needed quantities. Bangladesh, Nepal and Sri Lanka will require special assistance to avert widespread hunger and malnutrition. It is unlikely that they will have the necessary foreign exchange to import large amounts of food. Neither is it likely that enough food aid will be forthcoming to make up the gap between supply and need. Lastly, the challenge is to both grow more food and assure that the food is accessible by all people at all times. Even though enough food is available to feed the world, which does not help the many people who cannot get access to it. We must focus on both better distribution of available food and increased production of food to meet the needs of the ever growing population and to generate the incomes needed by the poor to convert their food needs into effective demand, recognizing that available food will not be evenly distributed.

References

Ahmed, R., S. Haggblade and T–e-E Chowdhury (eds.) (2000), *Out of the Shadow of Famine: Evolving Food Markets and Food Policy in Bangladesh,* Johns Hopkins University Press/International Food Policy Research Institute, Baltimore.

Alexandratos, N. (ed.) (1995), *World Agriculture: Towards 2010, An FAO Study,* Rome: FAO. Available from http://www.fao.org/docrep/V4200E/V4200E00.htm.

Bhalla, G.S., Peter Hazell and John Kerr (1999), *Prospects for India's Cereal Supply and Demand to 2020,* Food, Agriculture, and the Environment, Discussion Paper No. 29, International Food Policy Research Institute, Washington, D.C.

Bhattacharjee, J.P. (ed.) (1958), *Studies in Indian Agricultural Economics,* Bombay, cited in Sudan, F. K., *Demographic Transition in South Asia,* Anmol Publication, 1992.

Bilsborrow, R.E. (1987), "Population Pressures and Agricultural Development in Developing Countries: A Conceptual Framework and Recent Evidence", *World Development Vol.* 15, No. 2, p. 183-203.

Blaxter, K. (1986), *People, Food and Resources,* Cambridge University Press, Cambridge.

Bongaarts, J. (1994), "Can the Growing Human Population Feed Itself?" *Scientific American,* March, pp. 36-42.

Bongaarts, J. (1996), "Population Pressure and the Food Supply System in the Developing World", *Population and Development Review,* Vol. 22, pp. 483-503.

Boserup, E. (1965), *The Conditions of Agricultural Growth,* George Allen and Unwin, London.

Boserup, E. (1990), *Economic and Demographic Relationships in Development,* Johns Hopkins University Press, Baltimore.

Brklacich, Mike (2000), "Food Security", *IHDP Update,* No.2, Bonn, Germany.

Brown, L.R. (1988), "The Changing World Food Prospect: The Nineties and Beyond", *Worldwatch Paper 85,* Worldwatch Institute, Washington, D. C.

Brown, L.R. (1991), "The New World Order", in L. R. Brown, C. Flavin and S. Postel (ed.) *State of the World 1991,* Earthscan Publications Ltd., London.

Brown, L.R. (1993), "A New Era Unfolds", in L. R. Brown, C. Flavin and S. Postel (eds) *State of the World 1993,* W. W. Norton, New York.

Brown, L.R. and Kane, H. (1995), *Full House: Reassessing the Earth's Population Carrying Capacity,* Earthscan Publications Ltd., London.

CIA (1998), *The CIA World Fact Book, 1998.*

Daily, G.C. and Elrlich, P.R. (1990), "An Exploratory Model of the Impact of Rapid Climate Change on the World Food Situation", *Proceedings of the Royal Society of London, B 241,* p. 232-44.

Dreze, Jean, and Amartya Sen (1989), *Hunger and Public Action,* Oxford: Clarendon Press.

Dyson, T. (1996), *Population and Food: Global Trends and Future Prospects,* Routledge, London and New York.

Dyson, T. (2003), "Food Supply and Population", In: *Encyclopedia of Population.* New York: Macmillan, pp. 431-435.

Ehrlich, P.R. and Ehrlich, A.H. (1990), *The Population Explosion,* Simon B. Schuster, New York.

Ehrlich, P.R., Ehrlich, A.H. and Daily, G.C. (1993), "Food Security, Population and the Environment", *Population and Development Review*, Vol.19, No.1, pp.1-32.

FAO (1996a), *Rome Declaration on Food Security and World Food Summit Plan of Action,* Rome.

FAO (1996b), "Food Requirements and Population Growth", In: *World Food Summit, Technical Background Documents 1-5, Vol. 1.* Rome: FAO. Available from http://www.fao.org/wfs/index_en.htm.

FAO (1997), Gender: the Key to Sustainability and Food Security, Rome: FAO. Available from http://www.fao.org/sd/WPdirect/WPdoe001.htm.

FAO (2003a), *The State of Food Insecurity in the World 2003: Monitoring Progress Towards the World Food Summit and Millennium Development Goals.* Rome: FAO. Available from http://www.fao.org/documents/show_cdr.asp?url_file=/DOCREP/006/J0083E/J0083E00.HTM.

FAO (2003b), *World Agriculture: Towards 2015/2030, An FAO Perspective,* J. Bruinsma, ed., London: Earthscan.

FAO (2000), *New Dimensions in Water Security,* United Nations, Rome.

FAOSTAT (2000), (Online FAO Statistical Database – *http://apps.fao.org,* Rome.

Flew, A. (ed.) (1970), Malthus, T. R., *An Essay on the Principle of Population and a Summary View of the Principle of Population,* Penguin, Harmondsworth.

Fogel, Robert (1997), "The Global Struggle to Escape from Chronic Malnutrition since 1700," in *Ending the Inheritance of Hunger,* World Food Programme, United Nations University Seminar, Rome: World Food Programme.

Grigg, M. (1993), *The World Food Problem,* 2nd edn, Basil Blackwell, Oxford.

Haller, A. (1999), "National Food Surpluses and Food Aid in India," *Mimeo,* World Food Programme, Regional Office for South Asia, New Delhi.

Harrison, P. (1992), *The Third Revolution: Environment, Population and a Sustainable World,* I. B. Tauris, London.

Hayami, Y. and Ruttan, V. R. (1987), "Population Growth and Agricultural Poverty", in D. G. Johnson and R. D. Lee (ed.) Population Growth and economic Development: Issues and Evidence, University of Wisconsin Press, Madison.

Islam, Nurul (1996), "Growth, Poverty and Human Development: Pakistan", *Human Development Report Office, Occasional Paper 31,* New York: United Nations Development Programme, New York.

Kellman, M. (1987), *World Hunger, A Neo-Malthusian Perspective,* Praeger, New York.

Kuznets, Simon (1966), *Modern Economic Growth,* New Haven, CT: Yale University Press.

Mahbub Ul Haq Human Development Centre (2000), *Human Development in South Asia, 2000,* Oxford University Press, Karachi.

Malthus, T. R. (1798), *An Essay on the Principle of Population as it Affects the Future Improvement of Society with Remarks on the Speculations of Mr. Godwin, M. Condoecet, and Other writers,* St Paul's Church-yard, London.

Mathema, Sudarshan B. (1999), "Strategy of Sustainable Rural Livelihoods and Social Exclusion for Nepal: A Review of the Literature," *Mimeo,* Department for International Development, Kathmandu.

McNicoll, G. (1992), "The United Nations' Long Range Population Projections", *Population and Development Review,* Vol.18, No. 2, pp. 333-40.

Myers, N. (1991), *Population, Resources and the Environment: The Critical Challenge,* United Nations Population Fund, New York.

Pasha, H.A., S. Jafarey and H.R. Lohano (2000), "Evaluation of Social Safety Nets in Pakistan," *Research Report,* No. 32, Social Policy and Development Centre, Islamabad.

Pingali, P. and Binswanger, H.P. (1991), "Population Density and Farming Systems", in R. D. Lee, W. B. Arthur, A. C. Kelley, G. Rodgers and T. N. Srinivasan (ed.) Population, Food, and Rural Development, Clarendon Press, Oxford.

Population Action International (1992), Population and the Environment: Impacts in the Developing World, Population Action International, Washington, D. C.

Postel, S. (1992), Last Oasis, Facing Water Scarcity, W. W. Norton, New York.

Ravallion, Martin (1987), *Markets and Famines,* Oxford: Clarendon Press.

Ravallion, Martin (1997), "Famines and Economics", *Journal of Economic Literature,* Vol. 35, No. 3, pp. 1205-1242.

Roest, C.W.J. (2000), "Water for Food Production in South Asia: An Overview of ICID Draft Country Papers," In Mollinga P. (ed.), *Water for Food and Rural Development: Approaches and Initiatives in South Asia,* Sage Publications: New Delhi.

Saether, A. (1993), "Otto Diederich Lutken: 40 years before Malthus?", *Population Studies,* Vol. 47, No. 3, p. 511-13.

Sen, Amartya (1981), *Poverty and Famines.* Oxford: Oxford University Press.

Simon, J. L. (1981), *The Ultimate Resource,* Martin Robertson, Oxford.

Simon, J. L. (1992), *Population and Development in Poor Countries, Selected Essays,* Princeton University Press, Princeton.

Smil, V. (2000), Feeding the World: A Challenge for the Twenty-First Century, Cambridge, Massachusetts: MIT Press.

Sudan, F. K. (2001), "Water Scarcity and Food Security: Some Policy Issues", Paper Contributed for Second Biennial Conference of Indian Society for Ecological Economics, at Indian Institute of Forest Management, Bhopal, during Dec. 2001.

Timmer, C. Peter (2000), "The Macro Dimensions of Food Security: Economic Growth, Equitable Distribution, and Food Price Stability", *Food Policy.* Vol. 25, pp 283-295.

United Nations (1994), *World Population Prospects: The 1994 Revision – Annex Tables,* United Nations, New York.

United Nations (2003), *World Population Prospects: The 2002 Revision.* Sales No. E.03.XIII.10.

World Bank (2001), *World Development Report, 2000-2001,* Oxford University Press, New Delhi.

World Bank (2003), *Gender Equality & the Millennium Development Goals.* Washington, D.C.: World Bank. Available from http://www.worldbank.org/gender/resources/gendermdg.pdf.

World Food Programme (WFP) (1999), Assistance to Internally Displaced People: Country Case Study on Internal

Displacement—Sri Lanka, Displacement in the North and East, Rome.

World Food Programme (WFP) (2000), *Food Aid Flows to SAARC, 1987-99*, Regional Office for South Asia, New Delhi.

World Food Programme (WFP) (2001), *Enabling Development: Food Assistance in South Asia*, Oxford University Press, New Delhi.

Wrigley, E. A. and Schofield, R. S. (1981), *The Population History of England 1541-1871: A Reconstruction*, Edward Arnold, London.

4

GREEN CONSUMERISM AND CORPORATE SOCIAL RESPONSIBILITY AS A PANACEA FOR UNSUSTAINABLE AND INEQUITABLE GROWTH PATTERN IN THE CURRENT GLOBALISED SCENARIO

V. Vijayalakshmi

Introduction

Globalization and knowledge society has led to a new enigma and iniquitous world leading to a few big beneficiaries and new paradigms disturbing all walks of life. Mainstream economists however contend that globalization is a 'win-win' formula where one big global market exists with trade flourishing unhindered. Poor countries are expected to grow faster than rich ones in a free global market because capital from the rich will flow towards regions with cheap labour. Global economic integration and freer international trade is also said to offer tremendous benefits to consumers. It has resulted in lower prices, better-informed shoppers, wider choices and often better quality and product safety. Consumer sovereignty is effective in well-developed market systems, since it is the consumer's choice that directs the rest of the economy.

Globalisation, which allows efficient allocation of resources, also throws up challenges and contradictions of survival of the fittest. It is feared to create a single, elite business class networked across the globe that places markets above culture and politics. Disinvestment in the public sector has led to rampant corruption and state-capital nexus. While culturally globalisation poses problem of homogenization of culture, and replacing traditional values, identities, the greatest danger however is in economic and social globalisation, which promote an inegalitarian society and individualist and consumerist culture. The incongruity of modern lifestyles and consumerism is leading to environmental devastation, threatening the integrity of the biosphere and possibly life itself. Conservation of depleting resources is of great concern as doomsday predictions like the dangers of water wars and consequences of global warming ring alarm bells. The traditional society is disappearing and a seamless society is emerging with altering lifestyles. Internet technology has also largely influenced the culture of its users-net speak, net slang, advertisement, Spam mail, on-line trading etc. Satellite imaging eludes monitoring and regulation and poses problems of cheap portrayal of women, violence and crime. As *Mikhail Gorbachev* observed 'without direction globalisation may become a destructive process, and the first signs of such destruction are already starting to show.'

The causal links between globalisation and poverty, economic and environmental damage to the poor, limited access of the poor to technology, information, innovation and markets requires rethinking about surmounting the dangers ahead. This has brought about serious rural - urban divide in developing countries like India with prosperity in urban centers in contrast to the extreme poverty and helplessness of the rural poor. In India the average monthly percapita expenditure was 87% higher in urban areas compared to rural as released by MISH (2006, market information survey of households), by NCAER, (National Council of Applied Economic Research). Globalisation and economic reforms have resulted in dramatic changes in market dynamics and higher, superior, diversified consumption levels of urban consumers. No such progress has however been observed in rural India due to the high correlation between infrastructure deprivation and economic deprivation.

Within the urban centers itself the inequity is observed between the rich and poor on high valued manufactured goods with the poor spending Rs. 1 to Rs. 188 by the rich. (Indo Asian News Service)

The utopian idea of economic globalisation however considers that market regulation through politics is totally unwarranted. Demand and supply matrix are sufficient to control markets. This thinking is best articulated through a cliché, 'Governments have no business to be in business.' They vehemently refute the charge that globalisation is anti- people by citing China where the stupendous strides made are not solely due to FDI's but poverty alleviation measures like elaborate land reforms, agricultural growth, population control and educational reforms. As against this there is another alternate stream of thinking emerging based on 'alternative developmental strategies' which impose less strain on natural resources and corporate social responsibility drive among the big companies to eliminate poverty. This idea is different from conventional utilitarian economics and can be traced to Gandhiji who was again an early advocate of environmental protection. If markets work on efficiency and not morality, distributive justice will not be ensured. *Amartya Sen, Jean Dreze and Martha Nussbaum* have delved on the need for a normative, humane approach to radical growth policies.

The unhealthy practices of globalisation arouse pertinent questions as to why nations race ahead in the globalisation race despite sacrifice of environment, labour, health concerns at the altar of commerce. The pressure applied by private economic forces on national policy making and the desire not to be left behind in the race to progress is finally leading to acceptance of the fact that globalisation has come to stay. The next question that remains to be faced is, if unavoidable, the need arises to devise ways to mitigate its evil consequences. Here the role of consumer assumes significance, as customers in general are not only beneficiaries of, but also agents behind, and consequences that result from market efficiency. Delinking from global economy is not attractive for the producer either and hence measures to promote good corporate behavior are of primary concern now. Ecological democracy attempts to secure necessary conditions for the reintegration of society and nature and producers have to adhere to these norms and make suitable innovations. TNC's and market arrangements have to be modified to be pro-poor and environmentally friendly. Consumers have to be part of responsible shoppers and partner with companies in this global green shift. Large-scale deprivation requires resolutions, economically, socially, politically, and philosophically. (freedom from necessity). Concerted action to give recognition to traditional knowledge and practices, by curbing jurisdiction of international IPR, cultural movement to show the incongruity of modern lifestyles and consumerism and movement to sustain local markets is the need of the hour.

Consumer Sovereignty and Corporate Social Responsibility to Facilitate Sustainable Development

While environmental doomsayers warn of impending ecological catastrophes, consumer aspirations for both the rich and poor have expanded with globalisation. *Consumers unabashedly flaunt wealth* and happiness has become directly proportional to the sense of empowerment in the number of carry bags one gets back home. The whole premise of consumerism has to be questioned from the angles of alleviation of poverty and sustainable usage of resources. The ensuing debate lies in the role of government, corporations and individuals in maximizing social welfare by calculating the social costs and benefits of globalisation paradigm. Businesses able to defy conventional logic and combine social values with viable business ventures can provide a powerful moral counter point to the dominant logic of neo-liberalism. The whole logic centers on responsible consumption patterns through intelligent choices matched by socially responsible investment and good corporate conduct by producers.

In the US it is estimated that as much as 13% of total investment funds are managed according to socially responsible principles. Well-informed consumers are emerging as a new force in the global struggle to create an environmentally sustainable world, reports a new study by the World watch Institute, a Washington, DC-based environmental and social policy research organization. Aided by labeling programs, standards, and an expanding group of social and environmental certification organizations, the world's consumers are 'voting with their wallets' for products and services that promote sustainable development. Indian management should assume corporate social responsibility and move towards hybrid form of management incorporating Vedic management with Gandhi's Trusteeship doctrine combined with western principles. A number of foundations set by leading Indian firms in recent times, including Wipro, Tatas, TVS, Dr. Reddy's laboratory have taken keen interest in corporate activism to improve health care, education, and living conditions and reduce poverty.

As academicians the solutions seem apparent and straightforward. Realities however make the whole issue complex. Facts about global warming appear inadequate and dangers refer to diffuse effects on non-human individuals, species, and communities or future generations of humans. It is impossible to map a clear causal relationship between actions and harms and restraint simply does not emerge. Not withstanding the difficulties, consumer's choice becomes vital for it is the totality of such choices that dictate production patterns in an economy. Producer consumer relationships have to be redefined and be connected to global poverty and negative externalities of the environment. The government can certify the brands bearing the label of high ethics and moral values of its creators. Due to their potential to impact the environment the areas that should come under close scrutiny are health care, renewable energy, *traffic snarls, water crisis,* biodiversity, agriculture and waste management. Public private partnership in these with well defined goals and processes for the best use of resources will ensure sustained economic development.

The role of intelligent consumers choices and conscious decisions questioning themselves about the anticipated and unanticipated impact of their choices on the planet, is important. The role of citizen and consumer should be rolled into one, public spirited and rational. A combination of aesthetically pleasing products combined with incorporation of ecological values should be supported. Green consumerism should lead producers to seek alternatives for products produced under fair conditions and respecting interdependencies of life. If alternate products perform to expectation and are easily available they should be chosen. All this means consuming in a *different way* and not consuming less. Clearly a dramatic reduction in consumption would be impossible without challenge to the *supremacy* of consumer sovereignty. Consumers should learn the difference between the final goods and services that any economy produces and the productive resources, including human resources, capital goods and natural resources that are used to produce these final goods and services.

The complex processes involved in production and dependence on limited natural resources makes it imperative to study the life cycles of a consumer's purchases-because a consumer does not just buy 'a' product, but also everything that went into its production, and everything that will happen in the future as a result of the products we buy. This will enable us to better understand the connectivity between environment and economics. Green consumerism strikes a balance between the prospects of consumer behaviour and businesses' profit motives-within the *trajectory of environmental* protection. We need to realize that all products have an environmental impact, however small.

Consumer decisions guide resource allocation and businesses must respond to the demands of consumer. Consumer sovereignty drives the market and sensible, ethico moral choices can positively influence the quality of life and our environment. Twentieth century moral obligations have to be altered to make right choices like solar water heaters, avoiding plastic diapers, and minimized usage of plastic bags. Individual citizens are also responsible for particulate matter discharged by wood burning stoves, indoor pollution from cigarette smoking and air pollution caused by high fuel consuming cars. Co-operation in promoting global energy security and the promotion of alternate energy technologies such as wind, biogas, and solar energy speaks of new dimensions to the growth process. The concept of green consumers also focuses on businesses, and their survivability as they respond quickly to demands of consumers for products and services that are also environmentally friendly. Pro-active and futuristic minded consumers make responsible shopping decisions by associating with companies working towards this global green shift. Ultimately the decisions of the educated middle-income consumers will have trickle down effects on the rural economy as well.

A few practical examples will give insights into how consumer choices have the power to reduce depletion and pollution of natural resources. This is largely true in the case of wood, which is a renewable resource, and when grown and harvested properly, forests have a tremendous potential to regenerate. Consumer behavior, habits that would help to conserve wood include: reusing scratch paper, using e-mail rather than paper to communicate more, printing and copying double sided, fitting more on to one piece of paper, using less wood in construction, recycling all wood products, etc. Newsprint, office paper, junk mail, magazines, wrapping paper, cereal boxes and so on can all be recycled. Consumers can also build houses and other structures with non-wood alternatives such as straw, bale/ agricultural waste, adobe, rammed earth, etc. Finally consumers can promote forest protection by buying wood products, if they are made from "certified sustainable wood." Sustainable wood comes from the practice of "sustainable forestry" in developed countries, which ensures that the rate of timber harvest does not exceed the rate of timber growth. Moreover, "sustainable wood" companies promote the long-term health and productivity of their forests, wildlife and water quality protection, and lasting community employment.

Brazil is responding to using clean, renewable, alternative sources of energy to an even greater extent. More than 40% of Brazil's energy comes from "green sources' in comparison with around 7% in rich countries. The ethanol Brazil produces from sugar cane is attracting worldwide interest, for it is one of the cheapest and most dependable types of fuel derived from renewable sources. Three quarters of the cars now being produced in Brazil have' flex-fuel' engines, capable of running on either ethanol or petrol, or any mixture of the two. The biodiesel projects bring social benefits and are produced from oil-bearing plants. Bio diesel is significantly less polluting than conventional petroleum based diesel.

Role of Citizen Consumers and Food Security to the Poor

Trade liberalisation and globalisation of agriculture is supposed to increase production of food, enhance efficiency of food production, ameliorate the economic situation of farmers and improve patterns of consumption. Instead food production in India declined by 7 millions, and marginalisation of small farmer is the consequence. Large companies and multi-nationals are being welcomed into agri-business and existing laws are bent to accommodate them. Since globalisation is based on utilitarian philosophy and maximizing profits it results in inequality only. Laissez-faire and Darwinism is on the rise and benefiting the winners only. Globalised monopolies are being promoted and small farmers in third world are more powerless than ever. They are unable to produce enough to support their livelihoods and are abandoning farming in search of urban employment. The number of suicides among farmers with rising debts and the governments of Karnataka and A.P losing power due to negligence of agriculture bear ample testimony to the harm done. This is mainly due to deregulating of inputs such as seeds and chemicals and imports by the removal of qualitative restrictions. Farm suicides in Vidarbha crossing 400 and Sensex crossing 11,000 have taking place simultaneously in March 2006 are only a tip of the iceberg of the alienation of the poor.

The corporate hijack of our food and agriculture by global corporations using WTO and World Bank has come in for massive criticism as being responsible for starvation and death of farmers. Corporate take over of agriculture made large companies the top gainers from distress sales of cotton in Vidarba this season. The admission of this in McKinley vision 2020 of Chandrababu Naidu in A.P. resulting in ousting of millions from farming seem to awaken no moral conscience and is being continued with renewed vigour, resulting in massive human displacement in Maharashtra also. The predicament of a person to circumstances over which he has no control requires Sen's freedom to achieve rather than actual achievements. Governmental intervention becomes necessary to correct the dire consequences. Consumers may benefit from globalised trade but righteous action requires self-restraint and non-support to development with dignity and centrality of full employment in our politics and economics.

Unequal access to natural resources and unequal distribution of the burden of pollution on the poor meant total disempowerment. Even privileged consumers have no food security in the sense of access to safe and nutritious food. The globalisation of corporate agriculture is aggravating the problems linked with the centralized system of food production and distribution. It is increasing chemical use through the conventional methods as well as genetic engineering. It is promoting the mining of water and soil fertility by putting profitability above sustainability. It is giving primacy to trade and undermining domestic production. It is putting exports above the food entitlements of domestic consumers and the modern food industry has become a threat to health. Food security without food safety is pointless and meaningless. As *S.M. Mohd. Idris* stated in his address: "Apart from creating food dependence, modern commercialised agricultural practices are mortgaging the world's scarce, non-renewable resources at the expense of future."

The institutions to manage the emerging global market like G8, and WTO were transnational and largely comprised the developed nations who could take advantage of the new marketing possibilities in the underdeveloped world-due to 'opening up' (liberalization) of their economies. New standards were put in place–ISO, IPR, Patent laws, etc–to safeguard their control. International agencies (World bank, IMF) and direct monetary assistance was tied to adherence to these standards. Intellectual Property Rights (IPR), in particular, assumed a crucial role in subjugating and undermining the genius of native knowledge. The stranglehold on the agricultural sector–in seeds, pesticides, fertilizer, prices; has led to the almost total destruction of native knowledge and practices. The monopoly of genetically engineered seeds has been ensured through dubious ways. The massive protests of farmers in the underdeveloped countries (and even in some developed ones) mark this aspect of globalisation. The media too caters to the fancies of the urban rich whilst issues like raising the height of Narmada dam, mass suicides of farmers receive scant attention.

Knowledge Economy as a Driving force in Optimal and Sustainable Production

Global democracy is facing deprivation of the poor and destruction of non-human world. While knowledge economy is responsible for accentuating globalisation the same knowledge economy can be used to find answers to these new ethical issues and arrive at proper ethical guidelines for dealing with them. Bridging the gap between ethics and action, between knowledge and real life, and making consumers exert influence on problems addressed by environmental ethics and poverty is the need of the hour. Knowledge about facts–even facts about clear harms is insufficient unless greater efforts are directed to enforce corrective measures.

As citizens and consumers, one can learn to use these knowledge tools to press for change, especially where consumption is leading to natural resource depletion and pollution. They can form a knowledge base that leads to an awareness of the interconnectedness between what we buy and the natural world. This sense can lead to a belief that conscientious consumption can make a difference and serve to empower the society at large. Consumers are to be educated to consume differently and not less. Spreading success stories of companies using renewable energy patterns will demonstrate that a company can balance eco-friendly production and the need to return profit to shareholders. Individual consumer decisions like green choices when it comes to everyday shopping choices, weddings, green buildings, fuel consumption, water recycling and working as a community towards a green and sustainable future. This is particularly applicable to India where we have 17% of the world's population but 2% of the land mass and 4% of water resources only.

Advertising and communication tools can be used to encourage better consumption patterns. The demands of the United Nations commission on sustainable development in 1997 sought the advertising industry to help promote new and most importantly sustainable consumption patterns. Press, media, newspapers, magazines, books, T.V, radio is the links between consumer, entrepreneur and government. The Internet is the largest self-governing organisation-it is all-pervasive, Even those opposed to globalisation depend on it to exchange ideas and mobilise support. While the Internet facilitates exchange of ideas, access to knowledge, communication between diverse peoples etc it also alters the 'structure' of knowledge and proves advantageous to those who have better access to it and emerging technologies. Through it the citizen consumer will have choices simplified according to trust in the corporate world.

An example of its usage in the marine environment would for instance reveal how solutions can be reached to tackle the worsening crisis of fisheries decline in the once abundant habitat regions in the ocean. Fisheries management in the Northeast Pacific at federal, state and provincial levels has taken up increasing reliance on spatial and/or sequential closures to manage fishery problems arising from the historic disregard for multi-species and ecological linkages that characterize the ocean environment. Communities and managers immediately require spatially integrated databases and tools that can incorporate and depict multiple layers of ecological, economic and socio-cultural information. This is of utmost exigency as the economic situation of coastal communities rapidly worsens alongside the declining health of the marine ecosystems of the region.

In the case of technology assisting the rural poor an example is the Maharashtra funded Kisaan call center which fields enquiries from rural farmers, who get advice from operators speaking their own language and whose directive is to treat every farmer as a customer. Knowledge economy should enhance consumer sovereignty in rural areas by empowering them with information about water control, better seeds, micro finance, rural public works and getting rid of transgenic seeds and toxic chemicals. Success of these measures would check urban poverty by preventing migration to urban areas.

Similarly the idea of Wal Mart entering the Indian market requires consumers to be alerted about the pitfalls and wiping away of small business. Behind Wal-Mart's "everyday low prices" lurk hidden costs—from the exploitation of workers in US and around the world, to increased sprawl and pollution that we end up paying as consumers, taxpayers, workers, and citizens. Though Wal-Mart is shifting its strategy and moving on to join the eco bandwagon by affordable organic food and clothing, rerouting trucks for cost and fuel savings, its impact on small business has to be viewed with caution. By marshalling the facts and popularizing them a powerful ethical case for government intervention can be made to make sellers behave in fair, competitive ways. But the "consumer-side" also needs new empowerment tools to assert its autonomous will, such as comparative product information (e.g., warning labels,) and new legal rights (e.g., the right-to-know about toxic hazards, procedural rights to participate in government proceedings, the right to initiate class actions). There is the need to expose the unconcealed disparity between obvious public wants (clean air, safe workplaces, honest competition, quality goods and services) and the failures of the marketplace, as constituted, to meet those wants.

The idea of new economy dependent on Internet usage and mobile phones is responsible for creating huge electronic waste. Unless recycling measures are adopted this becomes a matter of grave concern as consumers seek the latest technology and manufacturers introduce disposable models. Productivity has to be metamorphosed to incorporate environmental protection and community enhancement as a means to increase prosperity. Under the umbrella of Green Productivity, innovation, a key engine of economic growth, becomes part of a holistic strategy to move towards a sustainable future. Giving tax credits for companies following green norms, awards like Toyota energy

Star for sustained excellence, 2006, popularizing commuter benefits by Companies to avoid unnecessary burning fuel, traffic congestion, stress and work place productivity etc should be encouraged. Green buildings, both commercial and residential with water harvesting, recycling should gain momentum.

There maybe lurking doubts among ordinary consumers and producers and disdain at this kind of moral policing. While environmental activists and researchers realize the seriousness of global warming it is imperative for trickle down effects at the grass roots level that awareness should be created on these issues. Ecological services are merit goods whose usage benefits society. Allotting public goods to serve principles of ecological welfare must be complemented by such provision of private goods dictated and directed by consumer sovereignty.

In the context of potentials and pitfalls of globalization it is necessary to build alternative identities arising from conscientious consumption. Responsible consumption and empowerment of the rural poor is needed to achieve optimal and sustainable production. Hence it can be concluded that global economic integration is neither a panacea nor a curse. It cannot be halted but definitely altered to advance prosperity and values. *The imperativeness of taking into account the inconvenient truths of global warming and green house effects, growing inequities, into each one's consciousness be it the producer or consumer is best summed in M.S. Swaminathan"s words...*

"There's an old North American saying:

The sky is held up by the trees,

If the forest disappears, the sky roof of the world collapses

Nature and man then perish together."

References

Books

Josee Johnston (2001), "Consuming Social Justice", in "Protest and Globalisation: Prospects of Transnational Solidarity", James Goodman, (ed.) Pluto Press.

Joseph Stiglitz, (2002), "Globalization and its Discontent." Penguin Books, India; New Delhi. p. 24.

Rawls, J. (1999), 'A Theory of Justice' Cambridge: Harvard University Press, pp. 32-34.

Wilkinson, R.G. (2005), 'The Impact of Inequality'. New York: The New Press, Newspapers.

Aiyer Pallavi (2006), 'China Turns to Nuclear Power to Fuel Growth", The Hindu, 18, March.

Inancio Luiz, & Silva da Lula (2006), "Join Brazil in Planting Oil", *The Hindu,* and 8, March.

Konana Prahdev (2006), "Towards Corporate Social Responsibility", *The Hindu,* 9, March.

Nagamallika G. (2006), 'Urban Media—where are the Rural Audiences? *The Hindu,* 30, April.

Nataraj V.K. (2006), "Development Ethics,' *The Hindu,* 28, March.

Sainath, P. (2006), 'Where India Shining Meets Great Depression', *The Hindu,* 1, April.

Shah Mithir (2005), "Environmental Justice Movement and the Poor", *The Hindu,* 24, May.

Journals

Baker Mallen(2006),"Measuring Corporate Social Impact-art or Science, *Business Respect,* Issue No. 92,7, April, 2006.

Gorbacheu Mikhail (2005), "Threats of Social Darwin's—An Alarmed World," *World Affairs,* Jan-March, 5(!) 21, 2005.

Internet

CNN & Google dot.com

Bharadwaj Atul: "Man, State and the myth of Democratic Peace". *www.mafhoum.com/press3/112521* files/AN-APRO402-9.htm.

Burford Gemman &Ngila Ole Lesikar & Rafiki Yunus: "Education, Indigenous knowledge and Globalisation". *www.scienceinafrica.co.za/2003/march/ik.htm*

Cuomo J.Chris: "Getting closer: Thoughts in the Ethics of knowledge Production *http://environment.harvard: edu/religion/disciplines/ethics/.../ethcuomo.html*

Cogburn L. Derrick: 'Globalisation, Knowledge, Education and Training in the Information Age. *www.unesco.org/webworld/ infoethics* 2eng/papers/paper 23.htm.

Edney Julian: 'How capitalism threatens your health,' April 4, 2006. www.countercurrents.org.

Fotopoulos Takis: "Globalisation, through Reformist left, and the Anti-globalisation Movement". *www.democracynature. org/dn/ vo17/takis globalisation.htm.*

Human Rights Resource Centre: "Products, Environment and Consumer choices," Centre for Economic conversion, University of Minnesota." www/.umn.edu/humanrts/edumat/sustecon/ toc.htm.

Lijenburg Anders: 'From socialism to Electricity:" in "The evolution of the role of customers in the market," Social change project, Stockholm school of Economics, 2004. *http://www.mercatus.org/ pdf/materials/683.pdf*

Navdanya: "Food security and sustainable agriculture" *http:// www.navdanya.org/contact.htm*

Nissanke Machiko & Thorbecke Erik: "The impact of globalisation on the world's poor", Sustainable Economics Curriculum *wider.unu.edu/conference/*

OCEAN: Ocean community's 3E Analysis network. *ajscholz@ecotrust. org*

Scammel Margaret: "Internet and civic engagement: Age of the citizen consumer". *jsis.artsci.washington.edu/programs/cwesuw/ scammell.htm*

United States Mission to the European Union: "Larson on globalisation" *http://www.useu.be*

Wikipedia:"Corporate social Responsibility" *en.wikipedia.org/wiki/ corporate social responsibility*

Notes

Amartya Sen: 1998 Nobel prize winner in Economics for his contribution to Welfare Economics.

Idris, Mohd, S.M: President, Sahabat Alam Malaysia.(Friends of the Earth—Malaysia)

Jean Dreze: Visiting professor in Delhi school of Economics and an International authority in Developmental Economics.

Martha Nussbaum: One of America's renowned classist and prominent philosopher, teaching philosophy and Law at the University of Chicago.

Mikhail Gorbachev: 1990, Nobel peace prize winner, President of USSR.

Swaminathan M.S: India's Renowned agricultural scientist and father of Green revolution.

5

A MATHEMATICAL APPROACH TO THE ISSUES WHICH INCREASE DROPOUTS IN SCHOOL EDUCATION

T. Pathinathan, K. Thirusangu & M. Mary John

Introduction

Well being of children and proper formation at every stage of their growth lays the foundation for future development of any society. If there is no expected growth then there may be some hindrance or blocks in the process. When the enrolment rate in schools is very satisfying, the dropout rate is very disturbing [5]. Using various fuzzy models, the causes for school dropouts have been studied in the literature [2-4, 7-11].

Contrasting from the Fuzzy Cognitive Maps (FCM) introduced by Bart Kosko [1], Vasantha,W.B., and Yasmin, S., introduced the notion called Fuzzy Relational Maps [12] to study the Employee-Employer relationship. It has been widely applied to analyze problems in various fields. In order to bring out the existing strong relationship among the various causes, in this paper, we introduce a new model called Induced Fuzzy Relational Maps (IFRM).

This paper has been organized as follows: In section 2, we give the basic notions and definitions relevant to this paper. The description of the problem is given in Section 3 and Section

4 gives the Induced FRM model. In the fifth section, we draw the conclusions from our study and propose remedial measures. Opinion of one expert is illustrated in this article whereas the conclusion given from our study is derived from many experts.

FRM Model

As the data under analysis is an unsupervised one we felt only FRM can give us the hidden pattern of the situation. We proceed to state the definitions of FRM and the corresponding Induced Fuzzy Relational Maps.

In FRMs, we divide the very causal associations into two disjoint units, like for example the relation between the parent and children in the case of school dropouts. For us to define a FRM, we need a domain space and a range space which are disjoint in the sense of concepts. We further assume no intermediate relation exists within the domain and the range space. The number of elements in range space need not in general be equal to the number of elements in the domain space. In our discussion the elements of the domain space are taken from the real vector space of dimension n and that of the range space are from the real vector space of dimension m (in general m and n need not be equal).

We denote by R the set of nodes $R_{1,\dots,}R_m$ of the range space,

where $R_i = \{(x_1, x_2, \dots, x_m) / x_i = 0 \text{ or } 1\}$ for i = 1,..., m.

Similarly D denotes the nodes $D_1, \dots, D_n$ of the domain space

where $D_i = \{(x_1, \dots, x_n) / x_i = 0 \text{ or } 1\}$ for i = 1,..., n.

When $x_i = 1$ or $x_i = 0$ then the node R_i is in the ON state or OFF state respectively.

Definition: A FRM is a directed graph or a map from D to R with concepts like policies or events etc., as nodes and causalities as edges. It represents causal relations between spaces D and R.

Let D_i and R_j denote the two nodes of an FRM. The directed edge from D to R denotes the causality of D on R, called relations. Every edge in the FRM is weighted with a number in the set {0,1}. Let e_{ij} be the weight of the edge $D_i R_j$, $e_{ij} \in \{0.1\}$.

The weight of the edge D_i R_j is positive if increase in D_i implies increase in R_j or decrease in D_i implies decrease in R_j. That is, causality of D_i on R_j is 1.

If $e_{ij} = 0$ then D_i does not have any effect on R_j.We do not discuss the cases when increase in D_i implies decrease in R_j or decrease in D_i implies increase in R_j.

Fuzzy nodes: If the nodes of the FRM are fuzzy sets, then they are called fuzzy nodes.

Simple FRMs: FRMs with edge weights {0,1} are called simple FRMs.

Relational matrix of the FRM

Let $D_1,\ldots,D_n$ be the nodes of the domain space D of an FRM and $R_1, \ldots, R_m$ be the nodes of the range space R of an FRM. Let the matrix E be defined as $E = (e_{ij})$ where e_{ij} is the weight of the directed edge D_iR_j (or R_jD_i), E is called the relational matrix of the FRM.

It is pertinent to mention here that unlike the Fuzzy Cognitive Maps (FCMs), the FRMs can be rectangular matrix with rows corresponding to the domain space and columns corresponding to the range space.

Let $A = (a_1,..,a_n)$, $a_i \in \{0,1\}$. A is called the instantaneous state vector of the domain space and it denotes the ON-OFF position of the nodes at any instant. Similarly let $B = (b_1,\ldots,b_m)$, $b_i \in \{0,1\}$. B is called the instantaneous state vector of the range space and it denotes the ON-OFF position of the nodes at any instant.

$a_i = 1$ or 0 if a_i is ON or OFF respectively, for $i = 1,\ldots, n$. Similarly $b_i = 1$ or 0 if b_i is ON or OFF respectively, for $i = 1,.., m$.

Cycle of the FRM

Let $D_1,.., D_n$ and $R_1,\ldots,R_m$ be the nodes of an FRM. Let D_iR_j (or $R_j D_i$) be the edges of an FRM, $j = 1,\ldots, m$, $i = 1,..,n$. The edges form a directed cycle if it posses a directed cycle. Feed back in FRM: An FRM with cycles is said to have a Feed back.

Dynamical System

When there is a feed back in the FRM, i.e. when the causal relations flow through a cycle in a revolutionary manner the FRM is called a dynamical system.

Hidden Pattern: Consider D_iR_j (or R_jD_i), 1<j<m, 1<i<n. When R_j (or D_i) is switched ON and if causality flows through edges of the cycle and if it again causes R_i (D_j), we say that the dynamical system goes round and round. This is true for any node R_i (or D_j) for $1 < i < m$, (or $1 < j < n$).

The equilibrium state of this dynamical system is called the hidden pattern.

Fixed Point

If the equilibrium state of the dynamical system is a unique state vector, then it is called a fixed point. Consider an FRM with R_1,.., R_m and D_1,..., D_n as nodes. For example let us start the dynamical system by switching on R_1 or D_1. Let us assume that the FRM settles down with R_1 and R_m (or D_1 and D_n) on ON state i.e. the state vector remains as (1 0...0 1) in R [or (1 0...0 1) in D], this state vector is called the fixed point.

Limit Cycle

If the FRM settles down with a state vector repeating in the form $A_1 \rightarrow A_2 \rightarrow \ldots. A_i \rightarrow A_1$ (or $B_1 \rightarrow B_2 \rightarrow \ldots B_i \rightarrow B_1$) then this equilibrium is called a limit cycle.

Determination of Hidden Pattern

Let R_1,.. R_m and D_1,..,D_n be the nodes of a FRM with feed back. Let E be the relational matrix. Let us find a hidden pattern when D_1 is switched ON i.e. when an input is given as vector A_1= (1000...0) in D the data should pass through the relational Matrix E. This is done by multiplying A_1 with the relational matrix E. Let $A_1E = (r_1,..,r_m)$ after thresholding and updating the resultant vector we get $A_1E \in R$.

Let $B = A_1E$, we pass on B into E^T and obtain BE^T. We update and threshold the vector BE^T so that $BE^T \in D$. This procedure is repeated till we get limit cycle or a fixed point.

Description and Method of Finding the Hidden Pattern in Induced FRM

Let R_1,.. R_m and D_1,..,D_n be the nodes of a FRM with feed back. Let M be the relational matrix. Let us find a hidden pattern when D_1 is switched on. We pass the state vector C_1 through the Connection matrix M. A particular attribute, say, $D_1$is kept on ON state and all other components are kept on OFF state. Let C_1 o M yield, $C_1^{¢}$. To convert to signal function, choose the first two highest values to ON state and other values to OFF state with 1 and 0 respectively. We make each component of C_1' vector pass through M repeatedly for each positive entry 1 and we use the symbol ≈ .Then choose that vector which contains the maximum number of 1's. That is, which causes maximum attributes to ON state and call it, say, C_2. Supposing that there are two vectors with maximum number of 1's on ON state, we choose the first vector. Repeat the same procedure for C_2 till we get a fixed point or a limit cycle. We do this process to give due importance to each vector separately as one vector induces another or many more vectors into ON state. We get the hidden pattern either from the limit cycle or from the fixed point. We observe a pattern that leads one cause to another and may end up in one vector or a cycle.

Next we choose the vector by keeping the second component on ON state and repeat the same to get another cycle and it is done for all the vectors separately. We observe the hidden pattern of some vectors found in all or in many cases. Inference from this hidden pattern summarizes or highlights the causes.

Description of the Problem: Analysis Using FRM Model

We have interviewed more than 150 children who dropped out of schools, their parents and teachers in 25 villages around Kallakurichi, Villupuram District, Tamil Nadu. They have expressed their anxieties, problems and worries related to school, expenses and their inability to pay school fee due to lack of resources and job opportunities. From; what we have gathered from all of them, we build a mathematical model in the following way.

Let us consider the relationship between the parent and the child who drop out of the school. Suppose the we take the domain space as the concepts belonging to the parent say $D_1,\ldots,D_8$ and the range space denote the concepts belonging to the child say $R_1, \ldots, R_7$. We describe the nodes $D_1, \ldots, D_8$ and $R_1, \ldots, R_7$ follows:

Domain space: ((1 1 0 1 1 0 0 0), (0 0 1 0 0 0 1)).

D_1 – Money is the main criteria as the school expenses are always on the increase.

D_2 – Poverty and inability of the poor parents to meet the day to day expenses.

D_3 – Importance and value of Education not known

D_4 – Selfishness on the part of the parents or guardian.

D_5 – Family problem/broken families.

D_6 – No proper earning member in the family.

D_7 – Hereditary job

D_8 – Frustration on the existing educational system and many more.

Range Space

R_1 - Children not properly motivated

R_2 – Teacher is not good and insufficient in number.

R_3 – No school with moderate fee structure.

R_4 - Language problem

R_5 – Parents not educated enough to help the child.

R_6 – Laziness/wrong company/bad influence

R_7 – Looking after the younger children.

The expert gives the following relation between the domain and range attributes.

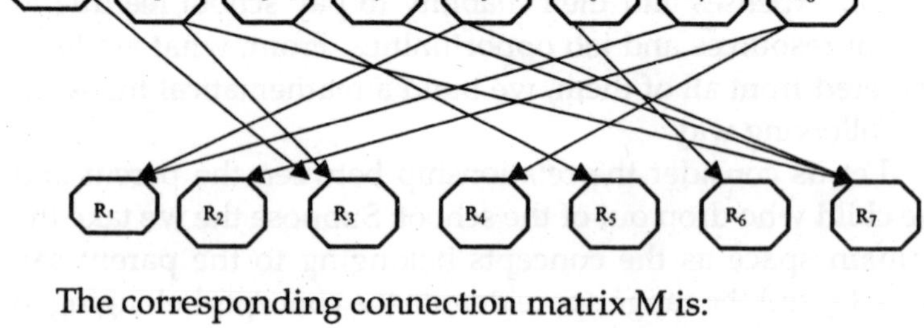

The corresponding connection matrix M is:

$$M = \begin{array}{c} \\ D_1 \\ D_2 \\ D_3 \\ D_4 \\ D_5 \\ D_6 \\ D_7 \\ D_8 \end{array}\begin{array}{c} \begin{array}{ccccccc} R_1 & R_2 & R_3 & R_4 & R_5 & R_6 & R_7 \end{array} \\ \begin{bmatrix} 0 & 0 & 1 & 0 & 0 & 0 & 0 \\ 0 & 0 & 1 & 0 & 0 & 0 & 1 \\ 0 & 0 & 0 & 0 & 1 & 0 & 0 \\ 0 & 0 & 0 & 0 & 0 & 0 & 1 \\ 1 & 0 & 0 & 0 & 0 & 0 & 1 \\ 0 & 0 & 0 & 0 & 0 & 1 & 0 \\ 1 & 0 & 0 & 0 & 0 & 0 & 0 \\ 0 & 1 & 0 & 1 & 0 & 0 & 0 \end{bmatrix} \end{array}$$

Analysis of FRM Model

Case (i): Let A_1 = (1 0 0 0 0 0 0 0)

A_1 M = (0 0 1 0 0 0 0) = B_1.

B_1 M^T = (1 1 0 0 0 0 0 0) = A_2

A_2M = (0 0 2 0 0 0 1) ↪ (0 0 1 0 0 0 1) = B_2.

B_2M^T = (0 2 0 1 1 0 0 0) ↪ (0 1 0 1 1 0 0 0) = A_3

A_3M = (1 0 1 0 0 0 3) ↪ (1 0 1 0 0 0 1) = B_3.

B_3M^T = (1 2 0 1 2 0 1 0) ↪ (1 1 0 1 1 0 1 0) = A_4

A_4M = (2 0 2 0 0 0 3) ↪ (1 0 1 0 0 0 1) = B_3.

B_3M^T = (1 2 0 1 2 0 1 0) ↪ (1 1 0 1 1 0 1 0) = A_4

((1 1 0 1 1 0 1 0), (1 0 1 0 0 0 1)) is the fixed point.

Similarly proceeding we get the following:

In Case (ii) we get ((1 1 0 1 1 0 1 0), (1 0 1 0 0 0 1)) as the fixed point.

In Case (iii) we get ((0 0 1 0 0 0 0 0) , (0 0 0 0 1 0 0)) as the fixed point.

In Case (iv) we get ((1 1 0 1 1 0 1 0), (1 0 1 0 0 0 1)) as the fixed point.

In Case (v) we get ((1 1 0 1 1 0 1 0), (1 0 1 0 0 0 1)) as the fixed point.

In Case (vi) we get ((1 1 0 1 1 0 1 0), (1 0 1 0 0 0 1)) as the fixed point.

In Case (vii) we get ((1 1 0 1 1 0 1 0), (1 0 1 0 0 0 1)) as the fixed point.

Except in case (iii), in all other cases we get the same fixed point ((1 1 0 1 1 0 1 0),(1 0 1 0 0 0 1)). This fixed point and the FRM reveals that D_1, D_2, D_4, D_5, D_7 and C_1, C_3, C_7 get on ON state at the equilibrium.

Analysis IFRM Model

We retain the same attributes and the same connection matrix M.

Step 1: Let C_1 = (1 0 0 0 0 0 0 0)
C_1 M = (0 0 1 0 0 0 0); (0 0 1 0 0 0 0) M^T X (1 1 0 0 0 0 0 0) = C_1^{ϵ}
C_1^{ϵ} M ≈
(1 0 0 0 0 0 0 0) M = (0 0 1 0 0 0 0); (0 0 1 0 0 0 0) M^T = (1 1 0 0 0 0 0 0)
(0 1 0 0 0 0 0 0) M = (0 0 1 0 0 0 1); (0 0 1 0 0 0 1) M^T = (1 2 0 1 1 0 0 0)
↪ (1 1 0 1 1 0 0 0) = C_2
C_2 M = (1 1 0 1 1 0 0 0) M = (1 0 2 0 0 0 3) ↪ (1 0 1 0 0 01);
(1 0 1 0 0 0 1) M^T Ξ (1 2 0 1 2 0 1 0) X (1 1 0 1 1 0 1 0) = C_2^{ϵ}
C_2^{ϵ}M ≈
(1 0 0 0 0 0 0 0) M = (0 0 1 0 0 0 0); (0 0 1 0 0 0 0) M^T = (1 1 0 0 0 0 0 0)
(0 1 0 0 0 0 0 0) M = (0 0 1 0 0 0 1); (0 0 1 0 0 0 1) M^T = (1 2 0 1 1 0 0 0)
↪ (1 1 0 1 1 0 0 0) = C_2
(0 0 0 1 0 0 0 0 0) M = (0 0 0 0 0 0 1); (0 0 0 0 0 0 1) M^T = (0 1 0 1 1 0 0 0)
(0 0 0 0 0 0 1 0) M = (1 0 0 0 0 0 0); (1 0 0 0 0 0 0 0) M^T = (0 0 0 0 1 0 1 0)
((1 1 0 1 1 0 0 0), (0 0 1 0 0 0 1)) is the fixed point.

Using the row representation of M, namely D_1,D_2, ... we get the following triggering pattern when the first attribute is kept on ON state

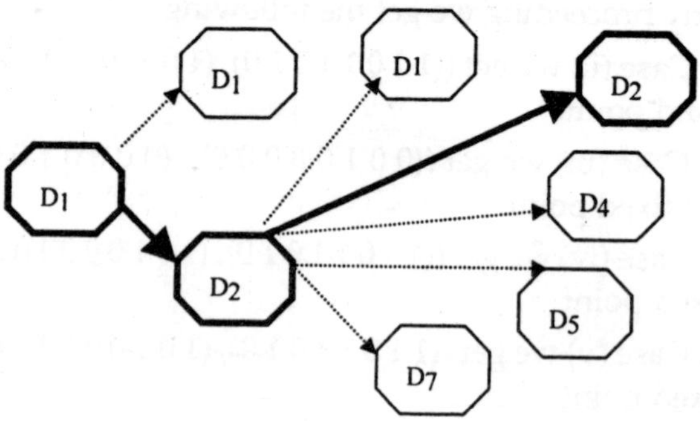

We get the triggering pattern as $D_1 \Rightarrow D_2 \Rightarrow D_2$
In step 2, we the triggering pattern as $D_2 \Rightarrow D_2 \Rightarrow D_2$
In step 3, we the triggering pattern as $D_3 \Rightarrow D_3$
In step 4, we the triggering pattern as $D_4 \Rightarrow D_2 \Rightarrow D_2$
In step 5, we the triggering pattern as $D_5 \Rightarrow D_2 \Rightarrow D_2$
In step 6, we the triggering pattern as $D_6 \Rightarrow D_6$
In step 7, we the triggering pattern as $D_7 \Rightarrow D_5 \Rightarrow D_2 \Rightarrow D_2$
In step 8, we the triggering pattern as $D_8 \Rightarrow D_8 \Rightarrow D_8$
Merging all these induced paths on a single graph we get

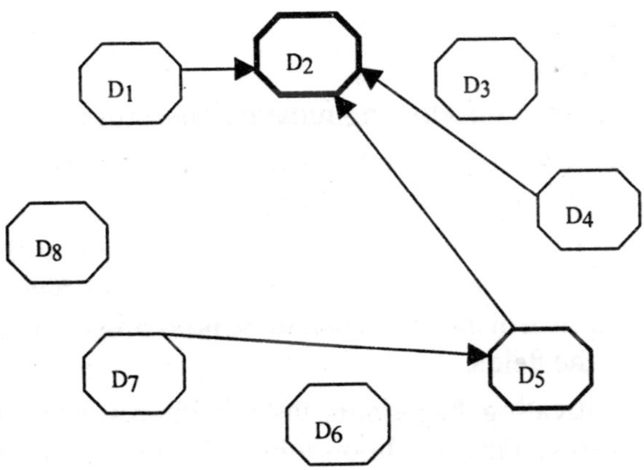

From our study and from the above graph, we observe that D_5 (family problems and broken families) is the intermediary node and D_2 (Poverty) is the terminal node.

Except in steps 3, 6 and 8 the fixed point is ((1 1 0 1 1 0 0 0), (0 0 1 0 0 0 1)).We conclude that the attributes D_1 (Problem of money to spend), D_2 (Education is not given its due importance), D_4(selfishness on the part of the parent or guardian), D_5 (Family problems like broken families) and R_3 (No school in the nearby vicinity with moderate fee structure) , R_7 (baby sitting) play a major role in increasing the school dropout rates. In FRM model, except in case (iii), in all other cases we get the same fixed point ((1 1 0 1 1 0 1 0), (1 0 1 0 0 0 1)).

Conclusion

The gap between the rich and poor widens day by day and the earning capacity of the poor decreases tremendously. Due to competitive market forces, the cost of living goes up along with the cost of good education. It has become the natural consequence that all cannot afford to have good school education. The very person who opened the Indian gates to the global traders, has said this: " In order to be ethically neutral in the context of inequality, *you have to be partisan towards the poor,* the weaker sections, minorities, women, the Scheduled Castes and Scheduled Tribes and all such disadvantaged people who need the support of the State" (PM's speech to the District Collectors during their two day conference at New Delhi on May 20, 2005) [6].

We suggest the following remedial measures:

1. Education must be made free at least for the very poor in the schools in their locality.
2. Increased employment opportunities will surely provide more income to the parents. They need to have a source of income when there is no possibility to work in the fields.
3. Motivating the parents, their children and the teachers involved in the schools where dropout occurs most, is an important step to retain the children in the schools once they come back as the 'Prodigal Sons'.
3. Opening of crèche and free residential schools will surely decrease school dropouts.

References

Bart Kosko (2003), Neural Networks and Fuzzy Systems, 4th ed., New Delhi–110 001, Prentice Hall of India Pvt. Limited.

Klir G.J. and Folger T.A. (1988), Fuzzy Sets, Uncertainty and Information, Englewood, Cliffs. N.J. Prentice Hall Publication.

Pedrycz, W. (1995), "Genetic Algorithms for Learning in Fuzzy Relational Structures". Fuzzy Sets and Systems, Vol. 69, 37-52, 1995.

Pathinathan, T., Thirusangu K., and Mary John, M. (2005), "On Causes for School Dropouts-A Fuzzy Analysis". Acta Ciencia Indica, XXXI M, No. 4, 1279-1299, (2004).

Policy Note: School Education Department, Government of Tamil Nadu (2001-2002).

The Indian Express, May 20, 2005 "DMs Seek Security of Tenure: PM Positve".

Vasantha.W.B. and Pathinathan T. (2002), "Child Labour and BAM Model" in V.K. Kapoor (ed.), Mathematics and Information Theory, Recent Topics and Applications, New Delhi, Anamaya Publication.

Vasantha, W.B. and Pathinathan T. (2002), "Dropouts in Primary Schools: Using FRM Model". Paper Presented at the Symposium on Mathematical Methods and Applications at IIT Madras, Chennai, December 22, 2002.

Vasantha W.B. and Pathinathan T. (2003), "The Impact of Missionary Interventions on the Education and Rehabilitation of Deprived Children–A Fuzzy Analysis", in T. Thrivikraman, S. Dunny Kuriakose and A. Mathew (ed.), Proc. of the National Seminar of Kerala Mathematical Society on Graph Theory and Fuzzy Mathematics, Catholicate College, Pathanamthitta, 151-162.

Vasantha, W.B., Pathinathan,T. and Mary John, M. (2005), "Migration of Parents and their Children Dropping out of School–A Fuzzy Approach". *Ultra Scientist of Physcial Scicences,* Vol. 17, No. 3 (M), 449-460, 2005.

Vasantha W.B., Pathinathan. T. and Mary John M. (2005), "School Environment: A Cause for Increase in School Dropouts–Fuzzy Analysis" in Proceedings of the State Level Seminar on Industrial Mathematics, Islamiah College, Vaniyambadi, 127–136.

Vasantha, W.B., and Yasmin, S. (2001), "FRM to Analyze the Employee–Employer Relationship Model", *Journal of Bihar Mathematical Society,* Vol. 21, 25-34, 2001.

6

TELEDOC PROJECT: A SOCIAL ENTREPRENEURSHIP VENTURE FOR SUSTAINABLE HEALTHCARE IN RURAL INDIA

Naresh Singh

Health Status in India

According to the Human Development Report 2004 published by United Nations Development Programme (UNDP) India ranks on 127 out of 177 countries and is under the category of medium human development index.[2] One of the major criteria for ranking under human development is life expectancy at birth and its related health indicators. Compared to the developed countries health status in India is very poor. Life expectancy at birth is 63.7 years. According to the statistics of World Health Organization (WHO) related to health status in India, child mortality under the age of five is more than 90 on 1000 births. Because of the poor health of Indian population 11.3 per cent (for male) and 13.6 per cent (for female) of their age are lost in sickness and morbidity. Maternal mortality ratio is 540 on 100,000 live births. The percentage of total expenditure of health as a percentage of GDP is quite low i.e. 5.1 per cent. The Government health expenditure is quite low at 17.9 per cent and the remaining 82.1 per cent is the private health expenditure.[3]

The scenario of health sector in India is quite alarming. The situation is worst in rural India which consists of almost three-fourth of the country's population. Extreme poverty, illiteracy, ignorance about healthcare, lack of transportation and communication and poor health infrastructure are the main factors behind it. Access to health services by villagers in India become more difficult because of unaffordable services and clinics and doctors being located in faraway towns. It leads to the problems of mortality and morbidity in rural India. For examples life expectancy in villages is eight years less than city dwellers and even diseases like malaria and tuberculosis are not treated properly. A study conducted by Singh (2003) show that poor referral system from bottom to top and lack of forward-backward feedback in health system in India leads to the problem of infant and maternal mortality as well as morbidity among the women in rural areas in India. The study also reveals the fact that proper improved referral system from bottom to top, documentation of the history of cases and forward-backward feedback can reduce infant and maternal mortality as well as morbidity.[4]

Poor health status is the direct consequences of poverty. There are many diseases like; Tuberculosis, AIDS, Malaria diseases caused by nutritional deficiency, poorly managed deliveries of pregnant women etc. common in Indian village due to poverty. According to the study conducted by Muniyandi & Ramachandran (2002) India accounts for nearly 30 per cent of the Tuberculosis cases in the world. Nearly 38 per cent of people of all ages are infected with the disease. Two million people in India develop the disease annually. Majority of the patients are from poor socio-economic background and are under indebt due to disease. The projected economic burden caused by Tuberculosis in India has been estimated more that 13,000 crores very year.[5] According to Sharma (2003) Malaria is rural disease in India. Poverty linked health issues in rural areas include lack of access to safe drinking water sources and sanitation, under nutrition, viral disease like Japanese encephalitis and acute respiratory infection. This causes Malaria and deaths due to Malaria. Malaria treatment can cost US $3

TO 10 and complicated Malaria US $300 to 600. According to him the key to Malaria control lies in understanding local Malaria with a primary attack on poverty and Malaria receptivity.[6]

Though as mentioned earlier, percentage of total expenditure of health as a percentage of GDP is quite low 5.1 per cent but the Government health expenditure is quite low at 17.9 per cent and the remaining 82.1 per cent is the private health expenditure. The Government health expenditure is only 0.9 per cent of the GDP on health care which is quite low even against an average of 2.2 by other developing countries. There are two clear segments of the population availing private health services. The largest one of the poor people who do not have any health insurance coverage, seek low quality of private services for health care and ultimately die or leave on the mercy of God. The other is the affluent segment of the people who not only have insurance coverage but also avail very high quality of private services by spending very big amount for health care. This is agony of the Nation State like India which is proclaimed as democratic socialism by our political leaders. Since the State has not been so successful in providing health care services to the people of India; especially to the poor, private players in health care services has exploited this market failure situation and ultimate sufferer are the poor people of this country.

This situation of health care services in India can best be understood by the theoretical framework of institutional change and political behaviour by using new institutional economic (NIE) approach in a holistic way. Not much has been done in independent India under institutional initiatives for health care services. Policies of the Government remains in contents and functions as like British rule in India only forms has been changed what Williamson (2000) says going beyond the rules of the game (affluent class) to include the play of the game (affluent and high cost private hospitals).[7]

Under this process we see a clear strategic conflict where political leaders were reluctant to provide health care services to all because being by themselves rich, they can afford private treatments. This explanation can be substantiating by the generalisation of Hegedorn (2003) on different models of rationality. According to him, "*The conception of rationality meeting the interest of politicians is one which accord equal weight to quality and legitimisation. By contrast means-ends, schemes represent only the criterion of quality. In other words, there are basically two ways of reacting to the requirements for rationality: disintegration or integration of the aspects of quality and legitimisation.*[8]"

In the entire process of health care delivery, powers and sources of actors were big political leaders. The power and sources of actors never wanted to provide cost-effective health care services to the poor people and they legitimised this power into authority by opening the health care services for the private players. Further to quote Hegedorn (2003), "*From these particularities we can conclude that all the black-box approaches which only consider the input and the output of the political decision-making system, rather than analysing the processes of decision-making and consensus building within the political system, can only be of limited value. This refers to all functionalist approaches of policy analysis patterned after the old systems theory and this also applies to some politometric approaches.*[9]"

Role of medical doctors and private hospital owners in the entire process has not been very positive. Their role was just like what Hegedorn (2002) called "bandits" while explaining political economy of transition countries who extract the maximum resources from the public.[10]

This difference between formal and effective health care services can be understood very well by applying Coase Theorem. It would be worthwhile here to lament the views of Coase (1988: 154)[11]. To quote,

> "In a state of laissez faire, is there a monetary, a legal, or a political system, and if so, what are they? In an ideal world, would there be a monetary, a legal, or a political system, and if so, what would they be? The answers to all these questions are shrouded in mystery and every man is free to draw whatever conclusions he likes. Actually, very little analysis

> is required to show that an ideal world is better than a state of laissez faire, unless the definitions of a state of laissez faire and ideal world happen to be the same. But the whole discussion is largely irrelevant for questions of economic policy since, whatever we may have in mind as our ideal world; it is clear that we have not yet discovered how to get to it from where we are. A better approach would seem to be to start our analysis with a situation approximating that which actually exists, to examine the effects of a proposed policy change, and to attempt to decide whether the new situation would be, in total, better or worse than the original one. In this way, conclusions for policy would have some relevance to the actual situation."

The problem of health care services for the poor people is gradually becoming issue of human rights in India. In a National Public Hearing on "Right to Care" organized by National Human Right Commission in December 2004, Union Health & Family Welfare Minster Dr. Anbumani Ramadoss regretted that despite the large infrastructure existing in the country in terms of human resources and physical infrastructure, nearly 90 per cent of India's population has no access to good health care.[12]

In nutshell we can say that the health care services in India can be best understood by applying the approach of NIE. Being predominantly a rural society and agriculture economy, there is a need to re-look the theoretical bearings on empirical explanations for economic development and social change in India in past 50 years after independence. Of course economists, sociologists, social scientists and management gurus have to break the blocks of their academic disciplines and need to work together. Objectivity of any academic discipline cannot be maintained at the cost of poor people and poverty and therefore, they also need to brainstorm the political elite, decision-makers and policy planners.

The Way Out-social Entrepreneurship Venture Models

This is paradox in India that affluent people have very high quality health care services and the common man suffers with lack of basic health care. Common man should not be left to die on the mercy of public health services and the false promises of political leaders and Government. The way out is to search a middle path of social entrepreneurship.

Several best practices of social entrepreneurship can be found world over. For example, Ashoka Fellow Veronica Khosa was frustrated with the system of health care in South Africa. A nurse by trade she saw sick people getting sicker, elderly people unable to get to a doctor and hospitals with empty beds that would not admit patients with HIV. So Veronica started Tateni Home Care Nursing Services and instituted the concept of ýhome careý in her country. Beginning with practically nothing, her team took to the streets providing care to people in a way they had never received it—in the comfort and security of their homes. Just years later, the government had adopted her plan and through the recognition of leading health organizations the idea is spreading beyond South Africa. Social entrepreneurs like Veronica redefine their field and go on to solve systemic social problems on a larger scale.[13] According to Jackson & Kelly, *"A Social Entrepreneur utilizes social capital to mobilize financial, human, knowledge, physical capital to acquire resources (social and conventional) in order to create a social enterprise which then delivers social dividends/ returns."*[14]

According to Dees (2001), *"Social entrepreneurs play the role of change agents in the social sector by adopting a mission to create and sustain social value (not just private value), recognizing and relentlessly pursuing new opportunities to serve that mission, engaging in a process of continuous innovation, adaptation, and learning, acting boldly without being limited by resources currently in hand and exhibiting heightened accountability to the constituencies served and for the outcomes created."*[15]

Prahalad (2004) in his seminal work "The Fortune at the Bottom of the Pyramid" has document exemplary cases of social entrepreneurship across the globe and of different sectors. Jaipur Foot and Arvind Eye Care System in India are worth quoting examples of social entrepreneurship in health sector. In these cases he pleaded logic of known problems and their unique solutions. To quote *"The problems at the BOP are not new.*

However, they represent a new challenge. They demand innovations in how these traditional problems are addressed. For example, the solution must be affordable. That means dramatic cost reductions from the solutions available to the top of the pyramid consumers in developed countries. Second, BOP consumers have unique demands based on the circumstances of their lives–poor infrastructure, lack of trend manpower, and lack of access to raw materials (page 241)."[16]

The most powerful force for change in the world is a new idea in the hands of a leading social entrepreneur. The job of a social entrepreneur is to recognize when a part of society is stuck and to provide new ways to get it unstuck. He or she finds what is not working and solves the problem by changing the system, spreading the solution and persuading entire societies to take new leaps. Identifying and solving large-scale social problems requires a social entrepreneur because only the entrepreneur has the committed vision and inexhaustible determination to persist until they have transformed an entire system. The above said philosophy has been materialized in TeleDoc Project of Jiva Institute which is a social entrepreneurship venture for sustainable health care in Rural India.

Jiva-A Social Entrepreneurship Initiative[17]

Background: Founded in 1992, Jiva Institute is a non-profit research and development organization that aims to foster sustainable development by producing innovations that improve practices of education, health, and social enterprise. Jiva has independent offices in India, the United States and the United Kingdom. The founders of Jiva define social enterprise as a business with social objectives that combines entrepreneurial skills with a strong social purpose. Returns on investment are demonstrated not just in terms of pure profits but also in the amount of social change impacted upon the target communities. The financial returns generated from such businesses are principally reinvested in the business or in the community, rather than being driven by the need to maximize profit for shareholders and owners.

Vision & Mission: The vision of Jive is to foster sustainable development by producing innovations that improve practices of education, health, and social enterprise. The mission of Jiva is (i) in the field of education to make high-quality learning resources and technologies accessible to students and teachers from low-income communities, (ii) in the field of health to create affordable health products and services that integrate indigenous and modern health systems, and delivery methods that use innovative technologies and (iii) in the field of social enterprise to help nonprofit and funding organizations achieve greater impact through the application of efficient management techniques, innovative income strategies, and enabling technologies.

Board of Directors: The Board of Directors is the strength of Jive. Among the Board of Directors, Rishi Pal Chauhan is founder President. A postgraduate in Mechanical Engineering, he has over 20 years experience in Quality Control Systems both in India and the USA. Mr. Chauhan sets the vision for the Institute, and works to expand the reach of Jiva products and services to the "bottom of the pyramid." He has led the establishment of Jiva's exacting quality processes. Steven Rudolph is an American educator who serves as Director of Jiva's Education and of Jiva International, a New Jersey-based nonprofit organization. He has pioneered education reform through curriculum design and the use of technology in India, establishing the Jiva Public School as an innovative K-12 test-bed for the use of technology and active learning, creating the India's Curriculum of Tomorrow series of textbooks, and developing software tools and training courseware for Jiva's support of Indian social enterprises. Mr. Rudolph has provided consulting to Media Lab Asia, UNESCO, the India Ministry of Human Resource Development, Apple Computer, Microsoft, Intel, the Royal Government of Bhutan, and Healing the Divide. Dr. Partap Chauhan, Director, Jiva Ayurveda, holds Ayurveda Degree from the University of Delhi, He has dedicated himself to popularizing Ayurveda across the globe. He established the Jiva Ayurveda Clinic and Panchakarma Center, and followed this by setting up a comprehensive online resource on Ayurveda (www.ayurvedic.org) that provides free consultancy, online courses, lifestyle advice and Ayurvedic products. In the Jiva pharmacy he has developed over 200 authentic Ayurvedic medicines, health and personal care products. Dr. Chauhan has conducted lectures and workshops in over 25 countries, and conducts regular videoconferences with students and with medical professionals. Shri Satya Narayan Dasa, Director, Jiva Institute of Vaishnava Studies, holds M. Tech. degree from IIT Delhi and a Ph.D. in Sanskrit, as well as eight additional degrees in various subjects. He has authored several books including "The Yoga of Dejection" and "In Vaikuntha Not Even a Leaf Falls". At his cultural center in Vrindaven, he conducts classes on ancient Indian sciences for scholars from around the world, and has initiated a program for preservation, translation and publication of ancient Indian works of science and wisdom. His library houses over 2500 texts dating back to the 13th century. Dr. Satya Narayan offers online courses in addition to books and audio/video tape recordings of the classes conducted at the culture center.

Advisory Board Members: Among the Advisory Board Members Naren Ayyar is IT Consultant. He served as the founding Managing Director of Dell India, and over the last 30 years has established and managed Indian-based businesses for multinational corporations including Apple Computer, Dell, IBM India, Hewlett Packard, HCL and NELCO (a TATA venture). Prof. Alex Pentland is a pioneer in wearable computers, health systems, smart environments, and technology for developing countries, is one of the most cited computer scientists in the world. He is the founding director of the Media Lab Asia, and is a co-founder of the Center for Future Health, the Wearable Computing Research Community, and the International Digital Nations Consortium. He was formerly the Academic Head of the MIT Media Laboratory, and is the Toshiba Professor of Media Arts and Sciences at the Massachusetts Institute of Technology. He has won numerous international awards in Arts, Sciences and Engineering, and was chosen by Newsweek as one of the 100 Americans most likely to shape the next century. He currently directs the Human Design research group at the MIT Media Lab. Dr. Terry Cole-Whittaker is a motivational speaker and best selling author, who has handled diverse portfolios as a television producer, business consultant, and celebrity counselor. She is a popular speaker on personal growth and organizational management. Over the years, Dr. Cole-Whittaker has been interviewed and featured in some of the most prestigious periodicals, radio and television programs including, Larry King Live, CNN, Good Morning America, Time Magazine, the New York Times, and the London Times. Dr. S. Sadagopan, Founder Director, Founding Director of The Indian Institute of Information Technology (IIIT), Bangalore is a Fulbright scholar and is listed in Who's Who in the World and Outstanding People of the Twentieth Century, published by the International Biographical Centre, Cambridge, England. Dr. Fred Mednick is a principal for almost 20 years, founded Teachers Without Borders to address the pressing need for durable educational change and solutions, worldwide, at the secondary level. He is the author of several books including "Rebel Without A Car: Surviving and Appreciating Your Child's Teen Years". He has received John Hopkins University's "California's Outstanding Educator" award.

Financial Resources: Jiva Institute and its affiliate office, Jiva USA, are nonprofit organizations. Jiva receives its funds through three main methods. These are: earned income activities by the sale of products and services, social investment by grants and strategic philanthropy and capital market financing i.e. loans. The majority of funding is through earned-income activities as Jiva operates financially more like a business rather than a typical nonprofit. The partners and associates of Jiva are: Apple India, Central Board of Secondary Education (CBSE), Cyber Media India Ltd, Educational Object Economy (EOE), The Public Affairs Section, The American Embassy, New Delhi, Ministry of Communications & Information Technology, New Delhi, The Flora Family Foundation, Healing the Divide, Hewlett Packard, Intel, Earn, Kala Raksha, Council for the Indian School Certificate Examinations (CISCE), Media Lab Asia, Natoma Group, Oneworld, Schlumberger, The Soros Foundation, Teachers Without Borders and UNESCO, New Delhi.

Programmes and Projects: There are mainly three areas Jiva has undertaken. These are education, health and social enterprise.

Education: Jiva's education division is dedicated to making high-quality learning resources and technologies accessible to students and teachers from low-income communities. To this aim, it conducts research, and develops innovative learning materials including textbooks, teacher training, web based learning resources and more. Jiva Education is constantly focused on finding solutions for creating a "learning society" that can apply its constantly upgraded knowledge and skills for socio-economic betterment and local, regional and global sustainability.

The Jiva Public School (a K-12 institution) was established in 1994 in a small residential building with only 8 students and 3 teachers on the first day. But today it operates from a large building on 1.5 acres with over 500 students and 40 teachers. It is located in a quiet alcove of Faridabad District, 15km from New Delhi. Every aspect of Jiva Public School has been designed to enhance learning from the use of innovative activities, to the study materials—even the furniture.

India's Curriculum of Tomorrow (ICOT) is a complete curriculum solution for schools. ICOT is the first curriculum of its kind to offer a comprehensive, well-organized solution for all subjects across all classes that includes textbook as well as digital resources for students, teachers and school administrators. It is so designed as to not only enhance learning and exam performance, but also to instill the love of learning.

In order help foster better teaching and learning practices, Jiva creates innovative products for students and teachers. These products have been produced from Jiva's own experiences at our Jiva Public School, as well as from the interactions we have had over the years with innumerable schools, teachers, principals, and others. Jiva has developed extremely efficient methods for content development. This, combined with our nonprofit business approach of social enterprise, has resulted in materials that are of international quality standards, while being priced affordably for Indian learners. These are: Textbooks, Digital Resources, Teacher Resources, Smart School Pro and Beat the Exam in 7 Days.

Jiva has given educational training and workshops to thousands of teachers and principals throughout India. These include seminars and workshops on using IT, teaching methodologies, and school management. We have provided our programs and have made customized programs and workshops for companies like Apple and Intel, for the ICSE Board, and different state governments.

Jiva also provides consultancy services to schools, boards, government bodies and organizations who are interested in making their learning programs more effective. Our distinguished team of educators works with you to identify your needs, establish an action plan, and ensure that goals are achieved.

Jiva enhanced learning for over 500,000 students across 350 schools through innovative learning materials. ICOT learning materials being widely used by both government and private publishers as a standard for revising and enhancing existing textbooks. Jiva developed the IT policy recommendation document for the Ministry of Human Resource and Development (MHRD) which has been used as a model by state governments, the central government, and UNESCO for other countries in South Asia. Jiva's IT curriculum adopted by the National Council for Educational Research and Training (NCERT) to set the national guidelines for IT curriculum. Central Board of Secondary Education's (CBSE) vocational computer training course for classes XI and XII developed by Jiva being used by over 300,000 students across all Indian states.

Health: Jiva's health division creates affordable health products and services that integrate indigenous and modern health systems and delivery methods that use innovative technologies. It runs its own website, clinic and pharmacy, conducts residential and online courses, organizes international seminars and videoconferences, and also publishes books and articles related to health and Ayurveda. Jiva developed world's first website on Ayurveda, founded in 1995. Ayunique is online Ayurvedic consulting service that enables you to get a consultation online. You can also have health remedies and products mailed to you wherever you are in the world. Teledoc is bringing Ayurvedic telemedicine services to rural villages in India. AyurBuyer: Jiva's online store where you can "Shop Ayurveda" beauty products, health items, books, audio and more. The Jiva College of Ayurveda: A place where you can take certificate courses on Ayurveda—both online as well as at Jiva Institute (India).

The first and most comprehensive Ayurvedic website with over 1800 pages of content. More than 10,000 patients treated online, More than 500 online registered students. Conducted workshops for over 5000 participants across 25 countries. More than 12,000 patients treated at 120 free health camps in India. Production of over 600 rare and classical Ayurvedic medical formulas. Over 100 patents for Ayurvedic medical formulas. Delivered a total blended value of over $ 230 million for 66,000 patients since 1995.

Social Enterprise: Jiva Enterprise works towards helping non-profit and funding organizations achieve greater impact through the application of efficient management techniques, innovative income strategies, and enabling technologies. It carries out grassroots ICT projects, provides consultancy, and develops effective tools for non-profit management and communication. Jiva provides training programs that help nonprofits make the switch—from old world non-governmental organizations (NGOs) to social enterprises. The Learning for Earning is a program developed especially to promote business and entrepreneurial skills among rural artisans. This innovative hands-on program equips organizational members and artisans with the necessary skills to enhance earnings and to improve marketing practices within cooperatives and artisan groups. Baatchit is a Jiva and Media Lab Asia (A partnership of Government of India's Ministry of Communication and Information Technology and the Massachusetts Institute of Technology) initiative for developing iconic multi-lingual community based software and establishing Community Learning and Information Centers (CLICs). Digital Bridges is an initiative of Jiva Institute to bridge the digital divide and empower people with low-cost tools and technologies that can lead to social, economic, and environmental sustainability. For the last several years, Jiva has experienced a need for software tools to improve efficiency, increase revenue and enhance communication within the organization. However, our quest for appropriate tools failed to provide us with viable cost-effective options. Therefore in order to fulfill our need we custom created tools such as Populog –a communications management tool, a social investment shopping cart and a Social Investment Portfolio, which are today an inseparable part of our operations.

An average 45 per cent increase in earnings for 500 artisans in 8 villages of the Bhuj region in Gujarat, through the Learning for earning program. Tripled attendance in the rural education program run by KalaRaksha in Gujarat by introducing constructive learning concepts.

Teledoc-A Social Entrepreneurship Venture for Sustainable Healthcare in Rural India[18]

Background: TeleDoc is a telemedicine program specifically designed to deliver healthcare services to remote villages of India. TeleDoc is a social entrepreneurship initiative of Jiva institute. Started as an experiment in Tikawali Village in 2001, so far the project has covered more than 50 villages. The development and pilot testing of TeleDoc project has been supported by Soros Foundation. Director of Jiva International, Steven Rudolf is guiding the TeleDoc team under the leadership of Dr. Pratap Chauhan, a world renowned authority on Ayurveda. Founding Managing Director of Dell India Naren Ayyar and development expert Edmond Gaible are the advisors of TeleDoc project.

Operation: Teledoc is built around two strands that are few thousand years apart: the ancient Indian medical system of ayurveda and the as recent as you can get phenomena of mobile telephony. Every day TeleDoc worker armed with a Nokia 6800 phone fan out to the 10 villages the project covers. At each village, villagers gather at a designated place to discuss their ailments with the TeleDoc field workers. The TeleDoc transmits this information through the GPRS enabled phone and a java based software to a team of five ayurvedic doctors at Jiva's Faridabad clinic. The doctors analyses the symptoms and prescribe medication, medicine are compounded at the clinic itself and delivered the following day by the TeleDoc health workers. Based on a franchisee model, TeleDoc is a sustainable social enterprise providing low cost and high quality healthcare services directly to the villagers. Under the project village-based health workers trained in Ayurvedic approach of healthcare record and transmit diagnostic data to an IT enabled central clinic using JAVA-enhanced mobile telephones combining off-the-shelf technology, GPRS network and J2ME. Jiva's expert Ayurvedic doctors analyze the data and then prescribe medication and treatment. Medicine are compounded at a regional office, picked up by field health workers and delivered to the patients at their homes @ 70 rupees per consultation. This cost is nominal when compare to any other clinic visits.

Application of ICT: TeleDoc uses java enabled mobile telephones and the GPRS data network to deliver traditional healthcare to India's rural poor. The TeleDoc mobile information system (MIS) uses off the shelf technologies and private sector mobile telephone networks to connect village field representatives and Jiva doctors to a central database where they exchange prescription and treatment information.

Financial Modeling: Jiva charges its TeleDoc patients Rs 70 per consultation including the medicine. This is much cheaper as compare to the cost of consultation by private Doctors and the medicine prescribed by them. A study conducted by Jiva shows that a patient from rural area visit on an average four times to city Doctor for consultation and in each visit s/he spends four hours, pays Rs. 100 for consultation, Rs. 280 for medicine and Rs. 50 for travel. Starting in July 2003 with 25 patients with the initial support of Soros Foundation, it has covered 7032 patients within a year till June 2004 with a cash surplus of Rs. 1,53,860. TeleDoc currently services 1500 paying patients that sum to Rs. 100000 in revenue every week. Encouraged by this response Jiva proposes to take TeleDoc national.

Impact: Starting from one village with 25 patients in July 2003 it has covered 50 villages with 7032 patients with success rate of 70 per cent curability by July 2004. These patients have saved total 112,512 man-hours, Rs. 42,192,200 against consulting fee/traveling and Rs. 7,875,840 against medicine by June 2004. Under TeleDoc project in case of serious diseases and surgical cases like Myasthenia Gravis, Tuberculosis, Cancer, Heart Diseases, Hepatomegaly, Cirrhosis of Liver, Emphysema, Leukemia, Deficiency Disorder of Nervous System, Rabies, Rickets, Caesarian Operation of Pregnant Women, Cholecystitis, Hernia etc. general herbs are given for improving the condition and the cases are referred to specialized hospitals. TeleDoc also organizes awareness camps for men and women in the villages at regular interval. The suggestions and advises provided to the pregnant women are about social and personal hygiene, anti-natal checkups, suggestions regarding diet and life style, vaccinations, advise for healthy and hygienic deliveries, advise for essential nutrients from locally available vegetables and fruits. For the women in general it provides suggestions regarding contraception, personal hygiene, care for child, care for common disorders of child with kitchen remedies, vaccination for child and awareness for sexually transmitted diseases. For the teenage girls it provides advice for menstruation, sex education and diet life style. For the elderly women it provides various types of suggestions and advises regarding how to maintain good health in old age and prevent diseases, personal hygiene, diet and life style. For the man in general it provides awareness for sexually transmitted diseases, contraception, personal and social hygiene and diet and life style. For the elderly men it provides advises as how to maintain health in old age and prevent disease, personal hygiene and diet and life style. For the teenage boys it provides sex education, contraception and diet and life style. Apart form these services TeleDoc also provides some special services like information about common available herbs and their medicinal properties and how to use them to treat various diseases. TeleDoc as a social entrepreneurship initiative offers numerous direct benefits to villagers. Credit goes to TeleDoc for providing common villagers access to affordable, effective medicine and treatment in their villages. Families get the benefits of increased saving and reduced stress due to less travel to town based clinic as the TeleDoc provides them comparatively cheap and locally available medication. The rural women are treated by female health worker of TeleDoc thereby encouraging discussion about birth control and other health issues. TeleDoc field representatives further provides educational materials on HIV/AIDS, sanitation and other health related topics. TeleDoc creates jobs in villages offering village men and women income opportunity and ensuring that a share of the health care revenues earned from the local areas remain in the local economy.

Future Plan: TeleDoc project intends to provide consultation to 9 million patients in 10,000 villages by the year 2006 through the franchisee model. For scaling up this sustainable social enterprise TeleDoc will provide franchisee to licensed medicine compounders who will be Jiva employees to achieve optimal quality assurance. The TeleDoc MIS will facilitate effective supply-chain management, billing and revenue sharing and oversight. One field worker will cover 10 villages by using Nokia 6800. One franchisee will cover about 100 villages consisting of 10 field health workers and one supervisor.

At this level of volume, financial projections show TeleDoc as a sustainable and cash positive with net profit of $ 1 million per year. The immediate concerns for the success of the future strategy are to expand training materials to address women's health issues, develop print based health education material for low literate adults and to recruits and train the prospective franchise.

Accolades for TeleDoc: In a very short time of its emergence and growth Jiva Institute and TeleDoc project have many accolades in their credit. To name few, Jiva Ayurveda Director, Dr Chauhan, honored with the Best Ayurvedic Physician Award. Jiva Ayurveda site awarded the Best of the Web Award. Jiva Ayurveda product stall awarded the Best Stall Award out of 187 stalls at the 27th Mind-Body-spirit Festival in London. TeleDoc project has been announced the winner of the world

Teledoc Statistics at a Glance

Month/ Year	Total No. of Villages	Total No. of Patients	No. of New Patients	No. of Old Patients	Patients with Chronic Diseases	Patient Cured from Chronic Disease	Percentage of Chronic Patients Cured	Patients with General Diseases	Patients Cured from General Diseases	Percentage of General Patients cured	Total Patients Cured	Percentage of Total Patients Cured	No. of Man-hours Saved	Money Saved by Patients Against Consulting & Traveling (Rs.)	Money Saved by Patients Against Medicine Rs.	Money Received by TeleDoc @Rs. 70 per Patient (income Rs.)	Cost of Medicine Incurred by TeleDoc @25% of Money Received (Rs.)	Salary of Health Workers (Rs.)	Salary of Doctors @Rs. 50 per Hour (Rs.)	Other Variable Costs (Rs.)	Other Fixed Costs (Rs.)	Net Surplus (Rs.)
Jul-03	1	25	25	0	18	11	61%	7	6	86%	17	68%	400	15000	28000	1750	437.5	5000	208	1860	36000	-41756
Aug-03	2	57	44	13	35	23	66%	22	20	91%	43	75%	912	34200	63840	3990	997.5	5000	475	1860	0	-4343
Sep-03	5	184	146	38	120	83	69%	64	61	95%	144	78%	2944	110400	206080	12880	3220	5000	1533	1860	0	1267
Oct-03	10	373	276	97	289	188	65%	84	81	96%	269	72%	5968	223800	417760	26110	6527.5	5000	3108	1860	0	9614
Nov-03	10	484	308	176	357	207	58%	127	112	88%	319	66%	7744	290400	542080	33880	8470	5000	4033	1860	0	14517
Dec-03	15	625	368	257	479	328	68%	146	133	91%	461	74%	10000	375000	700000	43750	10937.5	5000	5208	1860	0	20744
Jan-04	18	691	311	380	530	371	70%	161	158	98%	529	77%	11056	414600	773920	48370	12092.5	10000	5758	2260	6000	12259
Feb-04	30	783	592	191	623	324	52%	160	152	95%	476	61%	12528	469800	876960	54810	13702.5	10000	6525	2260	0	22323
Mar-04	40	850	630	220	710	454	64%	140	126	90%	580	68%	13600	510000	952000	59500	14875	10000	7083	2260	0	25282
Apr-04	48	920	723	197	780	523	67%	140	130	93%	653	71%	14720	552000	1030400	64400	16100	10000	7667	2260	0	28373
May-04	48	990	790	200	827	535	65%	163	158	97%	693	70%	15840	594000	1108800	69300	17325	10000	8250	2260	0	31465
Jun-04	50	1050	700	350	878	598	68%	172	164	95%	762	73%	16800	630000	1176000	73500	18375	10000	8750	2260	0	34115
Total 153860	50	7032	4913	2119	5646	3645	65%	1386	1301	94%	4946	70%	112512	4219200	7875840	492240	123060	90000	58600	24720	42000	

Contd..

Notes: 1. Salary of the Doctor has been calculated in view that the doctor is running his clinic and he works in TeleDoc as part time. To examine case of one patient, he takes approximately 10 minutes. The charge of the doctor is Rs. 50 per hour. Salary of Health worker is Rs. 5000/- per person)

2. Cost of one computer is Rs. 30,000/-
3. Cost of one mobile phone is Rs. 6,000/-
4. Electricity bill is Rs. 500 per month.
5. Telephone bill is Rs. 500 per month.
6. Running mobile expenses is Rs. 360 per month.
7. Rent of building is Rs. 500 per month.
8. The man hours, consultancy, travel and medicines expenses have been calculated assuming that the patient visits the city Doctors 4 times for one disease and for each visit the s/he spends 4 hours, pays consultancy fee Rs. 100, travel cost Rs. 50 and medicine expenses is Rs. 280. These figures are based on the finding of the survey conducted by TeleDoc.
9. The types of chronic diseases which are being treated under TeleDoc project are: Rheumatoid Arthritis, Ankylosing Spondylitis, Psoriatic Arthritis, Gout, Pyrexia of Unknown Origin, Diabetes, Epilepsies, Headache, Depression, Anxiety Neurosis, Bronchial Asthma, Chronic Bronchitis, Pulmonary Eosinophilia, Eczema, Discharge from Vagina, Sinusitis.
10. The types of general and seasonal diseases which are being treated under TeleDoc project are: Gastro Intestinal Infections, Conjunctivitis, Malaria, Flu, Chilblains, Generalized Dermatitis, Cold, Cough, General Debility.

summit award for e-health at the world summit on the information society (WSIS) conference held in Geneva in December 2003.

Conclusion

The Teledoc project of Jiva Institute will deliver effective, low-cost and immediate healthcare to rural villages in India. Appropriate and affordable technologies are used to create economies of scale, leading to real opportunities for social enterprise. The Teledoc field network is leading the investigation of new, scalable and sustainable ways of providing Indian villages with the social services that they need to achieve economic development. Social entrepreneurship ventures have to play important role in the socio-economic development of developing countries what C.H. Prahalad has pleaded in his famous book "The Fortune at the Bottom of the Pyramid" TeleDoc project is a reflection of it.

Acknowledgements

The author wishes to acknowledge name of Mr. Anshul Goel, MBA student of ICFAI Business School, Gurgaon for providing research support in preparing this article. This paper was presented as invitee speaker in Development Education Conference organized by Dublin City University, Dublin Ireland during 23-24 March 2006 and sponsored by Development Co-operation, Ireland. Thanks to Development Co-operation, Ireland for providing grants to participate in the seminar as invited speaker and presenting this paper. The author can be reached at *nspundir@hotmail.com*.

Notes & References

1. Bhattacharyya, Alokesh (2004), Distance Doc: GPs with GPRS, Business Today, 01 February.
2. United Nations Development Programme (2004): Human Development Report 2004: Cultural Liberty in Today's Diverse World (*http://hdr.undp.org/reports/global/2004/*)
3. World Health Organization (2004), The World Health Report 2004: Changing History (*http://www.who.int/whr/2004/annex/country/ind/en/print.html*)

4. Singh, Naresh (2003), Training Intervention for Improving Referral System: A Study of All India Hospital Post Partum Programme in Rajasthan, *Indian Journal of Training & Development*, Vol. 23, No. 1-2.

5. Muniyandi, M. & Ramachandran, Rajeswari (2002): Tuberculosis and Poverty, ICMR Bulletin, Vol. 32, No. 3.

6. Sharma, V.P. (2003), Malaria and Poverty in India, Current Science, Vol. 84, No. 5, 25 February, Pp.: 513-515.

7. Williamson, Oliver E. (2000), "The New Institutional Economics: Taking Stock, Looking Ahead". *Journal of Economic Literature*, Vol. XXXVIII (September), Pp. 595-613.

8. Hegedorn, Konard (2003), "Reasons and Options for Analysing Political Institutions and Processes". Discussion Paper, Summer Programme on Agrarian Institutions Analysis, 14-25 July 2003, Budapest: Central European University.

9. Ibid.

10. Hegedorn, Konard (2002), "The Political Economy and Institutional Evolution of Privatisation and Restructuring of Agricultural Land in central and East Europe". Paper presented in the Regional Conference on Land Issues in Central and Eastern Europe and the CIS, 3-6 April 2002, Budapest: Hungary.

11. Coase, R. H. (1988): "The Problem of Social Cost". in R.H. Coase, The Firm, the Market and the Law, Chicago: University of Chicago Press, Pp. 95-156.

    The article by Coase was originally published in The Journal of Law and Economics, Vol. 3, October 1960, Pp. 1-44. This articled developed the ground for Coase Theorem and it was the second of the two papers for which he received Nobel Prize.)

12. *http://nhrc.nic.in/disparchive.asp?fno=873*

13. *http://www.ashoka.org/fellows/social_entrepreneur.cfm*

14. *www.ipsm.org.uk/Cfairpaper.doc*

15. Dees, J. Gregory (2001): The Meaning of Social Entrepreneurship (*http://www.fuqua.duke.edu/centers/case/documents/dees_SE.pdf*)

16. Prahalad, C.K. (2004): The Fortune at the Bottom of the Pyramid: Eradicating Poverty Through Profits, Wharton School Publishing & Pearson Education.

17. See additional information at:

    http://www.ayurvedic.org/

    http://www.jiva.org

    Life Positive (2004): Promoting Authentic Ayurveda With Hi-Tech: Interview of Dr. Pratap Chauhan, March.

18. See additional information at:

    Jiva's TeleDoc Uses IT for Rural Healthcare (2003) 01 December (*http://www.expresscomputeronline.com/20031201/indiacomputes02.shtml)*

    Outlook (2003): Making a Difference: Jiva Medicine Byte By Byte, 15 December.

7

PARTICIPATIVE MODEL OF ORGANISATIONAL DEVELOPMENT IN GOVERNMENT[1]

Madan Mohan Upadhyay

Introduction

In India, interventions by the government for public welfare have increased steadily over the last fifty years. The increase in population over the period and subsequent reorganization of old districts and formation of new districts narrowed the gap between the administration and the community. The liberalization steps coupled with e-governance initiative, growing information technology and the all round socio economic and infrastructural expansions have increased the expectations of common man from the government. With the introduction of right to information and transparency act, citizens in India are better aware about their right as compared to last one or two decades.

In-spite of the technological changes, the government organizations are facing pressures from all fronts-informed citizens, own personnel, politicians and development agencies. The administration is finding it increasingly difficult to cope up to the situation due to lack of capacity in adopting Organization Development (OD) strategies and hence depending on external agencies for consultative support.

International financial institutions such as the World Bank and the Asian Development Bank are insisting upon the government to place in position systems which make the delivery of services efficient, transparent and cost effective. In this direction, it is necessary that all the government organizations in India adopt OD strategies for effective delivery of services. Most of the major municipal corporations and state owned public sector undertakings are using the services of experts in OD to achieve the desired changes with right perspective from their employees.

The healthy changes taking place across all the sectors require changing work culture among the bureaucratic machinery. The past decades have brought in new changes in the society, particularly the industrial and economic processes. It requires dedicated and enthusiastic personnel willing to update knowledge based on the current needs and implement the changes as required which needs OD interventions at all levels.

Understanding of OD

Experts define OD as an effort planned across the organization, managed from the top to increase organization effectiveness and health through planned interventions in the organizations process using behavioral science knowledge. Max Weber pointed out in the early 20th century that the then emerging rational bureaucratic forms such as charismatic or traditional leadership was an 'ideal' type of authority. The basis of this authority vested on a belief in the legality of patterns of normative ruler, and the right of those devoted to authority under such rules to issue commands. Since this authority was derived from law, there was no arbitrariness in its functioning. The bureaucracy depended on institutional memory (carefully preserved written records) of works implemented. Hence there was continuity and consistency in work regardless of who was performing. The principles of office hierarchy and levels of graded authority meant that there was a clear division of labour and proper supervision at all levels. The official enjoyed a lifetime career with a fixed salary and pension benefits. There were legal guarantees against arbitrary dismissal or transfer so that strictly objective and impersonal discharge of duties was possible.

This Weberian model is not the preferred model in western countries where performance contract, deregulation, and privatization are the current trends. Here the bureaucratic model is considered to be pro-inerta and anti-innovation, full of red tapism and undue delay, and more suitable to mediocre administration than efficient management. In developed countries, there has been a lot of experimental movement away from the Weberian to post bureaucratic organizations. These organizations have an empowered and participative work force which aims at maximizing efficiency & effectiveness and competitiveness with the private sector for survival.

Citizen Charter is a development of the recent years. It has helped in making the organizations more responsive, accountable, transparent, and decentralized and people friendly at all levels with the objective of restoring faith of the people in the fairness and capacity for administration against the prevailing frustration and dissatisfaction. With these in mind the citizen's charters were drawn by various departments and ministries wherein deadline has been given for various activities relating to public. These charters aim at affirming the commitment of an organization to the people that it will deliver its particular services promptly, maintain quality and that redressal machinery would be available.

Models of OD

The three popular models of OD are the Kurt Lewin's Unfreezing–Changing and Freezing Model (Kurt Lewins), Griener's Sequential Process Model and the Leavitt's Systems Model.

The Lewin's Model prepares the organization to change, disturbing the existing equilibrium and then introducing the change. The change moves the organization to a new equilibrium at which the organization has to be stabilized so that it does not revert to the earlier equilibrium. Refreezing refers to this process of stabilizing and integrate the change into behavioral pattern.

Griener's sequential process is in terms of certain sequential stages. The change process is initiated by external process and it is motivated to take action. The succeeding stages of intervention by a change agent are-diagnosis of the problem, invention of a new solution, experimentation with new solution and reinforcement from positive results.

The Leavitt's model focuses on the interactive nature of various sub-systems in a change process. Here the organization is a mix of four interacting sub-systems namely the Task, Structure, People and Technology. Change in any one of the sub-system tends to have consequences for the other sub-systems. Hence OD efforts should not only focus on the intended change but also the effects of change on the other sub-systems. The planned change may be interpersonal training of the required sort for a technological change or task modification. The intended changes in OD programmes may be done at any of the sub- system level such as Organization structure, Task accomplishment, Work climate, Method of decision-making & problem solving and Technology.

HRD Model in Government Sector

Organization Culture is the basic framework of values at work, the principles of which will guide our action. The issue is that can we build culture in government set up through human resource development concepts? The very idea of building culture through HRD presumes that a conscious attempt will be made to inculcate values which are probably more relevant or more desirable and then effect a change which will result in a change in the culture of the organization. Even though government organizations may have a greater degree of stability and consistency, it is a fact that the society is changing rapidly. It is therefore ideal that the government organizations are in tune with the needs of what government should do and then inculcate those values.

In the ultimate analysis of organization work culture it is government and governance which distinguish between anarchy and order. Even after the experience of the market friendly policies in Reagan's United States or Thatcher's Britain, it is being increasingly recognized that in the ultimate analysis, there are some functions that only the government can perform. Maintaining law and order is one example. Further government has to ensure that educations, public health as well as the basic infrastructure for the economy are provided for the public. Therefore one must appreciate the significance of the human dimension in the basic governmental function.

We must see whether HRD techniques can be adopted to build a new culture which will make the government to become more responsive and effective and above all ensure that the benefits of the government policies are brought to the common man. There is a need to bringing a change in the mind-set of the people who are operating in government organizations. Government is vested with power. After all, government is the authority that maintains law and order and this power orientation in turn leads to a culture of the government servant presuming himself to be a purveyor of patronage rather than a person serving the public. The HRD technique that should be used is to inculcate a value for integrity and honesty.

Current Efforts in HRD

Not all OD programmes contain all the possible intervention activities, but a wide range of activities are available to the practioners. Education and training activities form one such group. In the effort to improve the internal efficiency of the organization, training and development has a very crucial role to play. In M.P. such trainings are provided at two places namely-RCN MP Academy of Administration Bhopal and the State Institute of Rural Development, Jabalpur. There are training institutions located at various districts which are catering to subject specific training needs of various departments such as Foresters colleges, Rangers College, Police Training School, Training centers for Health workers etc. These centers give subject specific input to the trainees. A holistic on the job or hands on experience approach is lacking. Generally the participants for such courses do not participate voluntarily but are forced to come due to various compulsions which the departments have to follow in respect of various programmes under implementation in their areas.

Gaps in the Current Efforts

(a) In all departments of government HRD and OD are not priority areas, which are also reflected in the budget allocations provided to various departments.

(b) Different departments follow different norms regarding HRD needs. There is no uniform and well thought policy.

(c) The bureaucrats at all levels are generally under pressure to implement various programmes and to achieve financial as well as physical targets. The OD role is lost sight in that target oriented approach.

(d) Within government there is a wide diversity of work environment and diversity of work scenario spread over very large areas which make the OD work difficult.

(e) Government servants generally have low motivation levels with limited perception about their work. Their role in a wider network is not appreciated. In short one can observe that very rarely motivational interventions are carried out for them.

(f) The senior government officers are the main change facilitators in the bureaucratic set up with a mind set of theory X of McGroger. They believe unless the person is subjected to fear he will not carry out the desired functions. For effective organizational approach the team approach is lacking. At sporadic cases here and there good team approach may be observed.

Problem Identification

The problem areas were first identified using the OD diagnosis concepts and a new approach for OD was designed. It was called *Hamara Daftar–Hamara Ghar* model. It was designed keeping in view the following aspects of organizational climate & work environment in government offices:

(a) There is general apathy about the work place environment among the employees in the offices;

(b) Staff has very little or no role about taking decision on issues related to their place of work;

(c) The level of discipline among employees is not up to the mark;

(d) They generally come to work to just pass 7 or 8 hours and have no specific performance to look forward to;

(e) The response to public services lacks warmth and concern;

(f) They see little opportunity to individual growth besides one or two promotions that they may get in their career spread over 30 to 40 years;

(g) They are not abreast with the latest skills relevant to their jobs;

The sum total of above scenario produces a disinterested, lethargic and indifferent administration which is guided by external pressure of yearly financial and physical targets rather than some internalized factors.

Hypothesis for Interventions

The Hamra Daftar–Hamara Ghar model was introduced in eight district offices and the office of Divisional Commissioner Jabalpur. The model is based on the Hypothesis that:

- If employees give the same degree of importance to their offices as they give to their homes, the current gaps can be reduced significantly in government offices;
- If all the employees in an organization are made direct stake holder in the office matters, it would lead to improvement in the work place;
- If the organization becomes a model of individual development it would lead to better employee growth and also better organization;

Interventions Carried Out

Based on the above hypothesis a model was designed and developed. The various stages of this model are:

Open House Discussion by the Head of Office

The purpose of this was to have an open discussion with all employees on what they feel about the office, their concerns, their fears, their priorities, the organizational priorities, the role of office, the role of individual, their growth needs, the needs of citizen, the role of office as service provider etc. etc. This discussion highlighted the importance of the office in his life, what office means to him and his family. The office vis-à-vis home was put in perspective specifically the more significant role of office vs. job. This intervention helped in developing a climate for change.

Our Office has the Following Unique Features

(a) It provides us the means of livelihood.

(b) Our job provides us opportunity to serve the public and thereby making ours a laudable goal.

(c) Our job provides us an opportunity to grow both in terms of pay as well as in status and position.

(d) Our job provides us a platform to contribute something more meaningful in life i.e. Self Actualization

A Resolve to Change for Better by all Involved

They pledged, after coming to a consensus among all the employees that they all would join hand in bringing out the changes in the organization so that they all enjoy whatever they are doing. In other words they decided to create a work environment conducive to their working.

Make Every Individual Direct Stakeholder through Financial Partnership

To make the OD process participatory in active and sustained sense every individual at all levels in the organization contributed a portion of their monthly salary to a fund called the Hamara Daftar–Hamara Ghar fund.

Problems Identification

This was achieved by administering a questionnaire & forming a small committee to analyse the opinions expressed. The questionnaire was given to all to identify the issues, problems that the individual employee feels insignificant in respect to himself and in respect to the office. This could be related to discipline, service matter, work place & infrastructure, rules & procedures etc. These were documented and categorized.

Workout a Strategy to Address the Problems

Small groups of 6 persons were formed from the employees to discuss the problems and suggest the solutions and strategies that need to be adopted.

Discuss the Feedback

The feedback and the strategy were discussed with the group as a whole and minor corrections were made whenever felt necessary.

Draw an Action Plan

An action plan enumerating the time and cost was worked out and put to action. Here too the decisions were arrived through a participatory process.

Review Implementation on a Monthly Basis

The action plan was reviewed on a monthly basis by the head office. Where ever the deviation from the action plan was observed the factors causing the deviation were identified. The solutions were obtained for these deviations in the participatory problem solving approach.

The model was driven by the motive that our office should be a model of excellence and every individual will be a stakeholder in it as well as an active participant to make the plan successful. The fund created through monthly deductions from salaries was utilized in project aimed at individuals growth, their training needs, their work place improvement, improvement of work culture, promoting brotherhood among employees etc. etc. This being an employee fund, it was not subject to any constraint whatsoever. The only condition being that it should be spent on OD only.

The system of feedback was very strong as the employees were direct stakeholders. They also wanted to know how the funds were put into the cycle of new need. New need assessment and fulfillment can be repeated over and over any number of times. It may choose new area in every cycle. Thus with passage of time a work force was created:

- Which has a system of constant empowerment;
- Where every passing day the commitment of the individual towards participative process increases;

The model also impliedly included the principle of management by objective. The objectives being decided by the need assessment exercise and then the implementation started with these needs as the objectives.

Perception of Respondents on OD

The current satisfaction over the working environment plays a key role in carrying out any intervention on organizational climate. The responses to the working environment were obtained after the interventions made at the Commissioner's office in Jabalpur. The perceptions of the respondents indicate that more than 90% of the respondents are happy with the working space and sanitary conditions available in the offices. However, availability of working facilities are concerned it is seen that less than 50% have responded positively. In regard to availability of lighting facilities, 75% of the respondents have expressed satisfactory to good levels, while nearly one fourth of the respondents are not satisfied. It shows that working space & sanitary conditions have improved in the offices but much focus is to be paid towards improving the working facilities & lighting arrangements. Taken together it reveals that much needs to be done as these indicators are the basic requirement that increases the employees motivation level and hence efficient service delivery.

Training contributes positively to OD. During the survey it is found that nearly half of the respondents are not satisfied with the training needs. This is a serious issue which the organization has to focus for better delivery of services.

Therefore it was asked from the respondents whether their training needs met & to what extent.

Majority of the respondents (99%) have expressed a positive impact of work environment on their performance. This indicates that good working environment is essential for change in organization culture.

Forty two per cent of the respondents were of the opinion that working condition has an impact on performance improvement to the extent of 25%. Nearly 40% have expressed that up to 50% performance improvement is possible. Thus 97% of the respondents felt that improvement ranging from 25 to 75 % can be achieved under better work place facility condition.

About 51% people were of the opinion that the present OD Interventions efforts are not satisfactory.

There are different types of forums where employees can participate and express their needs. It is seen that more than half of the respondents have expressed that Employees Committee and the Joint Consultative Committee at official level are the two forums where the employees participate to express the needs. Only 10% of the respondents participate in meetings at the district level. There are employee informal groups which are attended by 18% of the respondents.

It was assessed from those who responded affirmatively about the existence of participatory forums on the adoption of team approach. Majority of the respondents (88%) expressed that the joint meetings were held by their bosses in problem solving mode. Thus a large number of offices have an arrangement in place where the head of office is sensitive on problem solving.

The status of percolation of team approach at lower level was also assessed. It is revealed that 75% of the respondents have expressed that their HOD discusses with the staff on a regular basis. While 25% of the respondents have expressed that the committee is involved in problem solving & then consulted with bosses. Thus, leaving lesser scope for autocracy. This too is a good local innovation where the staff initially works out the possible solutions within the staff committee and than brought to the head of office.

The possible methods of increasing employee participation were assessed. The responses were very encouraging as described in Table 1 below. These findings are extremely significant as it has put up same new alternative models to OD. If these methods are tried in the bureaucratic setup the OD Intervention will succeed to a large extent.

The survey also tried to elicit the awareness level of any OD Interventions in their office. About 52% responded affirmatively indicating that people could appreciate these interventions. However, there is still a large proportion of respondents who are not aware of any OD interventions prevailing in their offices.

Table 1

Possible Method	*Percentage of Respondents*
Contributing a portion of the salary on monthly basis for Office Development	62
Devote time in small groups for finding the ways of OD	26
Identify areas of individual growth needs & finding ways to achieve them	34
Contributing in the activities leading to capacity building of the organization	11
Others	1

Note: Total is more than 100% because of multiple responses.

The survey tried to assess which of the factors contributing for the success of OD interventions and their priority for each factor was sought. It was found that the majority (53%) sees that the involvement of HOD in OD interventions plays a crucial role. Collective involvement of employees is the second most important factor for successful OD interventions. Nature of work is the least priority for the respondents. The details are presented in the Table 2 below.

It is assumed that in bureaucratic set up giving incentives is one of the most difficult tasks. The promotion and increments are considered the only motivational tools applicable in bureaucracy. These two tools are very procedure oriented and follow strict rules like seniority cum merit. It was then tried what other incentives can be provided to involve the employees in better work culture and improve their performance. Table 3 below gives the respondent's views on the types of appreciation required for better performance. It is seen from the table that written communication appreciating the employee contribution to the department or recognition by the state government or oral appreciation by seniors would suffice for better performance. Cash awards as a method of recognition of the employee contribution to the department is lower in the priority.

Table 2

Factors significant in	*6th P*	*5th P*	*4th P*	*3rd P*	*2nd P*	*1st P*
Involvement of Head Office	0	2	9	9	22	53
Motivational Level of Staff members	8	10	16	28	21	13
Collective involvement of employees	6	10	16	26	25	25
Academic & professional skills of the staff	5	17	32	17	14	4
Physical Environment at Work Place	8	30	18	9	13	9
Nature of Work	53	11	4	2	2	3

Note: P = Priority.

Table 3

Methods of Appreciation	*6th P*	*5th P*	*4th P*	*3rd P*	*2nd P*	*1st P*
Oral Appreciation by seniors	0	17	21	13	14	26
Written Communication for appreciation/Certificate	0	2	9	21	34	24
Cash Award	2	37	16	21	6	4
Recognition by State Government	0	1	13	26	32	18
Physical Environment at Work Place	0	14	26	11	6	20

Note: P = Priority.

Conclusion

This study focusing on the OD issues at the government level is first of its kind in Madhya Pradesh or probably at the all India level. OD in government is still in its infancy in Madhya Pradesh and other parts of the country. How ever, it is essential that OD initiatives are necessary in government offices from the following perspectives:

Sensitization about OD Issues

In a typical government setup, OD is generally left to the senior officials who are located in state capital as Heads of the Department. Implementation of all activities is carried out by the subordinate staffs at the district and tehsil level with lack of exposure to OD concepts. A well thought out plan on workplace aesthetics, its physical needs, the work place architecture etc. are not seriously thought and every thing is left at the discretion of the field staff.

The project Hamara Daftar-Hamara Ghar sensitized the government officials and subordinate staff on the OD concepts. It also highlighted the role of the leader and the element of participative involvement. The study showed that a very large number of offices are adopting the Hamara Daftar-Hamara Ghar model of participative development, which has created a high degree of awareness about the individual training needs in the organizations.

Role of Environmental Factors

The study showed a very positive and high degree of correlation between the individual's performance and his working environment. While various studies are available in the industrial world, this type of study in government organization was first of its type. A good pleasing environment at work place and good infrastructure facilities go a long way in sustaining the employee's interest in their work. This is a very significant finding as the opinions have been unanimous on this account. This finding was found among all respondents irrespective of the department or the organization.

Employee Participation

This study has thrown open a new chapter in participative OD in terms of direct financial participation of all employees towards issues related to OD. Data from districts revealed that government employees are contributing every month a part of their wages towards the Hamara Daftar-Hamara Ghar fund.

The data for the division as a whole and the divisional commissioner office in particular shows very interesting organizational behavior changes which are highlighted in the following graph.

Hamara Daftar-Hamara Ghar model is a unique contribution of the study because no where else in Government sector in the country employees participated in OD activities in such an active manner that they contribute a portion of the salary back to the organization. This type of participative involvement in OD activities is not reported anywhere else in any OD literature. It was generally believed that the employees would not donate back their wages but this study has revealed that this model has been able to bring a revolutionary change in employee's behavior.

The visit to offices and discussion with employees has shown that this model has shown phenomenal results and employees have become truly committed partners in making their organization grow. Some interesting innovative interventions made from the Hamara Daftar-Hamara Ghar fund in different district offices are:

(a) *Mandla:* Diesel generator is installed in the collector's office so that staff could work un-interruptedly during power failure. Also, recreational facilities for employees are developed and regular health check up camps is organized at the work place. In health camps hypertension and heart ailments are diagnosed.

(b) *Jabalpur:* Special training course on accounts keeping and computerization were organized for all staff to empower them with latest tools. In collector's office extensive cleanliness campaign was initiated and old official correspondences were sorted and sent to record room. Work place furniture was redesigned to suit to their requirement.

(c) *Katni:* Computer system installed in PWD office as an effort to modernize office work. Extensive cleanliness campaign was initiated in zilla panchayat and collector's office. Old official correspondences were sorted and sent to record room.

(d) *Commissioner's office:* Extensive environment and infrastructural improvement work carried out apart from providing new job related training and regular health check up. It became the first court in the state where all caseworks were computerized.

(e) *Jabalpur:* Employee committees work as committee on Discipline in office. This has salutary effect on office discipline. Large quantity of old waste materials was disposed.

(f) *Dindori:* Training course on accounts keeping & computerization were organized for all staff. In collector's office extensive cleanliness campaign was initiated and old official correspondences were sorted and sent to record room.

(g) *Narsinghpur:* Employees committees were constituted to look into the matters relating to internal discipline, upkeep of office, infrastructure development etc.

The study thus revealed that there can be a working model to solve the OD issues wherein the employees themselves play a key role. Employees will become the prime movers instead of the passive participants in the conventional approach. As a contribution of this study the state government issued guidelines to all the offices throughout the state on 4th march 2003 wherein it directed them to:

(A) Initiate improvement in work place environment on a sustained and systematic basis.

(B) Evolve a participative process for creating a fund from the salary of employees for improvement of work place environment.

(C) A committee at district level under the chairmanship of district collector has been setup to review the mechanism at district level on OD initiatives in government offices. This committee would oversee the OD initiatives. Three best offices will be rewarded by this committee.

The study revealed that the participative model of training needs assessment is a very effective tool wherein the employees are not subjected to general training but employees are chosen for specialized training as necessary. This will create a facilitative environment training needs in the organization.

New OD Policies

The study provided data to government to formulate new policies on OD. The planning department, Government of M.P. issued on order that the government would make contribution on a matching basis where ever the employees make contribution under Hamara Daftar-Hamara Ghar yojna.

Similarly Commissioner of Income Tax, Jabalpur issued an exemption order under Income Tax Act on contribution made by the employees to the Hamara Daftar-Hamara Ghar fund. The exemption is valid up to March 2006.

Usefulness of the Study

The present study has been useful in the following context:

(a) Devising alternative strategies of OD in government offices;

(b) Identifying various environmental factors that contribute towards making the work place an excellent place.

(c) Identifying the employees training needs in a better manner so that suitable job specific trainings could be organized.

(d) Provided data to help the government formulate new policies on OD.

Future Directions

The Hamara Daftar Hamara Ghar model of participative involvement has emerged as a new innovative approach towards OD. It makes a paradigm shift from the traditional approaches. Every employee from top to bottom in the organization is directly responsible for the development of the organization in a new environment. Some of the future directions that can be visualized are:

- *Expansion throughout the State:* The participative model of OD has several distinct advantages over traditional approaches. The model could be replicated in other offices throughout the state.
- *New Areas of Research:* OD in government has been a much neglected area. Whatever interventions are made are done in the area of training. A holistic approach by giving the office a status similar to home with monthly deductions from their salaries on a voluntary basis is a new approach involving total participation at all levels. Again OD takes a much wider perspective and is not confined to the textbook arenas but the creative force of the entire organization is put towards OD. This makes everyday a day of new ideas. The days ahead can generate subsequent research projects into areas associated with various factors of OD.

Further Improvements

The Hamara Daftar-Hamara Ghar approach of participative OD works on a system of constant feedback and improvement. Thus it is a path which leads to improvements on a continuous basis thereby taking organization to newer heights.

Note

1. This paper is prepared from the study carried out by the author in the state of Madhya Pradesh (MP) in 2005 as a part of the desertation work for the MBA degree submitted to IGNOU.

8

TRENDS IN PRODUCTIVITY OF LABOUR AND CAPITAL IN DAIRY INDUSTRY IN INDIA DURING PRE-AND POST-REFORM PERIODS

Anil Kumar & Geeta Khurana

Given the welfare implications of enhancing productivity, substantial attention have been received from the economic and political communities in this area. It has been widely acknowledged in the economic literature that the economic growth, no matter how impressive, will not be sustainable without the improvement in productivity. In most of the developing countries, low productivity growth or its negative trend has been a commonly observed feature [Pardhan and Barik, 1999]. A drive towards higher productivity to generate economic growth, therefore, became more pressing in these economies. Besides this, the success of industrial development programmes to achieve pre-determined objectives implicitly depends upon the performance of their manufacturing sector on productivity front. The analysis of productivity growth by industrial sector provides an important tool for assessing how individual activities contribute to changing structure of the dynamic economy. In this paper an attempt has been made to analyze the productivity of labour and capital in dairy industry in India during pre- and post-reform periods.

The paper has been divided into two sections. Section I discusses the model for measurement of productivity of labour and capital and section two present results on productivity of labour and capital in dairy industry in India during pre- and post-reform periods.

SECTION-I

Measurement of Productivity Growth: The Model

Partial Productivity Indices

The most familiar concept of productivity is that of the partial productivity indices. Partial productivity indices refer to ratios of output to each of the categories of inputs for which separate data exist. The partial productivity index (P_i)of the input *i* can be computed as:

$$P_i = \frac{Y}{X_i}$$

where Y = Output; and X_i is Quantity of input *i*. The most popular partial productivity indices are labour and capital productivity indices.

The index of labour productivity for state "*i*" at time *t* is defined as a ratio of index of output to index of labour input. Symbolically, it can be expressed as:

$$LP_i(t) = \frac{Y_i(t)}{L_i(t)}$$

where $LP_i(t)$ = Index of labour productivity for state "*i*" at time *t*;

$Y_i(t)$ = Index of output for state "*i*" at time *t*; and

$L_i(t)$ = Index of labour for state "*i*" at time *t*.

On the same lines, the index of capital productivity for state "*i*" at time *t* can de defined as a ratio of index of output to index of capital input. Symbolically, it can be expressed as:

$$KP_i(t) = \frac{Y_i(t)}{K_i(t)}$$

where $KP_i(t)$ = Index of capital productivity for state "*i*" at time *t*;

$Y_i(t)$ = Index of output for state "*i*" at time *t*; and
$K_i(t)$ = Index of capital for state "*i*" at time *t*.

Growth Rates of Partial Productivity Indices

The average annual growth rates for the relevant productivity indices indicators have been computed for the entire study period (from 1980-81 to 2000-01) using the semi-log equation that takes the forms:

$$\log Q_t = \varphi + \gamma t + \varepsilon_t$$

where Q_t represents the value of the dependent variable under consideration in period *t*; *t* is a trend variable representing time and takes values $t = 1, 2, ..., 21$ and ε_t is the stochastic error term in period *t*. The growth rate of dependent variable Q for the entire study period has been obtained as:

$$g = 100\%[\exp(\gamma) - 1]$$

The impact of industrial liberalization and deregulatory policies on the productivity growth of dairy industry has been captured by computing and subsequently comparing the growth rates between sub-periods (*i.e.* pre- and post-reform periods). In literature, there are two basic approaches to obtain the growth rates for sub-periods: (i) discontinuous trend lines approach; and (ii) kinked exponential model. In the former approach, the separate exponential trend lines are required to be fitted by Ordinary Least Squares (OLS) to each segment of the time series for estimating the growth rates for distinct sub-periods. In case of kinked exponential model, we make use of information regarding the values of the dependent variable in question throughout the time series for estimating the growth rate for a given sub-period using dummy variables. For the estimation and comparison of past growth rates, kinked exponential model represents a distinct improvement over discontinuous trend lines method [Boyce, 1996]. Goldar and Seth (1989), Seth and Seth (1994) and Burange (2001) utilized kinked exponential models for estimating growth rates of sub-periods in their empirical studies. In kinked exponential model, we utilize a linear spline function as developed by Poirier (1974) for estimating the growth rates of distinct sub-periods.

Assuming that there are only two distinct sub-periods (Pre-reform and Post-reform periods), the following Piecewise Log-linear (PWLL) model has been utilized for estimating the annual growth rate for each sub-period.

$$\log Q_t = \alpha + \beta_1 Z_{1t} + \beta_2 Z_{2t} + u_t$$

where

$$Z_{1t} = D_{1t}t + D_{2t}t_1$$

$$Z_{2t} = D_{2t}t + D_{2t}t_1$$

Here t is a trend variable representing time and t_1 denotes the first break in the time trend. In present study, t_1 refers to the year 1991-92. The OLS estimate of β_i gives the exponential growth rate for the variable Q for the sub-period i. The annual growth rate, g_i, for the sub-period i can be obtained using the following equation:

$$g_i = 100\%[\exp(\beta_i)-1]$$

SECTION-II

Results and Discussion

This part presents an analysis of inter temporal comparison of growth of labour and capital productivity measures in the dairy sector of 14 major states. The analysis has been divided into two periods:

1. Pre-reform period (1980 to 1991)
2. Post-reform period (1991 to 2001)

In the present analysis labour productivity has been defined as gross real value added per employee Table 1 exhibits the average annual growth rate of labour productivity in dairy sector at both national and state levels.

The categorization of states on the basis of labour productivity trends into three distinguish groups.

Group I: Andhra, Karanataka, Maharashtra, Uttar Pradesh.

Group II : Assam, Kerala and Tamil Nadu

Group III : Bihar, Gujarat, Haryana, Madhya Pradesh, Punjab, Rajasthan and West Bengal.

Table 1
Growth Rates of Labour Productivity in Dairy Industry

State	*Pre-reform Period*	*Post-reform Period*
All-India	0.39	4.02
Andhra Pradesh	-1.17	6.54
Assam	0.25	-6.84
Bihar	1.52	3.35
Gujarat	1.47	10.14
Haryana	2.78	1.94
Karnataka	-0.60	6.45
Kerala	0.85	-8.66
Madhya Pradesh	0.94	5.25
Maharashtra	-0.50	6.77
Punjab	0.74	6.80
Rajasthan	1.47	10.77
Tamil Nadu	0.20	-1.76
Uttar Pradesh	-3.18	9.00
West Bengal	0.73	6.56

Source: Author's Calculations.

First group incorporates those states which have negative growth of labour productivity during pre-reform period but have achieved the positive growth pattern after post-reform period. The labour productivity followed a negative growth pattern in the states of Andhra Pradesh, Karnataka, Maharashtra and Uttar Pradesh during pre-liberalization period, but after deregulatory policy a significant u turn has been observed in the growth pattern of labour productivity in these states and the dairy sector of these states achieved the positive and high growth rates during 1991-2001 in comparison of realization of negative growth rates during 1980 to 1991. The labour productivity grew at an alarming rate of 9 per cent per annum in the state of Uttar Pradesh.

Group two comprises of those states which have low labour productivity pattern during pre-liberalization period but after reforms process states showed a downfall and negative growth of labour productivity. The labour productivity grew at the rate below 1 per cent per annum in the states of Assam and Tamil Nadhu in pre-liberalization period but in post liberalization period, the states of Assam and Kerala observed decline in the labour productivity in the tune of -6.84 per cent and -8.66 per cent respectively. State of Tamil Nadu also notice decline in labour productivity during post-reform period as compared to pre-reform period.

Group three includes those states which observed positive growth rates during pre-reform period. But these states observed improvement in term of labour productivity during post-reform period. All the states in this group achieved growth rate more than 5 per cent per annum except in the states of Bihar and Haryana. The highest growth rates have been observed in the states of Gujarat and Rajasthan (more than 10 per cent each).

In nut shell the Indian dairy sector at aggregate and disaggregate levels i.e. (state levels) registered increasing growth in labour productivity during post-liberalization period in comparison of pre-liberalization period.

In the present study, the capital productivity has been measured as the ratio of gross real value added to gross fixed capital stock at constant prices.

Table 2 highlights the intertemporal variations in capital productivity in Indian dairy sector at both national and state levels during the pre- and post-reform periods. It has been observed that the capital productivity followed a declining trend in Indian dairy sector during both the periods under consideration.

On the basis of the comparative analysis of growth pattern of capital productivity between pre-and post-libealisation periods at state levels, the 14 major states can be categorized into three distinct groups.

Group I : Gujarat, Karnataka and Punjab.

Group II : Andhra Pradesh, Assam, Haryana, Tamil Nadu and West Bengal.

Group III : Kerala, Bihar, Maharashtra and Uttar Pradesh.

Group one includes the states, in which the average annual

growth rate of capital productivity improved during post-liberalization period in relation to pre-liberalization period. The states are: Karnataka, Punjab and Gujarat. The growth behaviour of capital productivity exhibits a turn around in these states.

Table 2
Growth Rates of Capital Productivity in Dairy Industry

State	*Pre-reform Period*	*Post-reform Period*
All-India	–0.15	–1.50
Andhra Pradesh	2.50	–2.98
Assam	3.01	–11.05
Bihar	–4.55	–2.83
Gujarat	–1.53	2.25
Haryana	1.96	–2.65
Karnataka	–1.63	2.20
Kerala	–3.21	–4.67
Madhya Pradesh	0.38	0.78
Maharashtra	–2.97	–0.10
Punjab	–0.55	3.03
Rajasthan	1.04	4.63
Tamil Nadu	2.81	–6.00
Uttar Pradesh	–0.90	–1.54
West Bengal	0.49	–3.14

*Source:*Author's Calculations.

Group two consists of those states in which the capital productivity followed a negative growth pattern during post-reforms period as compared to positive trend in the pre-reforms period. These states are: Andhra Pradesh, Assam, Haryana, Tamil Nadu and West Bengal. The capital productivity declined at the alarming rate of 11.5 per cent in the dairy sector of Assam.

The third group involves those states in which deregulating policy has no impact and these states are: Uttar Pradesh, Kerala, Bihar and Maharashtra. The pattern of growth in capital productivity remained unaltered in the dairy sector of these states. State of Madhya Pradesh has been able to bring marginal improvement in the capital productivity of dairy industry during post-reform period. Only state of Rajasthan has been able to bring improvement in the capital productivity during post-reform period. On the whole, it can be concluded that the growth of capital productivity at both aggregate and disaggregate level did not respond well during liberal environment.

Suggestions and Policy Implications

The foregoing analysis reveals that labour productivity at national level has shown considerable improvement during post-reform period. But variations have been observed in case of growth rates of labour productivity at state-level. On the other hand, capital productivity has declined during post-reform period at national level and state level. To improve the labour productivity in different states, modern human resource management practices should be adopted by the industry. Reward system should be linked with productivity. Latest technology should be introduced in order to bring improvement in the dairy industry. Modern technology should be made available to dairy industry at reasonable prices. To increase productivity of labour and capital in dairy industry, financial assistance should be provided on liberalized terms and conditions. Encouragement should be given to rural youth to start dairy farming business to increase the supply of major input to dairy industry.

References

Boyce, J.K. (1986), 'Kinked Exponential Models for Growth Rate Estimation', *Oxford Bulletin of Economics and Statistics,* Vol. 48, No. 4, pp. 385-391.

Burange, L.G. (2001), "Liberalization and Employment in the Organized Manufacturing Sector of India: An Inter-Regional Analysis", *Journal of Indian School of Political Economy,* April-June, Vol. 13, No. 2, pp. 194-215.

Golder and Seth (1989), Spatial Variations in the Rate of Industrial Growth in India" *Economic and Political Weekly,* June 3, pp. 1237-40.

Pardhan, G. and K. Barik (1999), Fluctioning Total Factor Productivity in India: Evidence from Selected Polluting Industries", *Economic and Political Weekly*, February 28, pp. M25–M30.

Poirier, D. (1974), *The Econometrics of Structural Change*, North Holland, Amsterdam.

Seth, V.K. and A. Seth (1994), *Dynamics of Labour Absorption in Industry*, Deep & Deep Publications, New Delhi.

9

PERFORMANCE EVALUATION OF TEA INDUSTRY IN INDIA

R. Ezhil Jasmine

Introduction

Tea is a significant beverage crop of India. It is part and parcel of Indian social, economic and cultural life. It is the only industry where India has retained its leadership over the last 160 years. The global tea industry is dominated by India–the largest producer and consumer of black Tea. Around 32000 million kgs of tea is produced annually in the world and India accounts for 27.5% of it. Besides, it is also one of the major exporters of tea in the world. However India is facing stiff competition in the International tea market.

Objectives of the study

(1) To study the production performance of Tea industry in India.

(2) To study the export performance of Tea industry in India.

(3) To study the prices of Indian Tea at different auction centres.

(4) To study the problems of Tea industry in India.

Production of Tea in India

India has 39,700 tea estates (32000 in the south and 6700 in north) and a tea-producing workforce of over 1.1 million people. India produces varieties of tea grown in different regions of the country. The range of tea offered by India–from the original Orthodox to CTC (Crushed, Tear and Curl) and Green Tea, from the aroma and flavour of Darjeeling Tea to the strong Assam and Nilgiri Tea–remains unparalleled in the world.

Since independence, tea production has grown over 250% while land area has just grown by 40%. Tea is grown in 16 Indian states, of which Assam, West Bengal, Tamil Nadu and Kerala are the largest producers accounting for about 96% of the total tea production. The north Indian states have a larger share of land (77%) under tea cultivation and production. The principal tea-growing districts of northern India are in the Assam Valley and Cachar, in the districts of Darjeeling and Jalpaigure (more commonly known as the Duars) and in Terai in West Bengal. In southern India, tea is grown in the elevated region overlooking the Malabar Coast in Kerala and in the Nilgiris Hills.

Tea production in India has registered a slow growth rate over the last few years because of the closure of about 70 tea gardens in Assam due to the widespread recession in the industry.

Table 1
Production of Tea in India (Year-wise)

Year	*Production*	*Index (Qty. in M kgs)*	*Increase /Decrease 2000 = 100*
2000	846.92	100.0	–
2001	853.92	100.8	+ 0.8
2002	838.47	99.0	– 1.0
2003	878.13	103.7	+ 3.7
2004	892.96	105.4	+ 5.4
2005	927.90	109.6	+ 9.6

Source: Tea Board of India.

$$\chi^2 = \Sigma \left\{ \frac{(O-E)^2}{E} \right\} = 0.08$$

Table value at 5% for 5 degrees of freedom is 11.0. Hence the production of Tea is proved to be significant during the given years.

It is clear from the analysis that the production of tea in all the given years (except 2002) has recorded an increase as compared to the base year 2000. There is a Compound Annual Growth Rate (CAGR) of only 1.9 per cent in the Tea production during the period.

North India is the leading producer of Tea when compared to South India. Especially, Assam (North India) is the largest producer of Tea in India. Tamilnadu is the leading producer of Tea in South India.

The production of Tea in North India has recorded an increase of 39 m.kgs in 2005 (701 m.kgs of production i 2005 as against 662 m.kgs in 2004). But the production of Tea in South India has recorded a decline of 4 m.kgs in 2005 (227 m.kgs of production in 2005 as against 231 m.kgs in 2004). Tamilnadu and Karnataka are the areas where the production has declined.

India is the leading producer of Tea in the world followed by China, Srilanka, Kenya and Indonesia. But the share per cent of India in the world Tea production has reduced during the recent years. Though India is the topper in production, the growth rate of production is not as high as countries like China and Kenya.

India exports 15 to 20 per cent of its total tea production and the remaining 80 to 85 per cent is domestically consumed. Out of the 928 million kgs of Tea produced in India in 2005, the domestic consumption is around 750 million kgs.

It is apparent from the table that the Compound Annual Growth Rate (CAGR) of Indian Tea production (2002-2005) is 3.4 per cent as against 5.3 per cent in China and 4.6 per cent in Kenya. While India and china have a large domestic market, other countries mainly produce for export purpose. Therefore the international tea prices are closely linked with the prices in Srilanka and Kenya.

Marketing of Tea

Marketing of Tea in India consists of both Leaf and Dust Teas in the CTC and Orthodox grades. The consumption of tea is above 600 million kgs per year. Tea trading in domestic market

Table 2
Production of Tea in India–Area wise

(in Million kgs)

Sl. No.	*Area*	*2003*	*% share*	*2004*	*% share*	*2005*	*% share*	*Increase/ decrease 2005/2004*
1.	Assam	435	49.5	436	48.8	474	51.0	+ 38 (8.7)
2.	West Bengal	201	22.9	215	24.1	215	23.2	Nil
3.	Others	12	1.4	12	1.2	12	1.3	Nil
	North India.	648	73.8	662	74.1	701	75.5	+ 39 (5.8)
4.	Tamil Nadu	167	19.0	163	18.3	155	16.8	- 8 (4.9)
5.	Kerala	58	6.6	62	6.9	67	7.2	+ 5 (8.1)
6.	Karnataka	5	0.6	6	0.7	5	0.5	- 1 (16.7)
	South India.	230	26.2	231	25.9	227	24.5	- 4 (1.73)
	Total	878	100	893	100	928	100	+ 35 (3.9)

Source: Tea Board of India.
Note: Figures furnished in parentheses denotes per centage of increase or decrease of production.

Table 3
India's share of World Tea production

Year	*Production (Qty in M. kgs)*		*India's share %*
	World	*India*	
2000	2908.96	846.92	29.11
2001	3035.27	853.92	28.13
2002	3055.04	838.47	27.45
2003	3174.06	878.13	27.67
2004	3,305.97	892.90	27.01
2005	3,344.72*	927.90	27.74

Source: ITC Annual Bulletin & Tea Board of India monthly reports.
* Subject to revision.

Coefficient of Correlation between Indian Tea production and World Tea production is + 0.63. Hence there is positive relationship between them.

is done in two ways–Auction selling and private selling. The primary marketing of tea is conducted through public tea auction centres licensed by Tea Board of India which are located at Kolkata, Guwahati, Siliguri, Amritsar, Coonoor, Coimbatore and Cochin. Bulk trading is done through the auctions held in these centres. The Tea Board has partially introduced electronic auction system in Guwahati, Siliguri, Coonoor, Coimbatore and Cochin. The Board has also launched an IT portal (*www. indiateaportal.com*) for effective dissemination of information relating to tea industry.

Due to globalization, the consumption pattern of tea has remarkably changed in India, resulting in the growth of branded tea sector. New brands are therefore introduced in the market depending upon the tastes and preferences of the consumers. The best quality tea would now fetch Rs. 58 to Rs.65 per kg, medium quality Rs. 48 to Rs. 55 per kg and low quality Rs. 42 to Rs. 48 respectively. The branded Tea sector in India has two major players who take a lion's share in the industry. Hindustan Lever Limited (HLL) leads this segment with a market share of 31 per cent flowed by Tata Tea with a market share of 21.1 per cent.

Table 4
India among Top Tea Producing Countries of the World

(Quantity in Mkgs.)

Country	*2002*	*Rank*	*2003*	*Rank*	*2004*	*Rank*	*2005*	*Rank*	*Compound Annual Growth Rate*
India	838.47	I	878.13	I	892.90	I	927.98	I	3.4%
China	745.37	II	768.14	II	835.23	II	870.00	II	5.3%
Srilanka	310.60	III	303.25	III	308.09	IV	317.20	IV	0.7%
Kenya	287.10	IV	293.67	IV	324.61	III	328.58	III	4.6%
Indonesia	172.79	V	167.65	V	164.82	V	164.19	V	-1.69 %

Source: ITC Annual Bulletin & Tea Board of India monthly Reports.

Table 5
Prices of Tea at Indian Auction Centers

Quantity in M.kgs. Price in Rs/Kg.

Sl. No.	Auction centres	January to December						Increase/Decrease 2005 over 2004
		2003		2004		2005		
		Quantity	Price	Quantity	Price	Quantity	Price	Price
1.	Kolkata	133.87	68.13	119.32	80.34	140.27	70.02	-10.32
2.	Guwahati	138.67	59.01	127.09	68.78	121.63	60.03	-8.75
3.	Siliguri	87.09	54.58	91.99	64.13	90.42	58.38	-5.75
4.	Amritsar	0.19	28.62	0.15	26.04	NA	-	-
	North India	359.82	61.31	338.55	71.57	352.32	63.58	- 8.01
5.	Cochin	50.63	45.78	54.60	52.30	55.74	50.23	-2.07
6.	Coonoor	40.59	34.55	44.28	43.30	40.86	36.16	-7.14
7.	Coimbatore	22.33	38.30	18.40	46.50	18.14	40.90	-5.60
8.	Tea Serve	4.40	30.58	18.53	40.79	13.67	35.73	-5.06
	South India	117.95	39.93	135.81	47.01	128.41	42.89	- 4.12
	All India	477.77	56.03	473.36	64.54	480.73	58.06	- 6.50

Source: Monthly report 2005 & 2006, Tea Board of India.

Table 6
Price of Tea at Different International Auction Centers

Quantity: (in thousand kg) Price: (in US dollar/kg)

Sl. No.	*Auction centres*	*January to December*						*Increase/Decrease 2005/2004*
		2003		*2004*		*2005*		
		Quantity	*Price*	*Quantity*	*Price*	*Quantity*	*Price*	*Price*
	North India	359.82	1.32	338.55	1.58	352.32	1.44	-0.14
	South India	117.95	0.86	135.81	1.04	128.41	0.97	-0.07
	All India	477.77	1.20	474.36	1.43	480.73	1.32	-0.11
	Colombo	273.23	1.54	269.87	1.73	273.06	1.84	+0.11
	Mombassa	285.84	1.54	298.09	1.55	306.76	1.47	-0.08
	Chittagong	47.78	1.16	52.93	1.06	52.08	1.21	+0.15
	Jakarta	33.77	0.95	32.21	1.02	36.14	1.04	+0.02
	Limbe	15.90	0.95	17.22	1.00	11.93	0.92	-0.08

Source: Tea Board of India.

Hindustan Lever Limited produces tea brands namely Red Label, Taj Mahal, Taaza, 3 Roses and Lipton Tea. Tata Tea Limited produces Tata Tea, Agni, Kannan Devan, Chakra Gold, Tata Tetley and Gemini.

The Indian tea industry has been adversely affected by fall in prices during the last few years mainly due to supply and demand imbalances. Even though there was an improvement in average auction prices of tea during 2004, auction prices have been lower during 2005. The lower prices are dooming many plantations, especially in Assam, which accounts for more than half of India's tea production.

It is clearly known from the Table that prices of tea in all Indian auction centres have declined in 2005. Some of the estates are facing closure, while others have managed to survive by reducing wages with the co-operation of the workers' unions. The main components of cost of production in Indian tea industry comprises labour cost at 50 per cent, manufacturing cost 14 per cent and administration cost 12 per cent. Labour cost is generally fixed and if production suffers, the cost of production per unit goes up significantly. Cost of production in the competing countries like Kenya and Srilanka is lower due to labour cost advantages, better productivity from younger tea bushes and state support. Indian tea is not price competitive except for some niche segments. The tea industry veterans have predicted that prices could rise by 30 to 35 per cent and cross Rupees 100 per kg mark over the next 2 to 3 years, if the global tea production remains tight.

There is no single world price for Tea, but rather different prices at different auction centres. Tea prices across on all major international tea auction centres have remained soft in 2005 as against 2004. But price rises have been recorded in Colombo, Chittagong and Jakarta.

Import of Tea in India

In 2005, India imported 16.47 million kg of tea with the country's domestic consumption pegged at 805 million kg. The low import price is indeed a matter of concern particularly in the context that significant quantum of tea imported into the country is meant for re-exports.

Table 7
Import of Tea in India

Source Country	*2004 (in M.kg)*	*Rs/kg (in M.kg)*	*2005*	*Rs/kg*
Indonesia	2.65	57.73	2.26	62.52
Nepal	3.14	59.66	3.64	60.60
Srilanka	0.46	80.90	0.30	121.81
Vietnam	17.28	32.56	3.23	36.90
Kenya	3.29	82.25	3.17	77.73
Others	3.98	97.91	3.87	109.18
Total	30.80	45.88	16.47	58.65

Source: www.blonnet.com

Import of Tea has remarkably decreased in India in 2005 (16.47 m.kgs.) when compared to 2004 (30.80 m.kgs.). The Tea (Distribution and Export) Control Order, 2005 provides that no distributor shall carry on the business of distributing imported tea and no exporter shall export tea or export imported tea except under a business license obtained in accordance with the provisions of the order.

Imports for re-exports have two implications. First, re-exporting sub-standard teas in the guise of Indian tea would tarnish the image of Indian teas in the international market; and second import for re-export would result in additional pressure on supply position in the domestic market, as otherwise this tea could have been exported.

Export of Tea in India

Almost every major tea-drinking nation in the world imports some or other variety of Indian Tea. Despite India's historical success in the Tea industry, it is facing stiff competition in the international market. India has registered a decline in exports in recent years. Hence focus on the export front is necessary to promote Indian tea in domestic market through advertisement campaigns. The total net foreign exchange earned from Tea industry per annum is around Rs. 1847 crores. Besides, it also contributes revenue to the national exchequer by way of cess, sales tax, agricultural and corporate income tax.

Table 8
Export of Tea in India–Year wise

Year	*Export*	*Index 2000 = 100*	*Increase/Decrease*
2000	206.82	100	–
2001	182.59	88.3	–11.7
2002	201.00	97.2	–2.8
2003	173.68	84.0	–16.0
2004	197.60	95.5	–4.5
2005	187.60	90.7	–9.3

Source: Tea Board of India

$$\chi^2 = \Sigma\left\{\frac{(O-E)^2}{E}\right\} = 0.07$$

Table value at 5% for 5 degrees of freedom is 11.0. Hence the Export of Tea in India is proved to be significant during the given years.

It is clear from the Table that the export of Tea has decreased in all the given years as compared to the base year 2000. The Compound Annual Growth Rate (CAGR) of Tea Export in India is–1.94 per cent, which shows that there is negative effect in the growth of Tea Exports in India.

India ranks fourth in terms of tea exports in the world. However India's export share to three biggest international tea markets–Russia, UK and Pakistan has been on a decline. Srilanka and Kenya have been eating into India's market share. India's tea exports during January to December 2005 stood at 187.6 million kg. compared to 197.6 million kg. during the corresponding period in 2004. Quality is the major factor and that is why India's Exports are suffering.

The export of Tea from India has dropped by 10 million kgs in 2005 (8.1 m.kgs reduction in North India and 1.9 m. kgs reduction in South India). However, net exports from the country (export minus import) registered a growth which indicates a positive sign for the industry.

North Indian teas fetch twice as much as South Indian teas because of their quality and the markets they cater to. North Indian teas cater to the American and British markets while South Indian teas go to the Common Wealth of Independent States (CIS market), which offer lower realizations.

Table 9
Export of Tea in India–Area wise

Region	2004			2005			
	Volume	*Rs. Crore (M.kg)*	*Rs/kg*	*Volume*	*Rs. Crore (M.kg)*	*Rs/kg*	*% Increase/ Decrease 2005/2004*
North India	100.8	1203.85	119.43	92.7	1079.12	116.41	- 8.1 (8.0)
South India	96.8	637.28	65.17	94.9	618.55	65.18	-1.9 (2.0)
All India.	197.6	1841.13	93.17	187.6	1697.67	90.49	- 10.0 (5.1)

Source: www.blonnet.com & Tea Board of India.
Note: Figures given in parentheses indicate per centage of increase or decrease in export.

Table 10
India's Share of World Tea Exports

Year	*Production (Qty in M. kgs)*		*India's share %*
	World	*India*	
2000	1330.87	206.82	15.54
2001	1391.35	182.59	13.12
2002	1438.76	201.00	13.97
2003	1390.35	173.68	12.49
2004	1536.14	197.60	12.86
2005	1557.63	187.60	12.04

Source: World–ITC Bulletin
India's export–Tea Board of India

Coefficient of Correlation between Tea Export in the World and in India is 0. Hence there is no relation ship between them.

The share per cent of India in the world Tea Exports has reduced during the past few years. According to the Tea Board of India, India's earlier dependence on Russia's imports is of the main reasons for the drop in its exports. Besides big buyers like Iran and Iraq have also become inactive due to political reasons. Rising competition from Kenya is yet another factor affecting Indian Tea exports.

Decline is quality of Indian tea has been caused by mushrooming bought leaf factories which produce cheap quality tea by buying and processing green leaf from small growers. Further, blending of Indian teas with cheaper varieties and export of the same as Indian tea has also impaired the quality perception.

India is fourth in the row after Srilanka, Kenya and China with a world export share of 12.04 per cent in 2005. But all the major tea-exporting countries have reported explicit improvement in their export performance except India which has recorded a negative growth (Compound Annual Growth Rate of Indian Tea exports is –2.3 per cent).

At present due to drought conditions in Kenya, its tea production is expected to drop by 16 per cent. As such, the export of tea in India could do well in the days to come. India could export tea to United Kingdom due to lower projected output in Kenya. India could also tap

Table 11
India Among Top Tea Exporting Countries of the World

Qty. in Th. Kgs.

Name of the Country	*2002*	*Rank*	*2003*	*Rank*	*2004*	*Rank*	*2005*	*Rank*	*Compound Annual Growth Rate*
India	201.00	IV	173.68	IV	183.64	IV	187.60	IV	-2.3%
Srilanka	285.99	I	291.89	I	290.65	II	298.77	II	1.4%
Kenya	272.46	II	269.27	II	326.34	I	349.74	I	8.6%
China	252.27	III	259.98	III	279.50	III	295.00	III	5.3%
Indonesia	100.18	V	88.18	V	96.00	V	104.00	V	1.3%

Source: Tea Board of India & ITC Annual Bulletin.

the potential in Egypt as the latter has reduced the Import duty for Indian tea to five per cent. For the current financial year 2006-2007, Tea Board of India has set an export target of 100 million kg.

Problems of Tea Industry in India

The tea industry in India, which has an annual turnover of Rs. 10000 crores has been witnessing sea changes in the past few years. Despite some of the unique advantages, namely, largest production, huge domestic consumer base, diverse and unique climatic conditions, rich cultivation tradition, majestic art of tea making, the tea industry in India is ailing. The various problems are:

(i) Malt-based beverages such as Horlicks and Bournvita are the favourite type of hot drinks in the South, and are also growing at a faster rate. Besides, Soft drinks such as carbonates also represent a significant threat to the ongoing dominance of tea in India. Besides, the aggressive marketing campaigns of leading multinationals successfully persuade many young consumers to migrate from tea to soft drinks.

(ii) Stiff competition from the producing–exporting countries like Srilanka, China, Indonesia and Kenya pose great threat to the Indian tea industry.

(iii) Various tariff and non-tariff measures imposed by importing countries such as Russia, Egypt and Iran pose threat to Indian tea industry.

(iv) Land and labour productivity are two of the most serious banes of the Indian tea industry. The production, productivity and quality of tea are highly affected by the old age of tea bushes in India, with more than 30% of tea area being above the economic threshold age limit. The estimated life of a tea bush ranges from 80-100 years with the most productive age between 30-35 years. About 50% of the Indian tea bushes have crossed 50 years of age.

(v) Mechanization is one of the effective alternatives that can reduce costs. But in countries like India and Kenya where a large number of people are employed in the plantations, they feel that it is a major threat to their livelihood.

(vi) Lack of plucking standards among small growers is another problem in India.

Fresh investments and technology adoption are the primary vehicles to rejuvenate the Indian plantation sector and make it more competitive and viable in the current global scenario. For increasing labour productivity the industry is in discussion with the government and the Unions to go for piece-rate system instead of the traditional time-rate systems. There is also an urgent need to help the small growers in India to improve their plucking standards and to handle the plucked leaf in a proper manner so that the leaves could be transported it to the factories in a fresh condition.

With the slowing down in the rate of domestic consumption of tea, increasing competition from other beverages, particularly soft drinks and developments in the global arena, the tea Board has planned to go in for a massive advertising campaign to change the image of tea and increase its consumption. The TV commercials are a part of the first phase of the Rs. 10 crore internal promotional drive by the Tea Board of India that will be carried out throughout the 2006-07 fiscal year. Further, the Government of India has also planned for a series of initiatives to boost the plantation sector, which has been under rough weather due to growing global competition. A special insurance scheme for plantations, restrictions on import, new marketing initiatives and better compensation during price crash are some of the steps under consideration to boost the industry. Further, the Indian Government would continue to focus on the traditional Indian Tea markets such as Russia, the UK and UAE. "The future of plantation industry depends on research and development" said Mr. Jairam Ramesh, Union Minister of Commerce for state.

Findings

1. India ranks first in the world in Tea production followed by China, Srilanka, Kenya, and Indonesia etc. The compound Annual Growth Rate of Indian Tea production is 1.9 per cent.
2. North India is the leading producer of Tea when compared to South India. Assam is the largest producer in North India and Tamilnadu is the leading producer in South India.
3. India secures the fourth position in the world in Tea exports. But the Compound Annual Growth Rate of exports in India shows a negative effect of –2.3 per cent.
4. High cost of production is a fundamental problem of Tea industry in India.
5. The Indian Tea industry is widely affected by fall in prices during the past years.
6. Blending of Indian teas with cheaper varieties and exporting the same, has impaired the quality perception in the market.

Conclusion

In the era of globalization, the buzzword is competition and the bottom line is competitiveness. The road ahead for Indian Tea industry is not rosy, unless the industry drastically reduces the cost and improves its competitiveness. In order to revive the Indian Tea industry, the Central budget 2006-2007 has proposed contribution of Rs. 1 billion towards Special Purpose Tea Fund (SPTF) a 15 year programme, aimed at re-plantation and rejuvenation of Tea. The need for the hour is to increase the productivity of both land and labour. The Indian Tea Association (ITA) forecasts a high growth in 2006 for the recession-hit tea industry with more exports, production and domestic consumption. The Indian tea industry should gear up to meet the global challenges.

Reference

Monthly report of Tea, April 2005, Tea Board of India.

Monthly report of Tea, February 2006, Tea Board of India.

Performance Budget, Ministry of Commerce & Industry 2005-2006, Government of India.

www.agritrade.cta.int/tea

www.blonnet.com

www.commerce.nic.in/annual 2005-2006

www.dailypioneer.com

www.epwrf.res.in

www.hindu.com/2005

www.icra.in

www.indiabudget.nic.in

www.indiatea.org/ccpa

www.indiateaportal.com

www.Indiainfoline.com

www.newkerala.com

www.seattlecentral.org/faculty.

www.swannteas.com/abouttea

www.thehindubusinessline.com

www.teauction.com/industry/indiantea.asp

www.teaauction.com/statistics

www.teacouncil.co.uk

www.tribuneindia.com

www.voanews.com

10

PROMOTING FINANCIAL INCLUSION: AN ANALYSIS OF THE ROLE OF BANKS

Alpana Vats

The Eleventh Five Year aims to achieve a new vision based on faster, more broad-based and inclusive growth. While provision of basic economic services such as education, health, drinking water, gainful employment are the major planks to make growth more inclusive, financial exclusion of large segments in any society prevents them from effective participation in the country economic progress. Financial exclusion represents a situation in which people have no access to and so no usage of mainstream financial services in ways appropriate to their needs. It is characterised not just by a lack of affordable credit and savings but by having no bank account, no assets, no access to money advice and no insurance (HM Treasury 1999b, 2004). An effective response must address each element of financial exclusion in a co-coordinated, strategic and holistic manner. Significantly and challengingly for banks, it must begin by addressing the issue of banking and transaction services. Research has shown that accessing financially excluded groups to credit and savings products is often dependent on their having first access to bank account, which acts as a gateway to other financial services (Hogarth and O'Donnell 1997, Bridges & Disney 2004). Financial inclusion does not mean that everyone should be able to use each of the services, but they should be able to use them as and when need arise. In past a number of initiatives have been undertaken from time to time to bring in financially excluded people in financial net.

Financial inclusion is the endeavor of the formal financial system to outreach the vast section of the rural and urban population who are shackled by unorganized forces and trapped in the vicious cycle of poverty. Talking about financial inclusion, India is probably one of the pioneers in targeting inclusive growth. In past four decades, several government-sponsored schemes were launched for poverty alleviation and employment generation. Setting up Regional Rural Banks, introduction of Lead Bank Scheme and Service Area Approach to lending were some of the major institutional building measures initiated in seventies and eighties. Fixing targets for priority sector lending has been the hallmark of our policy intervention for achieving financial inclusion. Banking industry has shown significant improvements in the areas relating to financial viability, profitability and competitiveness, but it is still a cause of concern that banks have not been able to cover vast segment of the poor populance especially the down trodden and underprivileged section of the society. This paper examines the role of banks in removing the barriers for financial inclusion. The paper is organized as follows. Section I of the paper gives a brief overview of the extent of inclusion in formal sector in India. Section II of the paper discusses the various demand and supply side barriers of the inclusion. Various measures initiated to reach the goal of financial inclusion and the progress made in this direction has been highlighted in section III of the paper. Section IV highlights the international experience to confront the challenge with section V giving some random thoughts on microfinance bank linkage model, challenges and way ahead The paper concludes with section VI.

SECTION–I

Indian economy is at the growth trajectory of 8%-9% per annum. But the benefits are still to reach even the fringes of the rural population of India, at the bottom of the Pyramid. The poor are still left behind in the race for development and they are still unreached and continue to be excluded from all round development process.

The various forms of exclusion can broadly be classified as:

FINANCIAL - Lack of resources

PHYSICAL - Lack of shelter, Lack of place for business

ECOLOGICAL - Lack of sanitation, Lack of drinking water

SOCIAL - Lack of Education, health Care, Enhanced vulnerability of women and children

POLITICAL - Lack of choice and voice

In India still 54% villages do not have a Public Health Centre, but have to walk a distance of 5 Kms away and 27%villages have to walk 10 kms away for the nearest PHC. There are only 18 telephones per 1000 population. Basic facilities, like drinking water is available only for 18% of the villages. Only 10% of the villages have medical shops and just 20% have clinic. As regard to education facilities one third of the villages do not have pre primary schools and 28% do not have primary schools. Co-operative banks exist only in 30% of the villages.

For ensuring social justice in an equitable manner we need to include the hitherto excluded and unreached population of the rural and urban poor in all the above said aspect. Inclusion with regard to ecological, physical, social and political is largely related to the state. In this paper we will focus on the financial dimension of the inclusion.

Many official surveys and sponsored studies, carried out from time to time, have brought out the extent of outreach of the formal financial sector in rural areas. A brief overview of the findings of such studies is mentioned below:

As per 2001 census, 72 per cent of the India's population continues to live in rural areas. 60.4 per cent or 89.35 million out of 147.9 million rural households are farmers' households. 42 per cent of the total rural population was classified as main and marginal workers among whom 40.1 per cent of the total work force in rural India depends on agriculture for their major source of income. Between 1991 and 2001, the absolute number of cultivators and agricultural labourers increased in rural areas by 2 million and 21.7 million respectively. Among the total of farmers households, 74.97 million are small and marginal farmers (SF/MF). The Situation Assessment Survey of Farmers (SASF) conducted by NSSO shows that out of total (SF/MF) households, 40.27 million are excluded from the formal financial system and among other categories of farmers 5.66 million are excluded. 16 States, mainly in northern, northeastern and eastern regions in the country reported more than 50 per cent financial exclusion. The exclusion was the highest among marginal farmers at 55 per cent followed by small farmers 49 per cent. The acutest situation was manifest among agricultural labour households with 78.8 per cent remaining financially excluded.

Poor Outreach of Formal Sector: State wise Position

Despite substantial increase in agriculture credit, there are certain imbalances, which need to be addressed. One such imbalance is the reach of formal credit institutions in rural areas. According to NSSO Report: 498 Round (Situation Assessment Survey of Farmers- Indebtness of Farmer Households-NSS 59 Round, May 2005), the professional moneylenders had highest percentage of farmers' households (24.1 per cent of total) indebted to them. Next in order to come: Banks (22.5 per cent), co-operative Banks (21.7 per cent), Relative and Friends (15 per cent), Traders (10 per cent), others (4.2 per cent) and the government (2.5 per cent). It is rather disturbing to note that even after 37 years of nationalization of banks and about 15 years of credit targeting for agriculture lending, banks had still a smaller outreach of the Indian farmers as compared to rural money lenders.

The following table depicts the dominance of different agencies in different states.

Formal Sector and Exclusion of the Poor

The finding of the National Sample Survey Organisation (NSSO) 59th Round (2003) reveal the extent of indebtedness of the cultivator households. Out of 147.90 total million rural households in the country, around 89.35 million households

Dominant Agency	*Name of the States*
Professional money lenders	Andhra Pradesh, Bihar, Manipur, Meghalaya and Rajasthan
The Traders	West Bengal, Nagaland, Sikkim and Jammu & Kashmir
The friends and relatives	Assam, Arunachal Pradesh, Himachal Pradesh, Manipur, Meghalaya and Mizoram
The formal credit agencies particularly banks	Jharkhand, Orissa, Tripura, Uttar Pradesh and Uttaranchal
The co-operatives	Chattisgarh, Gujarat, Haryana, Kerla, Madhya Pradesh, Maharashtra and Punjab

(60.41 per cent) are the cultivator households. Of these households, approximately 49 per cent are indebted to either formal source of finance or non-formal sources or to both. This implies that about 51 per cent of total cultivator households who are free from debt are outside the perview of "Inclusive Growth". Further, of these 51 per cent non-debted category, majority of them (88 per cent) are households belonging to small and marginal farmers having land holding less than 2 acres. It has been observed that banks tend to have more bias towards cultivator households who possesses larger farm holdings. The NSSO data also reveals that in respect of small holdings of less than 0.25 acres, the system's outreach is of 65 per cent in case of big farm holdings up to 5-10 acres. The following table shows the land size and sources of loan:

Land in Hectares	*Formal Sources*	*Informal Sources*
Less than 0.01	22.6	77.4
0.010to 0.40	43.3	56.7
0.41 to 1.00	52.8	47.2
1.01 to 2.00	57.6	42.4
2.01 to 4.00	65.0	35.0
4.01 to 10.00	68.8	31.2
Above 10.00	67.6	32.4

(NSSO Report No. 498 Situation Assessment Survey of Farmers indebtedness of Farmer Households NSSO 59th Round – May 2005)

The above table indicates that:

- As the size of land holding increase, their dependency of the informal sector decreases and vice-versa.
- Poor farmers with less than 0.01 hectares of land depended largely on informal source of finance (77.4 per cent) and, in that too particularly, on the money lenders (47.3 per cent). The formal sector had little role by contributing 22.6 per cent of their total requirements. Bank's contribution was minuscule 15.4 per cent.
- On the other extreme, large land holders with over 10 acres of land accessed more from the formal sector (67.6 per cent of the total) as against 32.4 per cent from the informal sources. Bank's share in their credit access was as high as 42.7 per cent.

According to All India Debt and Investment Survey (AIDIS), 2002, over a period of 40 years, the share of non-institutional sources of credit in sources of credit for cultivator households had declined sharply from about 93 per cent in 1951 to about 30 per cent in 1991, with the share of money lenders have declined from 69.7 per cent to 17.5 per cent. In 2002, the AIDIS, revealed however, the share of moneylenders had again increased to 27 per cent, while that of non-institutional sources overall rose to 39 per cent.

Prominence of Informal Sector in Selected States

The findings of the Rural Finance Access Survey (RFAS) done by the World Bank and NCAER in Andhra Pradesh (AP) and Uttar Pradesh (UP) 2003 also reveals that only 24 per cent of the total rural households in AP and 19 per cent in UP had access to formal credit, while 56 per cent and 51 per cent of the households in these two states, respectively, depended on private credit sources. The small and marginal farmers accessed less credit compared to medium and large farmers indicating that the access to formal credit was poor and skewed in favour of the larger holdings.

Lower CDR in Rural Branches

Apart from the low outreach, another issue pertains to low Credit-Deposits Ratio of the rural and semi urban branches and the declining trend in CDR. Despite the RBI's norm for achieving a CDR of 60 per cent in rural and semi-urban branches, banks were not able to achieve the described norm. In fact, the CDR of rural offices in SCBs showed a continuous decline during the past 10 years between 1991 and 2001 from 60 per cent in 1191 to 50 per cent in 1994 to 41 per cent in 1999 and further to 39 per cent in 2001. As per the Report on Expenditure Committee on CD Ratio (2004), while the number of Deposits account with the rural offices of SCBs increased by 21 per cent between 1991 and 2001, the number of credit accounts (borrowal accounts) declined by 30.12 per cent in the same period and resultantly, CD Ratio continued to decline over the years. This clearly indicates that the resources raised by banks in rural areas are not deployed there but diverted to other areas.

Region wise Inclusiveness

A study by Ray and Singh (2006) on inclusiveness of Indian banks shows that there is only 31-account holder per 100 of population in 2005, which is increased from 29 account holder per 100 of population in 2001. Among the Regions, in 2005 Northern Region with 42 has the highest number of accounts per 100 populations, followed by southern Region (40)). The North Eastern Region has been showing a decline in number of accounts per 100 of population from 20 in 2001 to 19 in 2005. Large variation has been found between the states with Delhi having 92 accounts per 100 population, whereas Bihar having 16 accounts per 100 population. It is highlighted that in Bihar almost 79 per cent of the population does not avail banking services.

The main inferences drawn on the basis of the above survey/studies are as follows:

- Vast majority of rural population is beyond the purview of the formal financial system. The rich and the large farmers have greater access to the formal system while

Population Group wise Number of Bank Accounts and Amount

(In thousand)

Population Group	*Number of Accounts*							
	Current Number	*% to total*	*Savings Number*	*% to total*	*Term Number*	*% to total*	*Total Number*	*% to total*
Rural	2816	15.9	104922	32.8	34170	26.5	141908	30.4
Semi Urban	4000	22.6	88209	27.6	32989	25.6	125198	26.8
Urban	4872	27.5	65699	20.5	30805	23.9	101376	21.7
Metropolitan	6031	34.0	61168	19.1	31111	24.1	98310	21.1
All India	17719	100.00	319998	100.00	129075	100.00	466792	100.00

Report on Trend and Progress in Banking in India, RBI.

the smaller farmers are in the clutches of the village money lenders. The formal credit system has not been able to adequately penetrate the informal financial markets; rather it seems to have shrunk in some respect in recent years.

- Low income levels and irregular income are the major causes due to which the rural poor are considered non-bankable propositions.
- While deposits growth in the rural sector is increasing, the credit to rural sector is decreasing resulting in deceleration of CD Ratio over the years.
- The depth in growth of banking system varies from state to state.
- There is immense scope to extend the reach of banking system in rural areas through innovative methods.

SECTION–II

An analysis based on both the demand and supply side perspectives to understand the reasons for the exclusion may prove rewarding. Viewed thus, there are several dimensions for exclusion.

Demand Side Analysis

The Physical Dimensions

Vast numbers of the rural population resides in small villages, often located far away from the branches of formal financial system. If the several visits that are often required to secure a loan and the total time taken for transactions in the branch, and the availability of local transport facilities in rural areas etc. are factored, the overall transaction cost to the consumer in terms of both time and money proves to be a major disincentive for visiting financial institutions.

Lack of Literacy

The literacy rate reported under the census 2001 was 59.40 per cent in rural areas. The literacy rate in this context means the ability to read and write. However for participation in social and economic activities several other dimensions are required. One has to have functional literacy wherein it is possible to understand consequential implications of various documents, news, information etc. that one may read or sign up. There is also need, in increasing degrees, of trade, legal, financial and quality literacy in a dynamic economy on accelerated growth curve. Thus, literacy looked at from several other dimensions than the minimal approach may be highly lacking among the rural population. Even under the minimal read and write concept there is a high level of gender inequality with only 46.70 per cent of women being literate against 71.40 per cent of women being literate against 71.40 per cent males in India.

The Human Capacity Dimension

A large segment of the rural population suffers from low levels of social capital as well as skills and knowledge. In view of this, they are overwhelmed by the myriad of processes and documentation that are demanded by formal financial institutions. As a result, they are often required to make multiple visits to complete the transactions. The information asymmetry tends to create rent-seeking intermediaries also. The RFAS reports that rejection rates are high in the case of loan accounts and that the average time taken to obtain a loan varies from 24 weeks in cooperatives to 33 weeks in commercial banks. Leakages to the extent of 10 per cent to 20 per cent at the branch level is also is reported in the survey. The relatively lower social capital also results in exclusion. Empirically it is also seen that the financial exclusion of scheduled tribes is more than among other social groups.

High Transaction Costs

The transaction cost to the borrowers is also seen to be high due to above factors. The expenses related to multiple visits, the loss of wages, the costs that may be incurred to procure various documents as large number of rural folk may not have sufficient documentary proofs required by banking sector, the rents that they may pay etc. tends to drive up the real cost of borrowing far above the nominal interest rates charged by the formal financial system. An empirical study in Utter Pradesh shows that non-interest transaction cost incurred by a borrower for a loan of Rs. 5000/- with a two year monthly repayment schedule worked out to 8.4 per cent (where no leakages was involved).

Affinity for Informal Credit

The high costs, the uncertainties in obtaining loans, the negative experiences etc. also tends to keep the rural population from approaching the formal system, and increases their affinity for the informal system. The report of the National Farmer's Commission states that only 27 per cent of all cultivator households receive institutional credit. The all India Debt and Investment Survey 2002 reports that only 27 per cent of the total rural households were indebted and that 57.1 per cent of the total cash dues in rural India was accounted by institutional agencies and 42.9 per cent by non-institutional agencies with professional and agricultural money lenders together accounting for 29.6 per cent . It is alarming to note that dependency on the informal financial sector increased from 36 per cent as reported under AIDIS 1991 to 42.9 per cent in 2002.

Uneconomical Production System

As per the available information from the Agricultural Census division, Ministry of Agriculture, New Delhi, 61.6 per cent of total operational holdings in the country are marginal farmers with average size of holdings of 0.40 ha. In addition to this, 18.7 per cent are small farmers with average holdings size of 1.42 ha. In some of the larger states in the country like UP and Bihar, 75 per cent are small farmers with average holding size of 0.39 ha and 0.34 ha., respectively. The number of total operational holdings as well as number marginal farmers has been showing an increasing trend due to fragmentation of land aggravating the problem of low productivity due to poor scales and the disinclination for capital investments. Thus, the total cost of production and the value of the production from large number of operational holdings is very small. Both the farmers as well as the financial institutions may have a low propensity to access or service such credit.

Supply Side Analysis

Unbankable Rural Population

There exist a perception that large numbers of the rural population are unbankable as their capacity to save is limited. This perception is indeed borne out by the fact that most of the small and marginal farmers cultivate only a single crop with low yields. As a result they do not have a steady stream of income, but have an income spike after harvest. They often slip into informal borrowings to meet regular consumptions expenses or do not liquidate and entire production, keeping a significant portion for future consumption and food security. Only an encouraging thrift and empowerment through social engineering shall result in the creation of savings and thus equity to leverage credit from the formal system. This is amply proved by the large-scale induction of poor women into availing microfinance services.

Small Volumes

The loan amounts are too small to attract attention. It is seen that the number of loan accounts of less than Rs. 25,000/- decreased from 58.8 million accounts in 1991 to 19.5 million accounts 2005. As on March 2005, the average outstanding per account under this category was only Rs. 11658/-. As in the case of the borrower reported above, a study estimated the total cost to the bank of a small loan of Rs. 5000/- at 15.72 per cent and the bank had a negative margin on such loans.

Outreach Issues

Very often, even if the person may be bankable, the distances are too long for servicing and supporting the accounts at reasonable costs, even with the large number of rural branches that exist in India. The population base of large number of villages are very small for the bankers to aggressively market their services and products. As per census 2001, out of the 6.38

lakh villages in India, 4.29 lakh villages have population of less than 1000 persons (67 per cent). The situation is acute in 17 states accounting for 66 per cent of the total villages in India and 50 per cent of rural population as the average per village population of less than 1250.

Uncertain Cash Flows

The disadvantaged segments among farmers have an uncertain cash flow on the one hand and the banking system may not have the ability to evaluate and monitor rural cash flows, leading to a dependency on improper repayment schedules. There is lack of data base and absence of credit history available for farmers with small means. Such information asymmetry also results in a lower propensity to reach out.

Human Resources

There are also several human resources related constraints that hamper financial inclusion. The total number of officers working in rural branches of SCBs (including RRBs) was 59,276 which means that the ratio of population per officer is 12,512 in rural while this ratio is 1,120 in urban India (the ratio for all employees was 2,134 and 396 respectively). The average age of employees in the banking system is also skewed towards 50 years, and they may have greater propensity to rely on walkin customers.

Disinclination towards Repeat Transactions

The two most important factors that determine positive client behavior in micro finance are the ease of short tenure transactions and the assurance of repeat loans/withdrawals. However, the high vouching and processing cost at branches, and the highly stretched, aging human resources do not provide a fovourable climate for the fulfillment of these expectations. Consequently, the true outcome of even well designed products like KCC/GCC etc. may remain sub-optimal.

Identification Problems

Often the marginalized section does not have an identity proof to be able to open an account. KYC norms further alienate them.

SECTION–III

After discussing the demand and supply side hurdles in the implementation of financial inclusion in the previous section this section delves some recent initiatives taken by the regulator and regulated in the industry to address the issue of inclusion. The Reserve Bank of India, in its mid term review of the monetary policy, has envisaged that the banks should make available to all sections of the society a basic banking account with nil or low minimum balances and low maintenance and service charges. Such accounts are known as "no frills" accounts. The concept of basic bank accounts is not really new for some public sector banks. The features of the "no frills" account are practically identical with those of the popular, no cheque book, Ordinary Saving Bank (OSB) accounts (as distinct from the normal Special Savings Bank Accounts) that the State Bank group had introduced at all branches across the country in the mid 1970s.

While stringent Know Your Customer (KYC) norms are stipulated for opening normal bank accounts, the procedures for opening "no frills" accounts have been simplified to enable the underprivileged sections of the society in both urban and rural areas to access basic banking services. The mid term review of the annual policy policy for 2006-07 KYC procedure for opening of account has been simplified for those persons who intend to keep the balances not exceeding rupees fifty thousand (Rs. 50,000/-) in all their accounts taken together and the total credit in all the accounts taken together is not expected to exceed rupees one lakh (Rs. 1,00,000/-) in a year.

The other step initiated by banks is revolving credit through the GCC facility at their rural and semi-urban branches. The GCC may be in the form of passbooks and will provide the rural customers ease in operations and flexible source of liquidity. The Kisan Credit Card (KCC) scheme as part of financial inclusion was introduced in the year 1998-99 to enable farmers to purchase agricultural inputs and draw cash for their production needs.

Recently announced Union Budget 2007-08 proposes establishment of Financial Inclusion Fund with NABARD for meeting cost of development and promotional intervention and also a Financial Inclusion Technology Fund is proposed to be established to meet the cost of technology adoption, each fund having a corpus of Rs. 500 crore.

In order to extend the coverage of financial inclusion, State Level Bankers' Committee (SLBC) convener bank in all states /union territories were required to identify atleast one district in each state/union territory for achieving 100 per cent financial inclusion by providing (no frills) account and GCC. The SLBC bankers were advised to identify a suitable district in each state/ union territory, allocate villages to various banks for taking on responsibility for ensuring 100 per cent financial inclusion and monitor the progress in this regard. SLBC may form sub-committee for this purpose and based on the experience gained consider the scope for providing 100 per cent financial inclusion in other areas/districts. Palakkad District in Kerala recently became the first district in the country to achieve 100 per cent coverage for financial inclusion.

With the objective of ensuring greater financial inclusion and increasing the outreach of the banking sector, it was decided in January 2006, to allow banks to use the services of NGOs/ SHGs, MFIs and CSOs as intermediaries in providing financial and banking services through the use of business facilitator and business correspondent models. The guidelines issued in January 2006 mainly related to: (i) eligible entities and scope of activities under business facilitator and correspondent models; (ii) payment of commission/fees and other terms and conditions for these entities; (iii) redressal of grievances; and (iv) compliance with the ëKYCí norms. A group has been set up by RBI in order to examine the issues relating to (i) allowing banks to adopt agency model by using infrastructure of civil society organization (ii) appointment of banking correspondents' to function as intermediaries between the lending banks and beneficiaries and (iii) identification of steps to promote MFIs. Based the recommendations of the group and with the objective of ensuring greater financial inclusion and increasing the outreach of the banking sector, banks have been permitted to use the services of specified intermediaries and also post offices as business facilitators and correspondents. Many banks have introduced the innovative concept of Village Knowledge Centres in rural areas to cater the needs of the rural population in general and farmers in particular. These centers impart knowledge to farmer on improved methods of cultivation/technologies, proper use of fertilizers, pesticides, latest information on price of inputs and agriculture produce for better yield and higher income. Village Knowledge Centres also provide the farmers information about the current market prices of various commodities, various agricultural loan products/new innovative schemes of our Bank. These centers also serve as focal point for effective marketing of rural business.

SECTION–IV

Internationally, the financial exclusion has been viewed in a much wider perspective. Having a current account/savings account on its own, is not regarded as as an accurate indicator of financial inclusion. There could be multiple levels of financial inclusion and exclusion. Thus, it is worth while to have a look at the international experience in tackling the problem of financial exclusions that we can learn from the international experience.

United Kingdom

Among initiatives taken by UK, 7 deserve mention :

- Identification of 3 priority area for the purpose of financial inclusion namely,

  (i) access to banking services

  (ii) access to affordable credit

  (iii) access to free face-to-face money advice
- Establishment of Financial Inclusion Fund to promote financial inclusion
- Assignment of responsibility to banks and credit unions to remove financial exclusion
- Introduction of "no frills" bank account
- Creation of Post Office Current Account for those unable or unwilling to access a basic bank account

- Introduction of 'Savings Gateway' for those on low-income employment. Under this agreement, for every BO 1 saved by those on low-income employment, the state will put an equivalent BP 1 up to BP 5.
- Setting up of Community Finance Learning initiatives to promote basic financial literacy among housing association tenants.

Bangladesh

Grameen Bank in Bangladesh has done pioneering work in including hitherto neglected population through targeted credit. Infact to make targeting more effective and inclusive the Bank made it a point to target women more than men (women constitutes 97% of the total borrowers). Often, Banks feel shy of extending credit to marginal section due to fear of adverse selection. To overcome this fear, Grameen Bank evolved and enforced the practice of group lending. With this approach many hurdles were overcome in coordinated manner. Not only this enabled access to credit, it also developed a self-regulatory mechanism among the borrowers to effectively utilize the credit for the purpose it has been extended. Previously bad choices started turning into good economics. the loan recovery rate went upto 98.85 per cent. On the profit front Grameen Bank earned profit every year except three years i.e. 1983,1991 and 1992 since its inception. Besides it also included the savings habit among the borrowers thus making them more financially sound. This approach turned out to be sustainable. In fact the bank made special programme to include beggars in its fold. Approximately 81,000 beggars have already joined the programme.

Canada

In 2003, legislation entitled "Access to Basic Banking Services Regulations" was introduced to ensure that all Canadians could obtain personal bank accounts as well as cash most government cheques at no charge (even to non-customers) for any individual that meets basic requirements. The Federal Government also introduced legislation-requiring banks to offer a standard low cost bank account with the basket of services. Memoranda of Understanding were signed between the Federal Government and eight financial institutions to ensure that the Canadians have acess to affordable banking services.

United States

Between 9.5 and 20 per cent of U.S. households lack a bank account. 22 per cent of low income families (over 8.4 million families earning under $25,000 per annum) do not have either a current or savings account, although some states place an obligation on banks to provide accounts to all citizens.

The community Reinvestment Act and Home Mortgage Disclosure Act require banks to disclose details of people and groups to whom they are currently offering services. Originally introduced as a response to banks 'redlining' areas (refusing to do business with residents of certain neighborhoods) the Acts ensure that deposit services and credit services serve the convenience and credit services serve the convenience and needs of the communities in which financial institutions are chartered to business. This is a key part of ensuring that banks meet their social objectives and serves to encourage access by community of banking services.

France

The 1984 Banking Act made access to a bank account a legal right in France: people refused one can apply to the Bank of France, which will nominate an institution to provide the bank account. In addition, in 1992, French banks signed a charter committing themselves to opening a bank account at an affordable cost with related payment facilities.

South Africa

In many countries where bank-account use is low, such as South Africa, there is emergence of system like smart cards and pre-paid cellular telephony, which allow transactions between individual and between them and commercial entities, without the need for banking infrastructure. The state has promoted these channel as a means of democratisation, using them to deposit public transfers such as pensions, tax rebates, and conditional transfers to low-income population groups, among others. It goes without saying that the corresponding transaction costs are much lower than for payments using credit cards or cheques, which do not reach the low income population groups. This is the future of remittances.

South Africa has also been pioneer in establishing universal access fund, similar to that used to promote cellular telephony, to which banks make a contribution and in exchange receive fund resources as they expand access.

The international experiences of successful inclusive banking indicate that it is useful for banks to deal with groups of customers organized in the form of Self-Help Groups rather than trying to approach and attract customers individually. In Bangladesh, Gramin Bank offers small-sized loans to groups of customers. This helps in better recovery as the group ensures that its members maintain the credit discipline. The developments in computing and indicative technology provide another avenue by which products & services can be distributed among widely dispersed categories.

SECTION–V

The concept of Micro Finance includes a broad range of services viz. credit savings, insurance etc., to cater to the diverse and various needs of the poor and very poor who lack access to traditional formal institutions. Since then, the mission of the big players is to empower the unreached population. The most popular model in the country today is Self Help Group (SHG) banking model. Since the debut of several players in micro finance a decade and half ago, they have joined hands with informal channels to give microfinance movement the necessary momentum. The system is slowly and painfully transforming from infancy to childhood stage. Many milestones have been crossed in its journey and the impact is felt by the poorest of the poor and also by some corporate. For eg., companies like Hindustan Liver has made in-road in to the rural market for several of its products using novel credit delivery mechanism to derive mutual benefits.

The data published by NABARD indicates that as of March 2006, 22,38,565 groups have been assisted since the inception of SHG programme and the financial assistance provided thus far amounts to Rs. 113,975.50 million. Preliminary estimates from the latest National Survey (NSS), sample conducted in 2004-05 shows that the percentage of population below the poverty line in 2004-05 was about 28 per cent. The actual population below the poverty line, as per this estimate works out to be approximately 288 million. In other words only less than one tenth of the below poverty line population has been fortunate enough to have formal access to the credit in the novel system, leave alone the other financial requirements like insurance etc. In 2006-07 budget, the Finance Minister asked the banking sector to link another 3,85,000 SHG in 2006-07. SHG is not the only means to achieve the goal of poverty reduction and Millennium Development Goals but no doubt that this is one of the best systems that have evolved to achieve the inclusion. However, it may not be possible to cover all excluded poor and attach them to the main stream if the microfinance system grows at the present rate. The solution lies in accelerating the growth rate of microfinance through other means.

The study on the progress achieved through microfinance also throws up another interesting fact, which is about the inclusion. The state wise data of groups mobilised as on March 2006 is furnished in the table below:

It can be observed that the SHG movement is highly skewed in the geographical distribution, both in numbers and credit assistance. More than half of the groups are in southern region. In the regions falling under the backward states, popularly known as BIMARU, the spread is minimal. High illiteracy, poverty and unemployment are above the national average in these states. There is an urgent need that people of these states should be migrated to the mainstream within a reasonable time frame. Making the microfinance to penetrate fast in these geographical areas is the best means to achieve the objective of financial inclusion.

By the fiscal year end, the country has surpassed the goal set for doubling the flow of credit to agriculture, which began

Region/ State	*March 2001*	*March 2002*	*March 2003*	*March 2004*	*March 2005*	*March 2006*
NE Region	477	1,490	4,069	12,278	34,238	62,517
KBK Region	4,192	9,869	18,934	31,372	45,976	64,550
Orissa	8,888	20,553	42,272	77,588	123,256	180,896
West Bengal	8,739	17,143	32,647	51,685	92,698	136,251
Bihar	4,592	3,957	8,161	16,246	28,015	48,138
Jharkhand	0*	4,198	7,765	12,647	21,531	28,902
Uttar Pradesh	23,152	33,114	53,696	79,210	119,648	163,439
Uttaranchal	0	3,323	5,853	10,908	14,043	16,060
Rajasthan	5,616	12,564	22,742	33,846	60,006	98,171
Himachal Pradesh	2,545	5,069	8,875	13,228	17,798	22,920
Madhya Pradesh	5,699	7,981	15,271	27,095	45,105	58,912
Chattisgarh	0*	3,763	6,763	9,796	18,569	29,504
Maharashtra	10,468	19,619	28,065	38,535	71,146	131,470
Gujarat	4,929	9,496	13,875	15,974	24,712	34,160
All India	263,825	461,478	717,360	1,079,091	1,618,456	2,238,565

Source: NABARD. NE = North-east, KBK = Kalahandi-Bolangir-Koraput.
*included in the undivided State.

three years ago. Majority of the banks have shown the required growth rate within the period of three years. It is also worth to note that almost all the banks have achieved the sub parameter target of assisting atleast 100 new farmers per each rural and semi urban branches every year. It is also worth to note that almost all banks have achieved the sub parameter target of assisting atleast 100 new farmers per rural and semi-urban branches every year. The paradox lies in the findings of the NSS 59th Round (2003) study. It reveals that out of the total number of cultivator households, only 27 per cent receive credit from formal resources and 22 per cent from informal resources. The remaining households, mainly small and marginal farmers, have virtually no access to credit. The finding has prompted the Finance Minister to form a committee on Financial Inclusion. The committee under the chairman ship of Dr. C.Rangrajan is expected to suggest a plan for designing and delivering credit to every household that seek credit from lending institutions. Will the banking system play the required role to achieve this inclusion or will it turn out credit proportion for the weaker section? This is something debatable but is certain is that schemes like Rythu Mithra Groups give hopes to ensure desired inclusion.

Microfinance has grown at an alarming rate over the years when financial products offered to clients have increased in number, range and sophistication. It has proved definitely as an alternative credit delivery system to reach the unreached and poor. Although this is to note the only magic solution for financial inclusion, no doubt that this will certainly act as one of the means and supplement the other mechanisms and players in hastening the inclusion. This definitely help to hasten the growth rate of this movement, ensure an equitable geographical growth and develop specialization in various areas to cover the different section of the population like small farmers, artisan and others in the bottom of the exclusion pyramid. The micro-finance transaction costs are high as the business involves making small loans to a large number of clients. One way to reduce these costs and take advantage of economies of scale is by standardizing products and operations. There is an urgent need to develop standards in the system and a national lever is required to ensure healthy competition and orderly growth of the different players.

These micro-finance organizations fund cost is also high and the thrift/savings of the group is kept out of the reach of the agencies other than banking system so as to ensure that the poor is not exposed to unnecessary risk. Non Banking Financial Company or even the local area development bank too needs lot of initial resources. The recently opened External Commercial Borrowing route may solve the issue to some extent however; it is not a complete solution.

Three major banks in the country have entered into an agreement for a joint business strategy with the future plan to of establishing a separate subsidiary, if required jointly, to harness the business growth. Subsidiary is not new to the banks. Why can't they begin with a subsidiary for microfinance? If the bank can venture into this growing and prosperous niche market, the return will certainly help them to improve bottom line . This is more so, as the market in the urban areas is fully saturated because of aggressiveness of different player and multiplicity of products for the retail segment. Further penetration in the urban retail segment is relatively risky in terms of bad loans and also high capital requirements as per the Basel-II norms.

The specific strength of the micro-finance sector is its expertise in developmental activities. Despite being an effective instrument for poverty reduction and employment, the aggregate efforts of all players put together runs to only Rs. 7000 crore, whereas the demand is in range of Rs. 45,000 to Rs.50,000 crore. Efforts should be made towards meeting the capital requirements of micro-finance sector. This would facilitate the growth of the sector by increasing accessibility of funds.

Rural Infrastructure Development Fund was established in 1995 for giving loan to state government and state owned corporations for quick completion of projects relating to medium and minor irrigation, soil conservation, watershed management and other forms of rural infrastructure. This fund has been established out of contributions from scheduled commercial banks, which have not met agricultural lending sub-target of 18 per cent of Net Bank Credit. Since the inception the fund has mobilized several thousand crores of rupees and invested the amount for the development of rural infrastructure.

On the similar lines Micro Finance Development Fund may be planned and put at the disposal of the micro finance subsidiary of the commercial banks. The shortfall in lending to the weaker section by the commercial banks may be the best source to supplement the capital of this fund.

Advances to Weaker Section as on March 2006

(Rs. In crore)

Banks	*Weaker section advances*	*% of Net Bank Credit*	*Shortfall of weaker section target*
Public Sector Banks	78373.90	7.7	23410.39
Pvt. Sector Banks	3909.26	1.6	20523.62
Total			43934.01

Report on Trend and Progress in India 2005-06, RBI.

Banks are expected to lend at least 10% of their net bank credit to weaker section. The list of the beneficiaries under this group largely refers to the poor and excluded section. Hence, the shortfall in lending to this group by the commercial banks may be used to augment the capital base of the micro finance subsidiary. It can be seen that about Rs. 44,000 crore may be mobilized in this manner and made available for the micro finance subsidiary for its immediate use to penetrate faster in all geographical areas of the country.

As a sequel to continuous reforms, Indian Banking Sector has been gearing itself to match the international benchmarks of Profitability and Operational efficiency. Greater use of multiple service outlets like ATMs, Internet and Mobile Banking, Sharing of delivery channels, swapping of branches, introducing co branded products, tie-ups, strategic partnerships; MOUs with other market players have become the order of the day. With 'profit' as the main motto, the present fulcrum of banking business is a profitable customer since profit is directly proportional to the number of profitable customers. As such, there is an inherent feeling among banks that Financial Inclusion and Profitability are mutually exclusive. It is quite natural to hold on to an initial impression that Financial Inclusion is servicing the Bottom of the Pyramid. However, it is to be realised that it is no longer mere extension of services; it is the value creation activity. The focus on Financial Inclusion comes from the recognition that this can serve the interest of both society and the banking system.

Our previous experience also shows that the lending methodologies specializing in micro finance reduced the risk, growing volumes of finance for consumption is generally targeted low-income groups and few recipients open or maintain a bank account through which those resources could be put to productive use,. Thus there are major opportunities for offering both deposits and loan products to this vast low-income population group provided the banking services are made affordable. Further, in the context of India becoming one of the largest micro finance markets in the world, especially in the growth of SHGs and the sustaining success of such institutions which has been demonstrated by the success of SEWA bank in Gujarat, inclusive banking is not necessarily an unviable proposition. It can be relooked as a new business opportunity that is capable of creating value across Indian social spectrum. There is very possibility that the relatively low margins on high volumes can make a good profitable proposition. The sophistication, convenience, speed and technology achieved in the banking business through reforms are to be utilized fully to make Financial Inclusion as potential business opportunity failing which the dire consequences of exclusion shall have to be encountered.

In coming days, with the implementation of Basel II focus will be more on capital planning. There is looming danger of further ignoring marginalized sections, as there will be more stress on secured assets for providing credit. Financial Sector has to take concrete steps. There is a need to understand clearly that it is not just un-availability of financial products, but inhibition, lack of confidence in system–at times fear and illiteracy that stop people from availing banking services. To overcome this block, Financial Institutions, Self Help Groups and Government at different levels have to work in coordination. Partnership between banks, post offices, NGOs offer great opportunities. Proper planning and adequate monitoring will help to overcome risk factors.

Banks can overcome the barriers of demand side and supply side of financial inclusion by making people aware of advantages they will have by having bank accounts, helping them out in opening accounts and ensuring the services/ banking products offered by them meet their requirements, besides giving them timely feedback to recover loan.

The benefits of having bank account should be advertised in local dialect, bank staff should have patience to understand the needs of customers. There is also urgent need of providing financial skills training to the deprived sections. Gram Panchayats, Nukkad Nataks, village fairs, local schools etc. could become forums for training. In such training more and more diagrams and pictures modules should be used to make it attractive and easy to understand.

One of the problems has been treating rural and urban branches on par. Instead, the segregation of urban and rural banking is urgently needed to cater different needs of the two segments. Bankers have to think of alternate banking structure to include sensibilities and necessities of rural populance with different financial needs and accordingly, concentrate on the marketing of suitable products. While planning products, we have to consider the income level of different segments of the population as well. It can be started by assessing the needs and behavior pattern of marginalized section, get their feedback by listening patiently that about their needs, their expectations. Afterwards banks should concentrate on developing appropriate products, which can fulfill their needs, and aspirations including providing similar comfort and control as offered by cash transactions.

Certain technical aspects also need relook, like developing a more users' friendly loan application form so that such sections do not feel intimidated and feel that their savings will be secured.

We can also think of something on lines of "Payroll Cards"– pre-paid debit card, for daily/marginal labourers to bring them into electronic payment system.

In fact we can use huge talent of IT simultaneously with the use of Self Help Groups very effectively to bulldoze all the hurdles. Some of the basic issues which kept away banks from providing access to banking services to marginalized sections like high cost of transactions, inadequate infrastructure in rural areas, lack of awareness etc, can be easily overcome by making use of technology. Centralised processing, telecommunication development, computer terminals, simputers, Biometric ATM/ Debit Cards etc. offer tools to convert lost opportunities to profitable ventures.

SECTION–VI

As stated by C.K. Prahlad, the future lies with those companies who see the poor as their customers. It is becoming increasingly apparent that addressing financial exclusion will require holistic approach on the part of the banks in creating awareness about financial products, education, and advice on money management, debt counseling, savings and affordable credit. The banks would have to evolve specific strategies to expand the outreach of their services in order to promote financial inclusion. Technology can be very valuable tool to promote financial inclusion. Technology can be very valuable tool in providing access to banking products in remote areas. ATMs cash dispensing machines can be modified suitably to make them user friendly for people who are illiterate, less educated or do not know English.

The formal financial system has to recognise the huge business potential coming from the unmet demand for financial services from those who normally tend to be excluded. The focus on financial inclusion comes from the recognition that financial inclusion has several externalities, which can be exploited to the mutual advantage of those excluded, the banking system and society at large. Banks need to understand the market and develop products suited to the clients. They need to develop data sets to evolve risk assessment models for proper rating and pricing. Financial inclusion has to be viewed as a business strategy for growth and banks need to position themselves accordingly. Further, improvements in rural connectivity, through roads, power, and telecom, can ensure greater penetration by the financial system into remote areas and provide safe and efficient financial services to large segments of the financially excluded. Use of IT, apart from speeding up transaction time and reducing cost, facilities building automatic safeguards by ensuring on-line identification, authorization, monitoring, transparency and accountability and in turn enables banks to deal with much larger numbers with minimum risks. The state governments will need to ensure such rural connectivity and also facilitate capacity building to use IT in a big way.

To sum up, banks need to redesign their business strategies to incorporate specific plans to promote financial inclusion of low-income group treating it both a business opportunity as well as corporate social responsibility. They have to make use of all available resources including technology and expertise available with them as well as the MFIs and NGOs. It may appear in the first instance that taking banking to the sections constituting " the bottom of the pyramid", may not be profitable but it should always be remembered that even the relatively low margins on high volumes can be very profitable proposition. Financial Inclusion can emerge, as commercial profitable business only banks should be prepared to think outside the box!

Refrences

All India Debt and Investment Survey, 2002, NSSO (2005).

Building Inclusive Financial Sectors for Development (June 2006), Department of Economic and Social Affairs, U.N.

Census of India, 2001

Financial Inclusion Taskforce, Financial Inclusion Deliberative Workshops, Prepared for HM Treasury/ Financial Inclusion taskforce by Opinion Leader Research, May 2006.

'Financial Inclusion and Millennium Development Goals'- Speech by Smt. Usha Thorat, Dy. Governor of RBI at the IV Progrmme on Human Development and State Finances at CAB, Pune on January 16, 2006.

Financial Inclusion Taskforce: Report on 'Progress towards the shared goal', U.K. HM Treasury, March 2006.

Financial Inclusion: the way forward', U.K., HM Treasury, March 2007.

Hogarth, J. M., and O'Donnell, K. H. (1997). Being Accountable: A Descriptive Study of Unbanked Households in the U.S. Proceedings of the Association for Financial Counseling and Planning Education, Phoenix, Arizona.

Leeladhar V. (2005), Dy. Governor, RBI 'Taking Banking to the common Man Financial Inclusion', Fedbank Hormis Foundation at Ernakulam on December 2.

Mohan Rakesh, Address at the Annual Bankers' Conference 2006, at Hyderabad on Nov. 3, 2006.

Punnathara, C.J. (July 31, 2006), No-frills Banks Accounts: Financial Inclusion in Good Economies, *Business Line.*

Report of the Internal Group on Rural Credit and Micro-finance (Chairman: H.R.Khan, CGM and Principal, CAB, RBI), *www.rbi.org.in.*

Report on Trend and Progress of Banking in India, 2004-05, 2005-06, RBI.

Situation Assessment Survey of Farmers Indebtedness of Farmers Households-NSS, 59th Round, NSSO, New Delhi.

Thorat, Y.S.P. (July 31, 2006), Speech by Chairman, NABARD at the Banking Conclave on 'Indian Banking: Shaping an Economic Powerhouse', organized by FICCI.

11

IMPACT OF INFORMATION AND COMMUNICATION TECHNOLOGY (ICT) ON E-GOVERNANCE

M. Chakraborty

Introduction

Over the last two millennia of human history, the society has evolved continuously from its pre-industrial to industrial and finally to post-industrial manifestation. Another way of looking at the evolving society is to divide it among the following sectors:

1. Primary Sector - with a focus on nature
2. Secondary Sector - with a focus on material
3. Service Sector - with a focus on community
4. Leisure Sector - with a focus on individual

While different section of human society have lived overlapping through the various sectors, there has been a perceptible shift of labour as well as capital from the primary society to the service society, and now to leisure society. This trend has been as much evident in the developed world as in the newly industrializing world of India.

It is interesting to note that technology has provided continually the underpinning in this social revolution. Alongside the technology, the role of information has been an increasingly predominant one from the primary society to the leisure society, so much so that many call it a gradual evolution towards information society. Computers have also been increasingly involved in this evolutionary process, thus almost metamorphosing even the primary, secondary, service and leisure.

In the backdrop of this change to the leisure society, the society has begun to realize the importance of information availability and have begun to explore the ways and means of maximizing their capabilities and potential through effective decision making by utilizing the information. The people have begun to expect more from the government and have come to view it rightly as a means whose very existence is justified as an instrument to further the end of improving their lives. They are now able to see it, to a large extent, as a means and not an end in itself, a means by which their collective and individual aspirations are to be given a concrete shape.

In the ensuing change, the government has also come a long way to view its responsibilities as a provider of service to the society and the right of the people to demand the services which are necessary to develop a context in which people can utilize their will and capabilities to the maximum. There is still a long way to go before the government is able to shed its self-proclaimed responsibilities of a provider of material to the society and the limited right of the people to know about it and its ways. But an evolution towards that realization is still on and if anything, it has gained momentum in the recent years.

It is no mere coincidence that in this process of the redefining the role of government by itself and the society and the gradually shifting equilibrium towards the latter, the thing that has acquired maximum visibility in terms of the demand of the society and also in terms of the resistance meted out by the government is the availability of information.

That "information is power" is not just a cliché but something the materialization of which is an important pre-requisite for a stage when people are going to be able to take informed and effective decisions about their life and how they choose to lead it has gradually started to cement its place in their sensibilities. And that is the reason the information has come to acquire an altogether new meaning in the modern times.

First, one can describe information and then technology related to information. To describe information, one starts with the low-level data linking with the environment, the circumstance etc.–events, occurrences etc which by themselves carry no meaning. At this point, all we have is essentially just data the analysis of which leads to information on which we can act; then esoterically, one talks about all that linkage from information to knowledge and then on to wisdom. Information has now a "place in the sun"; the new paradigm of management puts it as the prime resource (displacing cash) from which one can derive every other necessity.

The next logical question that arises is how do we juggle with information and to the rescue came technology of two Cs–Computers and Communication. These two Cs from two distinct streams have become highly interdependent, so that progress on either is mutually beneficial. A merger of the two is a happy marriage leading to ICT. The pace of progress in this area is so fast that what was achievable in the pre-chip era in a matter of years is now possible to accomplish in a matter of days or hours.

With a paradigm shift in the prevailing thinking and the availability of technology as a means to effect that shift, we are in the midst of two major changes:

- The transformation of the business of government–improving service to citizens as customers of government. The goal is to reach beyond current efforts to "reinvent government" by identifying breakthrough strategies that rethink the core value of key government services, dramatically improve service delivery, reduce costs and renew administrative processes.
- The transformation of governance itself–changing the role of the citizen as a shareholder in government. The goal is to reexamine the nature of democratic institutions, the role of the private sector, the relationship between the citizen and the state, the

future of the nation-state, and new requirements for governance in a global, networked economy.

We believe that technology will have a major role to play for the government to cope up with the pressure of bringing about these transformations.

Why ICT in Government

Government in the ultimate analysis is an information processing organization. All Government workers are knowledge workers. Whatever the area of activity, on one hand, every Government organization is concerned with collecting information or using information to administer the laws, rules and procedures so that the objective of the organization is achieved while on the other hand, it is concerned with supplying the relevant information to the citizens with a view to empowering them to take informed decisions and make informed choices. Introduction of electronic governance is the only way to make Information and Communication Technology (ICT) relevant to ordinary citizens in a country like India where at least 30 per cent of the population lives below the poverty line and nearly 50 per cent is illiterate. Electronic governance would help make life easier for people who have to constantly interface with the government on most matters, thanks to the largely socialist system that was adopted after independence.

In Government systems, the processing of information decides the culture of the organization. If we go to find the root cause of delay in administration, we will find that it is because of the delay in either collecting or collating or accessing information. The greater the speed with which information call be collected, collated and accessed, the less will be the time taken. The delay in turn leads to corruption. Speed money is a very common source of corruption. If we are able to eliminate delays, logically, to some extent, the speed money corruption can also be checked.

Another source of corruption is the limited access to information. These days, there is a lot of discussion going on about the Freedom of Information act. We have seen for example, in Rajasthan, that the NGOs were able to point out how funds are misused in IRDP and other poverty alleviation programmes by informing the beneficiaries about the funds allotted to their village. Providing information became a route for increasing awareness of the people and raising their conscientiousness.

Traditionally, Governments' have guarded the information access rigidity because there is another aspect to information across namely, security. The Official Secrets Act highlights the need for protecting the society and not compromising on the security issue. But this is a gray area where under the guise of security and national interests, a lot of information can and has been classified as secret.

Added to this is the power dynamics in the Government administration. Access to information, capacity for recalling the relevant information or controlling information in which a citizen may be interested are factors which give power to a bureaucrat. The bureaucrat who is either drunk on power or is after corruption can use this aspect of information dynamics in Government to line his own pocket.

Information and Communication Technology is going to be the decisive technology in the years to come. Its characteristics are such that if it is intelligently and imaginatively used, many of the negative aspects of the dynamics of information processing and information handling in Government can be overcome. It has features that appear as if they have been designed for handling a system like Government.

- ICT brings enormous speed in processing of information.
- Random access memory is characteristic of Information and Communication Technology and this is another important aspect of Government administration.
- Diffusion of information can be done on a much wider basis and much more effectively that what has been possible in the past. Everyone today is talking about the internet. After all, with 100 million people accessing a whole lot of databases, it is a classic example of the enormous diffusion power of ICT.

- The ICT can eliminate many middle level posts in management. The hierarchy is one of the factors that cause delay in the movement of papers and the processing. Information in Government and Information and Communication Technology can eliminate the element of delay caused by hierarchy. It can empower people because access to information can become easier.

Functions of ICT in Government

The managerial environment shaped by Information and Communication Technology is ambiguous and complex since Information and Communication Technology can support distinct function in government. Yet that environment should be jacketed in a clear objective–that public managers and administrators must learn to harness technologies as they emerge and as the expectations of public service change. The functions of ICT in government can be summarized as–(1) access engineering, (2) substantive policy, (3) public record retention and retrieval, and (4) administrative decision making.

Access Engineering–In an article on trends in Information and Communication Technology, some information industry leaders were asked, "What is the single greatest benefit governments can obtain from technology?" Beyond the familiar generalization about "increased productivity", the majority spoke about the opportunity to extend access networks between government and citizenry. The technology can provide a seamless transfer of both knowledge and information between government and citizens. It means a significantly improved access to information and ideas that will improve people's quality of lives. Such a technological function–sometimes associated with "electronic" or "kiosk" government–serves as a fundamental means for strengthening the consumer orientation in the movement to reengineer or reinvent government.

Substantive Policy Communication–Traditionally, file drawers in government departments contain correspondence and memos that support decisions or justify actions taken.

Whether those files contain relevant supplemental information (such as notes and summaries) is typically a matter of discretion. Such artifacts can now be made available to the public by effective use of ICT.

Record keeping–The electronic storage of data is basic to the success of ICT in any organization. With regard to record keeping as a technological function, fundamental questions focus on determining what constitutes a public record, and how that information is disseminated upon request.

Decision making support–Electronic information tools have a subtle but decided influence on the balance of political and administrative rationality in the management of public affairs. On the one hand, large scale information systems that guide and control government programs place more responsibility in the hands of technical experts. On the other hand, the ability to integrate information from a variety of sources can often lead to better informed decision making by elected policy makers themselves. That is, the power of large-scale integrated data systems can give both legislative and executive leaders access to much information concerning the detailed operations of government itself. In principle, it is possible for legislators to move beyond their traditional oversight and policy-setting roles to become involved with the "micro management" of program operations.

Government Information Management

The relationship between Information and Communication Technology and the management of public information can be characterized as an extension of the traditional view within public administration theory, with efficiency and performance as the benchmarks for success. Though there are radical possibilities for change that can be credited to the internet-based communication strategies, the public management systems in India should focus on two narrowly defined goals: (1) centralization of public data and (2) electronically based internal communication systems. The achievements of these goals can be followed by transforming public departments into externally oriented organizations which actively engage citizens in policy formulation and implementation. But first things first. The need of the hour in India is to get the government and its departments focus towards attaining increased productivity and a citizen friendly interface through the medium of ICT and this is precisely what we will try to focus in this section. The short-term goals we described above should be targeted by means of three strategies: (a) Data Warehousing, (b) World Wide Web, and (c) Intranets.

Data Warehousing

Data has to be collected and presented in a readable form before the question of managing it comes. Data warehousing represents a recent innovation in both corporate and public sector information management. A data warehouse is a centralized database of information accessible to a large number of organizations or a group of departments within a single organization that previously maintained separate data sources. In this context, there is a great need for the existence of a unified database on citizens. It might seem highly futuristic to expect the information about all the citizens contained in a centralized database but it is something we believe will happen and it is just a matter of time before the different departments are able to derive their own data requirements from such a database thereby reducing the problem of need for collecting same data multiple times by different departments and of consistency of data across different departments redundant. A data warehouse encompasses more than simply the store of electronic data itself. Instead, data warehousing for the management of public information includes five components: (1) the acquisition of pre-existing operational data stores; (2) procedures for converting these data sources into a standardized format for inclusion in the data warehouse; (3) creation of data warehouse; (4) the design of electronic tools which provide the user interface for data query and information retrieval; and (5) administrative tools and procedures for maintenance and system optimization. Data warehousing allows for increased efficiency and performance by reducing the costs of data collection and storage and by facilitating employee access to information. Such unified database is also desirable because of many other reasons. The population of this country is exploding in spite of sincere efforts by Governments all over the country. This increase in population makes the old manual system of databases of our citizen more and more unwieldy. The Government of Karnataka pays old age pension to about 4.5 lakhs citizens but Deputy Commissioner does not have a database of the beneficiaries. The state Government does not have any information on the nature of beneficiaries. How many are women, how many are between 65-67, how many have relatives but who don't support them, where do these relatives live and so on. Even if some information, which is available with department of treasury is picked up, it may not be of nay use except for getting the expenditure figures. The absence of a properly designed computerized database hampers any meaningful efforts to weed out ineligible or bogus beneficiaries or to remove dead people from the list.

These databases are, in most of the cases, manual and maintained on typical Government registers and ledgers. Extracting any information from these databases is not only difficult and time consuming but in many cases lead to wrong results. Even in cases where some of the enthusiastic officers have tried to create such databases, data does not match with corresponding databases of other departments either because of formats being different or the values of data for same item differing from one department to another department.

Some examples of databases maintained by different departments will be in order:

- The revenue department is the custodian of land records databases. These databases are manually maintained and have not undergone any major change since the time of British rule. The databases are village-wise and survey number centric(and not farmer centric). The structure of these databases was probably designed keeping in mind the Land Revenue which used to be the major source of income for the British Government. Even these manually maintained databases are village-wise databases again for the reason that land revenue used to be collected village-wise. Under the Centrally sponsored scheme of *Computerization of Land Records (CLR)*, all the state Governments is computerizing the land records. Unfortunately, these databases will also suffer from the above infirmity of being survey number and village centric. One of the problems, for example, of this database in its present form is as follows–under the Karnataka Land Reforms Act, a person cannot hold more than 54 acres of land, more commonly known as ceiling limit. Now as the ceiling has to be calculated with respect to the total holding of a person, which may be spread over whole state, there should be some mechanism to link RTC to the person. No such provision exists in this database. This means that in most of the cases, unless a person foolishly discloses his total holdings, it is just not possible to find out the total holding of a person.

- The Rural Development and *Panchayat Raj* Deptt. (RDPR) of Karnataka Government carries out periodic survey of people below poverty line for the purpose of eligibility under various schemes of the Department. Last such survey was carried out in 1998. As per the survey, there are 22 lakh families below poverty line. Extensive information about the details of such families like name of the head of the family, number of members, educational background, caste, religion, training undergone under rural development schemes, type of house owned, animals, expenditure etc. is all available. However, this information is only available at *taluka* level in traditional manual registers.

  The Food Department distributes ration at subsidized rates to the families below the poverty line who are supplied with green cards. Ideally speaking, the department should identify the eligibility for green card based on the BPL survey of RDPR department. As noted above, the BPL families are about 22 lakhs whereas 64.67 lakhs families hold green cards. As this database, again maintained manually, does not interact with BPL database of RDPR, the Government effectively have two sets of figures. It is roughly estimated that about Rs. 500 crores are overspent by food department and that many of the beneficiaries, as detailed above, are ineligible to receive ration at subsidized rates. It is therefore required that not only the two databases computerized but also that these databases "talk" to each other. Once this is done, the system can generate reports of beneficiaries above poverty line who are not eligible to receive subsidized food but have been included in green card list, helping the Government to save precious funds.

- The transport department data is centered around the details of the vehicles owned by people. The database is not only maintained manually but also does not allow search on a query like how many vehicles a citizen is having. The database here is again department oriented and not citizen oriented. This database, for example, should have helped the Government in filtering ineligible beneficiaries for the BPL survey of RDPR department as BPL conditions exclude such families for the inclusion in the BPL list who own a vehicle.

All these examples point to three fundamental flaws in the present system of collection and maintenance of information:

1. Databases are maintained manually.
2. Databases are department centric and not citizen centric.
3. The databases have the citizen name in the text form.

As we have already discussed, the solution of the first two problems lies in maintaining the information in a digital database which facilitate easy retrieval of information. Secondly, the information should be citizen centric.

An equally important problem is the non-standardization of a citizen's identity. The use of names of people presents obvious problems. There has to be a system in which every citizen has an identification code, called citizen ID. This ID should obviously not be same for two citizens and should never be changed even if a person moves to a new location. This ID, once there in a database, immediately makes it citizen centric. It is then possible to find out the total land holding of a person in while of the state using the ID of the person. The ID helps to find out if he is there in BPL list and also owns a vehicle and therefore ineligible for being included in the BPL list. Again, the names of such person can be removed from the green card eligibility list if he is not in BPL list. Citizen ID field allows all this automatically and naturally.

This ID would help in searching across the databases as one would never have to worry about how a person's name is pronounced. Citizen ID value of the person will be enough for any query on the database. This ID would help in knowing all about the citizens like Passport number, PAN no. of Income Tax department, electricity bills, water bills, telephone details, property tax, details of property held by him etc.

This experiment of assigning a citizen ID has been carried out in Andhra Pradesh in their survey known as multi purpose household survey(MPHS). MPHS is slowly being extended to all the *Mandals* there. This survey is a step in right direction and worth emulating by other states. Giving citizen and ID helps in delivering citizens the required services in a more friendly way. The Andhra MPHS will help the Government to immediately process the request for caste certificate, income certificate without any harassment and without being bounced from one department to another department.

One should go a step further and design a unified database for use of all the departments. Needless to say, the whole database should be citizen centric by way of primary key being the citizen ID. There is also a concept of "data mart" which can be used along with data warehouse to automate data archiving within individual agencies by state and local government agencies. Data marts deal with departmental data which is well understood, familiar to those who deal with it everyday, and much more limited in scope. Both data warehouses and data marts may contribute to efficient management of public information.

Every department would write to their portion of the database, say for example, the Food Department would write about the information about the ration card held by the citizen and his family. Many updations can even take automatically in this database. For example, as soon as a person turns 18, his name as voter gets checked. A person name is marked for deletion as a voter, as soon as birth and death registration authority updates the fact that a particular person is dead. The technologies allow site-wise storage of copy of portion of such databases and of replication with main database when the network traffic is slow.

Such databases would also avoid repetitive work and repetitive field survey by different departments. Once the basic survey is carried out by a department responsible for carrying out the survey to collect figures for an item in the database for which that department is authorized, no other department would carry out survey for collecting figures for those items as it is not authorized to update the value of that item. Hence there would be no contradictory figures for same items as all other departments would use the figures in "read only mode" in the unified database collected by the department who has been authorized for updating that item avoiding unnecessary embarrassment to the government.

Therefore, it can be seen that although difficult to plan in the beginning, such unified database or "data warehouse" would go a long way in providing citizen centric and effective service.

World Wide Web

Many of the government departments today have started to have an online presence on the world wide web. Some of them have useful content and others go to the extent of providing certain services to the people. An example of the latter is the railway reservation site which provides for services like train inquiries, ticket status, reservation rules etc. While this is a positive development, it requires the citizen to know the department and its web site address to obtain that service. This can be termed as a typical first generation government internet presence characterized by a proliferation of individual departmental Web sites each with a separate URL, offering its own department information and online services. There are some governments which had the foresight to create one Central Web site, from where a citizen could then link to any department. Unfortunately, bottom line, either approach has the same effect. It forces the citizen to have to know what department to go to for what service.

A competitive e-government has to move beyond providing one or two transaction services to a situation where hundreds and thousands of services are provided online and has to start thinking their web strategies from their citizens' perspectives. Instead of launching online services on a department-by-department basis, they are aggregating services across departments, accessible through a common portal.

A portal is a window to an array of Web based content. Portals are typically multifunctional which offer a variety of capabilities aggregated at one place. In other words, if you did not have the portal, you would have to go to a lot of different places on or off the web. In government, the portal will be the main web site. On this government portal, people are given a variety of choices. For example, when citizens reach the portal and see a category, "Online Citizen Services", they click once to access an alphabetized list of all available online transaction services, regardless of department. So whether one needs to see the status of his railway ticket, or to calculate his income tax, he simply clicks the desired transaction from the list. A form comes up which the citizen completes and gets confirmation right then and there. They don't need to know, nor do they care, what department actually processes the transaction. And, they do not have to surf down through multiple departments to find the service. The transaction is processed in the background using web-enabled tools which access, update and transfer data to and from disparate legacy systems and databases of the responsible department(s).

The first step in building a portal approach is to inventory services across the departments. Then apply a comprehensive set of selection criteria to filter out online candidates. Criteria should address questions such as: What is the annual volume of transactions associated with that service? Is the service routine in nature? Does the service require positive identification? Does delivery of service create staff or seasonal bottlenecks? Has this service process recently been reengineered? Are there any public policy issues which must be addressed? Is the service already online on a departmental web site? What is the current cost of providing the service? Using weights for these measurements, one can prioritize or rank the services and make their online presence available.

Intranet

Not all government operations consist of one simple form and one transaction. Many government services require nonlinear, complex collaboration among employees among departments. Those operations affect overall process, service quality and delivery time to citizens and businesses. Permitting and reasoning are examples which include multiple players–citizens, businesses, utilities, multiple government departments, and many times, boards and authorities up through the executive office or legislative body and frequently involve intergovernmental levels. What if all those players had common and high bandwidth access to each other, seamless processes, electronic work flow and data exchange?

The same technology infrastructure built for citizen services can host employees through an intranet. An intranet is just like the internet–same protocols and accessible through the web–except that it is not open to the public. Intranets typically require Ids, passwords and are completely separate and secure through firewalls. Through intranet technologies, employees as well as external authorized members can share information and collaborate across the boundaries of their work communities.

To achieve e-government, the quest is not so much for the "killer application" as it is for a set of "killer capabilities" and integrating strategies to leverage the power of the internet. Intranets definitely speak to the goals of efficiency and performance in public administration.

Steps in Managing Government Information

In this section, we discuss the various steps an organization needs to take to manage the information effectively.

Planning Agency Information Needs

Now when most of the required information is available within an organization's reach, the next and the most important question comes: How to manage that information? Information systems are large, complex and expensive, involving significant investments in human and physical capital over extended periods of time. Careful advance planning helps ensure an optimal return on these investments. This section reviews some of the many issues associated with planning for an organization's information needs.

As a matter of theory, good information planning involves forecasting the present and future information needs of an organization and designing information systems whose characteristics meet those needs. Very often, the information planning reduces to deciding about buying hardware boxes and seeing over time what they can do. This gap between ar d theory and practice of planning is not without explanation. It is hard to forecast information needs in a rapidly changing technical environment. It is often easier to see what use an existing system can be put to rather than establishing an abstract statement of needs. The most complex information systems have actually developed incrementally over time and put to use in ways that was not envisioned during the planning phase. But experience also tells us the strategic pitfalls of patchwork system solutions. Despite this, some amount of planning definitely helps and it would help to distinguish the overall planning of an organization's information system between strategic planning and operational planning.

Strategic Planning

Strategic information systems planning differs from operational or tactical planning in that it involves rethinking of an organization's basic goals or mission in light of new or changing demands, revised mandates, or the emergence of new services or programs to be provided. Strategic planning can and often does take place without an explicit information management component. But modern information technologies and their associated management potentials are increasingly seen as important instruments for helping agency managers respond to shifts in the environment, seize new opportunities for service, and meet their strategic program goals.

For example, the collector of a district or the SDM of a sub-division may be concerned about providing better services to the citizens in the area for birth/death registry, effective implementation of rural development schemes, health services for the poor, education for the poor, voters' list during the elections, payment of water and electricity bills, better access of the citizens to the grievances redressal systems and a prompt service of complaints, quick and hassle-free availability of land records etc. The collector's strategic mission is to enhance and integrate what he sees as a fractured service system. Each service organization in the district touches upon these areas, but none of them comprehends their interdependence. That is, service being provided by the birth/health registrar, DRDAs, electricity board, etc. must be integrated at a point where they are able to take the maximum advantage of their interdependence and to provide a more efficient and effective service to the people. The information management component of this strategic mission is to integrate the services provided by various departments in the district and to build a database that is accurate and up-to-date and provides data to different departments.

Figure 1 provides a framework for thinking about strategic information management in the public sector. Its is adopted from a similar one developed by Porter in 1980 where he defined the key components of strategic planning for private sector firms to be the interaction of buyer, sellers, new firms entering a market, and the possibility of substitute products and services within a market. All of these external forces combine to produce the key concept of rivalry or competition among firms struggling for market share or customer attention.

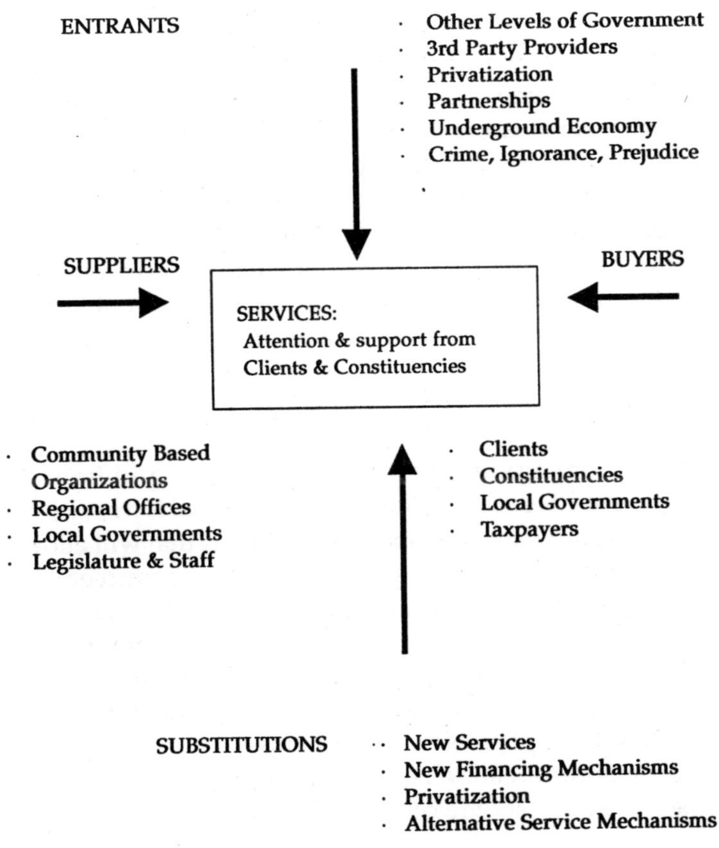

Figure 1 : **Public Sector Strategic Analysis**

However, as shown in Figure 1, the key focus of attention in public sector strategy is not competition or rivalry among similar units. Rather, the key strategic focus of the public sector is on providing services to clients and on receiving attention and support from the organization's various clients. In the public sector, the analog of Porter's customers or buyers consists of our clients, those members of the public that our organizations are designed to serve. Rather than having sellers or suppliers, public sector strategy analysts think in terms of providers–the community based organizations, other levels of government, or regional and local offices that are the means whereby we create and deliver services.

Whereas in the private sector, new entrants commonly refer to competing firms, the public sector strategic analysis of new entrants is broad enough to include notions of other levels of government, third party providers, or other units that may enter to assist with the delivery of much needed services. Again, in a market framework, substitutions refer to new products or services that might be developed or introduced by a competing firm. In the realm of public sector strategy, substitutions refer to new financing mechanisms, modes of service delivery such as privatization, or even new services that might be developed or nurtured by public organizations.

When engaging in strategic planning, public sector managers need to scan the full array of external forces sketched in figure 1 and search for policy innovations that will allow an organization to capture new energy or resources in its environment, to reach out towards new goals or missions, or find new ways of relating to clients and customers. Often information management techniques can become key instruments in assisting an organization to realign its strategic posture vis-à-vis its external environment.

An example can serve to highlight how information management can serve a central role in helping an organization redefine its operations and goals and reach for new levels of service. In responding to the call for new level of effective and efficient service delivery, many individual departments maintain their own databases, very often in manual registers, about different kinds of data pertaining to the individuals. By hammering out a single record definition and by sharing information, the birth/death registrar, revenue department, state election commission, transport department etc. can create and can better maintain more accurate records on all citizens in a centralized database from where individual departments derive their needs. Such information systems help to create a systemwide perspective on an integrated approach to the service delivery in a district.

Using information systems as a tool for achieving strategic goals will become more and more popular as a principle for good management in public sector. Good strategic information planning coupled with thoughtful and forward thinking operational planning is evidence of good management at all levels of government.

Operational Planning

The next step after strategic planning is what we are referring to as operational planning and it is closely related to such concepts as the systems development cycle, tactical information planning or an information planning cycle. As shown in the Figure 2, operational planning can be roughly divided into four phases–Design, Specification, Acquisition and Installation, and Operation and Maintenance. Each of these four phases involves a linked set of issues that build upon each other through the four phases. For example, in the design phase, questions of what decisions are to be made by whom leads in the specification stage to the definition of a data dictionary, which in turn becomes incorporated into a Request for Proposal (REP) in the acquisition and installation phase. Finally, during the operations and maintenance phase, changed circumstances predictably lead to new definitions of information needs, data dictionaries and so on.

In addition, a number of policy concerns, all of which are more fully discussed elsewhere in this volume, run through all stages of the operational planning cycle. Security, documentation, standards, privacy, access, information sharing and eventual record disposition must be planned for in the earliest phases and continue to be important considerations as the system moves through the acquisition, installation and operations.

Design. Good planning begins with a sound design phase. Often involving a user survey, the design phase asks the basic question, who are the clients for the system? What decisions must be made, by whom, based on what criteria to accomplish the program this system is to s support? What functions are to be performed by the information in the system? What is the useful lifespan of the information being collected and what is

Design/User Survey Phase
What is the client?
Who is the decision maker?
What functions are affected?
What is the useful life of the information to be produced?
What is the frequency of transactions?
What level of accuracy is needed?

Specification Phase
Develop data definitions
Develop data structure
How will information be collected?
What software functionality is required?
What hardware functionality is required?
What reports are needed?
How is staffing affected?
What training is needed?
How are physical space needs to be met?

Acquisition and Implementation Phase
Estimate life cycle costs
Decide whether to make or buy
Develop request(s) for proposal
Manage procurement process
Select hardware
Select software
Plan for conversion
Conduct training

Ongoing Operation Phase
Adjust to changes in operational demands
Respond to policy shifts
Stay abreast of hardware and software advances
Stay in step with changing agency mission and programs
Evaluate performance
Revise and retrain

Figure 2: **Typical Consideration in Operational Planning for Information System**

the necessary frequency and accuracy of that information? Planning should begin with an attempt to articulate the decision-making needs of the manager who will use the data. Questions of how to collect and structure data as well as what hardware, software, and staffing are required are necessarily and logically subsequent to the more important questions of who will be using the information for what purpose.

From the very beginning of the planning process, information system planners must remain aware of the policy issues sketched in Figure 2. For example, the proper time to think about designing procedures for ultimately disposing of outdated records and archiving those reoccurs with permanent value is before any records or documents are created. Too often, these questions of document life cycle are left as an afterthought, creating impossible-to-manage files of raw data many years into the future. The early design phases must also pay attention to issues such as ultimate public access to information, standards for managing the information system, and adequate documentation.

Specification: Only after the important prior questions of the audience and purposes of an information system have been clearly answered should the planning process move toward a more detailed specification of the information system itself. At this phase, the important questions are what data needs to be captured and how should the data be defined and structured? What type of reporting capacity will be needed? What type of hardware and software functionality will be needed (stopping short of trying at this phase to define what specific hardware boxes need to be purchased)? What will be the physical space and staffing and training requirements necessary to support the information system under design? In most government settings, this specification phase becomes rather formal, often culminating in a written plan for review at some control point within the government (a budget unit or information-planning unit). Usually these fully specified plans become the basis for requests for proposals subsequently drafted by the organization.

Of course, the policy concerns first surfaced in the design phase continue to be developed and elaborated during the specification phase. For example, questions of hardware, software, and standards become more fully fleshed out and issues of documentation standards must be completely specified.

Acquisition and Installation: During the acquisition and installation phases, other organizations usually become intimately involved in the planning process. Most governments maintain formal procurement and bidding procedures that must be observed in the acquisition of information systems. Open competition among various vendors is the commonly accepted basis for deciding what hardware and software will be selected to support the information system under design. Because of the relatively technical nature of purchasing and installing large-scale information system, most governments have special procurement standards and procedures. For example, in purchasing expanded memory for a server system, a low bid may be received by a vendor other than the one now supplying the agency's hardware. However, this bid may include only hardware costs and may ignore staff time necessary to modify numerous applications. To account for these non-hardware costs, organizations should be allowed to factor in conversion, training, and other non-equipment costs that they may incur in acquiring a piece of hardware.

The need for staff training and the dilemma of using external consultants versus in-house staff for installing major systems are two issues that all information plans must address during the acquisition and installation phase. Most implementation plans call for additional staff to be allocated to an operation during the installation phase and call for significant amounts of staff training. Often parallel systems are run side by side for some time when a new system is being installed to replace an older one. The details of all these installation issues must be clearly thought through in the operational plan.

Operation and Maintenance: A virtual rule of information system planning is that large-scale information system will be obsolete before they are fully installed. The pace of technological change is so rapid, policy environments change so quickly, and system development cycles are so long that something important must change between the first design phases and the final installation phases. Hence all operational plans should make some allowance for ongoing implementation or the continual revaluation of the implementation plan in the light of recent developments. The more we plan, the more we realize the difficulty of planning in the realm of information systems.

Finally, as systems mature and develop, new policy issues that may not have been anticipated in the design phase will inevitably surface. For example, another organization may learn that yours has created a valuable new data set and may wish to have access to it or to match its own records against it. Information managers must continually be alert to these emerging information policy issues.

Procurement

In an expanding economy like ours, the need for efficient and effective utilization of various resources like money, manpower and materials and implementation of projects in time can not be over emphasized. The Govt. of India has introduced various steps to promote the use of computers and evolved liberal policies for meeting the requirement. The result is that in addition to large number of imported systems which were available earlier, indigenous manufacturers have thrown into the market a variety of systems. Besides, the power of Personal Computers has been increasing to touch the boundaries of large system. Choosing the right type of computer system for the right application at the right time from the right vendor and at the right price/performance ration has become a very evolved process.

Planning for Computer System

Planning for new computer is complex and requires knowledge of a number of disciplines, besides the utmost understanding and support of the higher ups in the administration. The sequential process from concept to commissioning of a computer system constitutes a number of phases and decision-making based on several parameters. Broadly, the steps for planning can be identified as:

- Specification of requirement/Need analysis/identification, including feasibility study.
- Alternative selection-Purchase/Hire/Lease.
- System study and configuration.
- Invitation to tenders.

- Evaluating the tenders.
- Selection and ordering.
- Delivery and installation.
- Acceptance and takeover
- Post installation.

❖ **Need Identification**: The first step in the planning process is the feasibility study i.e., an analysis to determine that it is technically possible and economically useful to use a computer in an organization or to replace an existing computer. A properly conducted feasibility study provides the groundwork for the entire subsequent evaluation of actual performance. However, other objectives of the feasibility study should be:

- To access information requirements and determine whether data processing techniques can be applied to the process.
- To determine the economic consequences of the application of information processing techniques.
- To establish a complete plan of action for the implementation process after feasibility has been established: and
- To provide the management with requisite documentation for planning, control and ultimate implementation.

The feasibility study would be conducted by a multidisciplinary team with considerable experience in a number of skills. It is desirable that the team has experience in organizational planning. Operations research, economic analysis, statistics, and above all, a deep understanding of the organization, its management requirements, and its policies and long term objectives.

These days Computers are available in a wide range of cost, therefore, the management has to decide about a particular computer, keeping in view, besides other factors, the cost of hardware configuration as well as the cost element of other factors. Three major components of cost can be categorized as equipment cost, operating cost and development cost. The equipment cost includes the cost of the computer and peripheral equipment and may be considered amortisable over a three-year period. The operating cost includes the personnel cost, the people necessary to prepare input, handle peripheral functions and operate the computer itself besides cost of power, stationery etc.

The third major component of cost is the development cost or total planning cost required to install and to maintain the computer. This planning cost whose major components are system design and development may be considered amortisable over a five-year period. For the purpose of decision-making it is essential to analyze these costs under the assumption that a computer will survive for not less than five years from the date of its physical installation. This assumption is an important one; if the system does not last the five years period, the total annual cost of operation will be substantially higher. A longer life will simply provide the ability to reduce annual operating costs substantially and thereby increase the economic viability of the computer.

- **Alternative Selection:** The next step is to evaluate various alternatives available for using a computer system viz.-utilizing services of a software house, renting out computer time, getting a terminal from a an already installed computer systems or have an in-house computer center. The consideration involved are the total machine time requirements, infrastructure to coordinate with the software house, reliability of such agencies, criticality of the applications, security demands etc. Also worth serious considerations are the factors of cost benefit analysis for each of the alternatives and the human angles with reference to organizational policies.

Essentially, there are three financing alternatives for computer systems: Purchase, rental or lease. Usually all of them are available from manufacturers or their representative and rental and lease arrangements can also be made through a third party.

(a) *Purchase:* The primary advantage of purchasing equipment is the potential cost saving if the equipment is kept for its useful life, usually three to six years. Although purchasing equipment generally results in lower overall costs, the buyer assumes the risk of obsolescence and does not have flexibility of canceling the arrangement. Additionally, purchasing requires capital that may be better utilized elsewhere. Another consideration when purchasing computer equipment is maintenance. If the equipment is rented, the manufacturer usually provides maintenance services.

(b) *Rental:* Under the rental option, the company rents the equipment on monthly basis directly from manufacturer or third party. Most agreements have a minimum rental period, such as ninety days. After minimum period, the user can cancel the agreement with short notice - one to two months. This flexibility is perhaps the major advantage of renting. However, the value of this flexibility is often overestimated since the use may have large investment in training, preparation and implementation. Renting is the most costly approach in terms of overall cash flow. However the user does not need the large capital outlay required in purchasing equipment. In addition, the risk of obsolescence and the responsibility for maintenance are borne by the manufacturer.

(c) *Leasing:* Leasing is a compromise between purchasing and renting. Typically leasing costs less than renting but more than purchasing. Most risks of obsolescence can be transferred to the lessor through an option to purchase the equipment at the end of the lease. Moreover, leasing is as flexible as renting because the lessee is locked in until the lease expires, typically after two to three years. However, sometimes the lease can be terminated early through the payment of termination charges. Leasing offers substantial cost savings over renting for the users who is willing to forego the additional flexibility the renting offers.

The ultimate choice of financing involves a trade off between risks of obsolescence, flexibility and costs. The flexibility variable has become less important because computer system themselves are now designed to be much more flexible. They can be upgraded through additional primary storage, secondary storage or attached CPUs.

- **System Study and Configuration:** 'What' to buy is immensely important in the process of selecting right computer. The Organisation structure, information/ data flow, geographical disbursement of offices/ divisions, various existing application areas and future growth plans require a careful study. The points that need to be considered while configuring a system are Word Length, Memory, Auxiliary storage, terminal, Graphics, Printers, Plotters, Communications etc.
- **Request for Quotation/tender:** The request for proposal or quotation (RFP) document puts the requirements for the equipment and software in forms the vendor of H/W and S/W can respond to. It serves as a communication tool between the potential buyer and vendor. It is sent to each vendor that is asked to propose H/W and S/W for the system. This is the document which enables the vendor to respond to the inquiry and its importance needs no emphasis as the various terms and conditions makes the basis for final contract for supply of the computer systems.
- **Evaluation:** The exercise of evaluation of response has become tedious, time consuming and involved particularly because of the large number of systems which are available in the market. In order to eliminate commercial bias, it is better to segregate the technical evaluation from commercial evaluation. Performance evaluation of computer H/W & S/W is a major tool used in the selection of new equipment. For each

proposal buyer would like to know the performance characteristics (job run time, through put idle time, response time etc) when executing current and planned applications obtaining such information is obviously impossible. Planned applications have not been developed and current applications may not execute on various equipment involved without program modifications. However, techniques are available to provide the buyer reliable and extensive measures of a system's performance, these are benchmark programs, workload models, simulation and monitors.

- **Hardware and software demonstration**: In the first phase of proposal evaluation, vendors demonstrate their proposed system. They generally present the major features of their proposal orally. The complete system may be demonstrated at buyers' location, if the system is easily portable. If not the buyer may visit the vendor's facility for demo. The vendor's presentation enables several of the buyer's employees to gain an understanding of the features of the proposals. However, buyers must use more substantial techniques to evaluate these proposals than merely listening to oral presentations, watching demonstrations and reading proposals.
- **Selection and ordering**: A widely used method for ranking competitive system is to assign points based on the degree to which each system meets important criteria, and then to total the points to obtain a ranking. Maximum points are assigned, based on the relative importance that the buyer feels each system characteristics should have. Usually a team of two to four people independently rank each system being considered. Of course, the difference among the vendors on one or two factors can override the total score based on the ranking. For example, vendor support could be so poor that it precludes the purchase of an otherwise outstanding system. Communicating

with the vendors about the point ranking system can be effective tool for helping them respond more effectively to the Request for Proposal (RFP).

❖ **Delivery and installation:** As the process of delivery takes 4 to 6 weeks, the phase regarding training and S/W development can be started shortly after the issue of purchase order. Linked with the delivery of the system is the preparation of the installation site providing for the environment and other conditions as laid down by the vendor. Normally the clearance for dispatch of the system should be given only after completion of site.

Table 1
Outline of Point Ranking System

System Characteristics	*Maximum Points*	*Points assigned system* A	B	C	D
Hardware					
Memory Size	20	10	15	20	10
Data Channels	20	10	8	5	10
Disk Capacity	20	20	20	15	10
Modularity	30	30	10	15	20
Compatibility	30	30	10	15	20
Warranty	20	15	15	20	10
Maintenance	20	15	20	15	10
Backups	20	15	10	10	10
Bench Mark Results	50	30	30	20	20
Software					
O.S.	30	20	15	25	30
Compilers	20	15	10	15	20
Application Programs	50	30	40	20	25
Compatibility	30	30	30	25	25
Vendor Support	40	20	30	35	40
Cost	50	30	40	40	50
Bench Mark Results	50	50	40	45	30
Total	500	370	343	340	340

❖ **Acceptance and taking over**: The acceptance of system is the phase which needs most attention. The rigorous checking and testing of various components of the system often reveals "bugs". The system should be taken over after it has undergone the specified performance parameters and all supplies envisaged have been completed.

- **Post-installation**: The warranty maintenance corrective preventive maintenance would have been defined in the purchase order. The manufacturer's commitment can be obtained in regard to the schedule to preventive maintenance and it needs to be ensured that the same is fulfilled.

Existing Vendor versus New Supplier

Most units of government procure equipment and services according to competitive bidding procedures that are well defined in both statute and regulation. Often bidding and contracting process is overseen by a specialised central control agency rather than by the operating agency that is requesting or making the purchase. Most government procurement regulations tend to be risk averse, seeking solid value for government investments. They rely principally on the criterion of minimum cost (the lowest bid) for evaluating proposals that meet the stated specifications for the product or service sought. Government procurement is often a relatively slow process, often tied to multiyear planning cycles with lengthy procedures for preparation of Request for Proposals(RFPs) and extensive publication and notice procedures to ensure maximum vendor awareness and opportunity to respond.

In this kind of process, a number of apparent contradictions can arise. For example, a unit of government may bid a standard contract to purchase a certain popular type of computer. By purchasing such a machine in large volume, the government may plan to achieve considerable cost savings. However, if it takes several months to bid the contract and if the contract lasts for up to one or two years, it is very likely that by the end of the contract period, a better technological option will have been introduced into the market and that the bid item will be selling on the open market for less than the contracted price competitively set by the government. The pace of technological change is so rapid that it simply confounds the normal contracting process.

System upgrades and conversions are often difficult to handle within existing procurement guidelines. In a normal process of computerization of operations, the hardware accounts for five percent, and "orgware" (costs for training people, changing processes and systems, redefining missions etc) eighty-five percent, it than becomes immediately apparent that actual procurement cost are merely tip of the total cost iceberg. However, the procurement procedures for major equipment purchases do not often factor in personnel costs associated with running or converting that equipment in future years. If full "life cycle" costs are factored in, then the current vendor has a decided competitive edge in bidding process. To replace or upgrade while maintaining the same vendor is usually much less costly because most vendors maintain compatibility within their own lines of equipment. Hence, an organization must decide early in the acquisition process about whether and how to deal with these considerable but usually hidden "orgware" costs. Ironically, this apparently technical decision often determines whether the existing vendor receives the ultimate contract. So what happened to a competitive bidding process as mandated by statute?

The technical issues involved in procurement can become quite complicated and can often have significant implications for the line operations within the organization. For example, a decision by the library to acquire an automated catalog or circulation system or a decision by a social service agency to automate client claims can considerably alter both the volume and the type of work being performed by most employees of the organization. Because of the special nature of information-intensive procurement decisions, government should create special organisations, often within central budget units, to help analyse technology-intensive procurement decisions.

Maintaining Data Quality

Since so many public records contain personal information or control financial transactions, the importance of maintaining quality control over databases should be apparent. Incorrect entries (whether due to error, sloppy procedure or fraud) could lead to incorrect payments to ineligible persons. They could prevent people from receiving other rights or benefits like driver's licenses, rural development benefits, BPL cards, pensions etc. Government information is a building block of the physical infrastructure. Roads, bridges, airports and nuclear power plants all depend in one way or another on government information. Public data is also used to support broad policy decisions and specific programmatic ones. Businesses use it to help plan new ventures. Consumers rely on it to make informed purchases and exercise their rights. All of these are reasons to actively pursue data quality and usability.

Procedural controls are important tools for maintaining data quality. Measures designed to endure physical and electronic security automatically help to ensure data quality. Control over data entry and inquiry (passwords and other restrictions on persons who input data, dual verification by two or more employees of important entries, and electronic security measures designed into data entry protocols) can all help to achieve data integrity. In addition, routine and random audits of computer operations and records are an additional check on data security, as well as a deterrent to those who might otherwise consider tampering with government data systems.

Networks present special problems of data integrity. Since many users in different locations share data, protocols that specify when and from where information will be updated, how conflicts will be resolved, and how local information needs will be meshed with central databases are another tool that restricts the ability of users to see and manipulate information in accordance with their level of expertise or specific job.

The ever-declining cost of data storage can be a problem as well as a blessing. Since comparing and evaluating old information against new is expensive, there is a tendency to simply keep it all. This can contribute to "information overload", the chronic problem of finding the right information in an ever growing storehouse of useless data.

Not all quality control measures relate to technology. Laws give individuals access to records kept about them and specify procedures whereby errors can be identified and corrected. These are another mechanisms for enduring accuracy although these protections are not always easy to understand or implement.

Finally, most government information still begins with a person filling out a form. Clear instruments, explicit definitions and a source of human assistance all contribute to getting accurate data in the first place.

Records Management, Archives and Preservation

The problem of archiving and preserving public information resources is in principle simple to state. Figure 3 illustrates the life cycle of a typical document and record. The management of active records is most often limited to the processes of information creation imaging (whether in paper or copy, electronic form or other media), and immediate and near term use. The hidden costs of data and file management are illustrated in Figure 3 to the right of the domain of active management. Here the information is first placed into an active filing system where it is available for rapid, frequent access. Access files might include for example, the census data of the living individuals. The downgrading of active files requires either the destruction of the record or a transition to a long term resting place. For example, the census data related to a dead person might go in these longer-term files. The selection of specific records or data items to form the permanent archives of an agency is the final step in the life cycle of a record or a document. Selected for their intrinsic, legal or historic value, archived records need special, expensive handling if their preservation is to be ensured.

Information in electronic form offers several advantages in the archiving and preservation processes. First, it is typically stored in very compact form, significantly lessening the burden of physical storage. Second, using the technology with which it was created, electronically stored data can be more systematically sorted and evaluated for archival value. However, the existence of information in electronic form also poses some special problems. Primary among them is vulnerability to environmental factors and possible loss of data due to undetected or unexpected changes in the physical characteristics of the storage media. For example, tapes of disks can deteriorate in their magnetic properties over time, especially if exposed to unusual heat, humidity or magnetic fields. Even minor disruptions can make an entire file virtually unreadable. White paper records are subject to similar problems (loss due to fire or flood, or physical deterioration due to light or humidity), the possibilities of massive information from seemingly minor disturbances in the storage environment have not existed in the past.

A closely related problem is the rapid obsolescence of the equipment and media used to store and read information in electronic form. Tape drives, disk drives and the size and format of tapes and disks change every few years. Equipment and formats considered standards as recently as fifteen years ago are no longer in use. It seems like that fifteen (or one hundred) years from now, the brand new technologies like compact disks

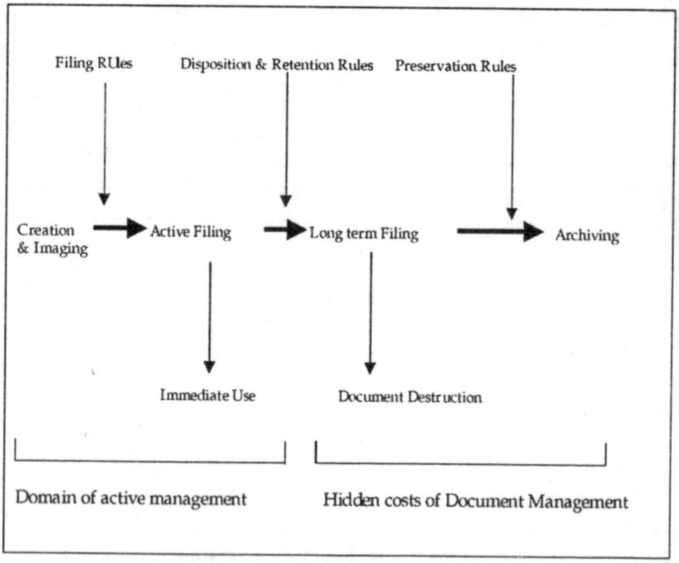

Figure 3: **Life Cycle of a Typical Document**

and optical storage devices necessary to read and interpret today's electronically stored information will no longer be used. Even twenty years from now the equipment needed to read today's government records may well be antiques. But twenty-first century libraries and archives need to have as good access to information preserved in electronic form as today's have to the nineteenth century's written records. Deliberate steps will have to be taken now to ensure continued access to electronically archived material in the future. This will most likely involve plans to build archival considerations into current record management activities, to periodically evaluate stored material and to record it in new media formats for continuing accessibility.

Information Sharing within a Organization

Most hardware and software issues, requiring considerable skill and often a considerable investment, are more amenable to solutions than many of the associated organizational problems. In large measure the question of information resource sharing within and between levels of government is more an organizational than a technological issue. We may have standardized hardware, operating systems, and telecommunications protocols supporting databases and software written in a common language. But the fundamental questions of data ownership, definitions, control, access, security, integrity and confidentiality all remain. These are issues technology cannot solve. Our managerial and political skills are the only tools we have to deal with them.

Information Sharing between Different Departments

Additional complications arise when information resources are to be shared between organizations or jurisdictions. Struggles for organizational turf are even fiercer than within agencies. Often ethical, legal, and even constitutional issues arise when data is shared across organizations. Consider a tax department using the data about the vehicles owned by a citizen maintained by the Transport Department to see if he falls under the presumptive tax bracket. Such a case involves competing goals: maintaining public access to public information, protecting the privacy of individual citizens, improving the accountability and credibility of public organizations, and achieving the policy objectives of the government.

Shared information resources can alter traditional balances of power in intergovernmental relations. For example, a statewide information system that supports *Panchayat* operated welfare programs puts the state in a better position to control and monitor the payment policies and practices of local units of government. It increases the state's power over the administration of public welfare and diminishes local discretion even though no laws or regulations have changed. On the other hand, such a system could set the stage for a successful local initiative to transfer more of the costs of welfare programs to the state. The loss of local policy control could be turned into a local fiscal advantage if laws regarding financing could be changed to reflect the de facto shift in power.

Information resource sharing between units and organizations is complicated. No one can say whether it is a uniformly good thing that should be consistently promoted or whether it should be subject to scrutiny at every step. Whether or not information resource sharing will work depends on what is being shared, how much each party benefits and at what cost, the nature of the applications, and the organizational culture of the units involved.

When different organizations share information resources, technical questions are interwoven with political ones-debates over common procedures and data definitions become proxies for the larger questions for power and program control. When the involved parties belong to the same organization, strong executive leadership is a key to successful resolution. When sharing is inter-jurisdictional, however, no common executive influence can be brought to bear. In these cases, both parties must see benefits flowing from the considerable resources they will invest in solving their mutual information problems.

The Role of Information Itself

Technological, organizational, and political issues are not the only constraints on information sharing. There are issues that arise from the content and meaning of the data itself. The nature of the information to be released or exchanged influences the technical choices that underlie data sharing. Copying and transferring information means databases must be easily formatted, duplicated and transported. These characteristics also make them more vulnerable to unauthorised disclosure, alteration or loss.

Other difficulties spring from the information histories of the organizations involved. It is unlikely that they have separately come to the same conclusions about identifiers, data element definitions, update schedules, and the like. Sharing information between them means changing things that may be working quite well for them individually. There are the associated problems of training, retraining, and documentation, which all arise even if there is complete agreement about the need for the changes.

Protecting Public Information Resources

Government data system must be reliable and secure. Both agencies and individuals are dependent on the reliability of government data systems. This means physical security and the ability to recover from disasters-important issues. Advance planning, working with simulated disasters, and other precautionary measures help secure the continuous operation of government information centers.

The range of possible failures (and their impact) varies widely. At the lower end of the scale are interruptions of the power supply, defects in a storage device, or programming problems. At increasing levels of severity are malfunctioning peripheral hardware components, loss of telecommunications links, loss of a hard disk, or ultimately, the loss of an entire data processing facility.

All these problems can be minimized by good advance planning. More difficult to plan for and avoid are human errors or intentional tampering. Ranging from innocent errors such as inadvertent erasure or alteration of a data element, human threats to data security can include "hackers" tampering with data or inserting "viruses" more or less as a source of amusement, theft of data by an employee or an outsider, deliberate sabotage of databases or, in extreme cases, of information processing equipment and facilities.

System users and managers, especially those with responsibility for critical operations, have long recognized the possibility (indeed, probability) of disasters large and small. In response they follow procedures designed to guard against failures in public information systems. Full-site backups may be put in place for some highly critical functions. Given the extreme reliance of government operations on some data processing functions, the cost of maintaining a fully operational reserve site might be justified.

For most systems, the key barrier to disaster recovery is inadequate planning. The procedures and technologies available for ensuring the security of information systems by far outstrip our managerial will to make use of them. The critical, and often missing, ingredient is the attention of the top management and budgeters within an organization. It is understandably often difficult to keep major disaster planning on the agenda of an administration concerned with the more immediate pressures of active operations. In this light, disasters are only hypothetical questions-until they occur.

Regardless of the amount invested in physical security, recovery will depend on organizational factors. Perhaps the most important and difficult is priority setting. Managers need to decide which applications must be recovered first. If program operations have been supported by automation for any length of time, manual procedures and associated paper processes may have been forgotten or may no longer do the job. Alternatives need to be thoroughly investigated and periodically reviewed as part of any good disaster recovery plan.

Malicious Threats to Security

Deliberate threats to information systems are more difficult to plan for and deal with because one must work against intentional, intelligent actions, not mere random events. This is the area where problems are most difficult to detect. Often they do not involve misuse or abuse of equipment, but rather fraudulent manipulation of a properly functioning system-such that benefits can be illegally authorised, services stolen, or selected information changed or destroyed. To tackle these problems, preventive measures are better than corrective ones. Thoroughly trained supervisors, carefully thought out procedures, and an organizational culture that gives security highly visible support are three of the best ones.

Many of the strategies for dealing with malicious threats, however, are similar to those for dealing with naturally occurring events. For computers, precautions against intentional abuse can be enhanced by securing the physical location of the equipment and by limiting access through such devices as security guards, badges, and entry check points . Electronic security may be enhanced with simple identification and password requirements (often sufficient to deter violations of data by non-technical staff or to prevent inadvertent data violations by trained personnel). More complex encryption techniques increase the level of sophistication needed to breach the security of protected information systems. Some of the techniques being designed for military systems are highly sophisticated and very difficult but not impossible, to breach.

Beyond measures aimed at physical and electronic security, procedural safeguards such as double verification of key entries by two or more employees, limiting input points for certain type of transaction s to physically isolated stations, requiring both pre-audits and post-audits of selected data entries, and system design and data architectures that conform to easily audited standards can provide for additional degrees of confidence. Specially organised security units can help detect, and in some cases prosecute, incidences of abuse and fraud .

Public Access to Government Information

Agency administrators must recognize and resolve many practical issues that arise from giving public access to Government information. These include creating and maintaining carefully designed classification systems for records and specifying access procedures and internal controls. Training and clearly articulated agency policy are necessary to ensure that requests that go through the collector's office, and across the desk of an operator in the data processing division will receive similar treatment and responses. An agency must also explicitly decide what purposes its information access policy actually serves. It may view itself as an aid to public access and understanding. It might help requesters to better define their needs, or it might simply respond to questions as they are posed. It may allocate specific resources to public access, or handle them within the limits of existing funds.

This is an area where many organizational issues come into play. For example, work unit, agency level, and jurisdiction wide policies need to fit together. An agency may intend to support broad access and citizen assistance, but its budget request for resources to carry out that kind of policy may be denied. Fees for information services is another sensitive issue. Some believe it is fair to charge fees high enough to cover the actual costs of access, arguing that they would allow agencies to give more public support, individual assistance, and responsive service. Others contend fees would be a deterrent. Public organizations will treat these issues in different ways. Some will lean towards greater access and public service, others toward consistently applied clear-cut rules that do not disrupt agency operations or drain away unplanned resources. Still others will put the agency's interest in protecting its discretionary powers first and other considerations later.

Routine Dissemination of Government Data

Another class of issues centers on the accessibility of information released as a matter of course. Some of the data routinely collected by government agencies have always been designed to inform the public. This information, largely statistical in nature, describes government operations and the condition and performance of the social systems in which we live. For example, census data, employment trends, and economic indicators such as national and regional computations of the cost-of living index are information "products" designed for public release. In addition, most government agencies collect data that, when released in functioning of government, the economy, and the society at large. Reports concerning state and local finances, schools, corrections, agricultural production, and health care fit this class of data. The primary problem with the publication and release of this kind of information is its low priority among the other routine operations of an agency. The missions of the agencies collecting this data seldom emphasize (or even recognize) the resource commitment needed to sort, analyze and prepare it for public release. The time and effort needed to locate and understand raw data, analyze it, prepare summary statistics, and publish statistical abstracts is, in fact, the key impediment to the dissemination of this kind of information.

Releasing information in electronic form creates additional complications. Most agencies are neither willing to provide free public access to their complete data files nor willing to tailor-made tapes or disks for each special request. Furthermore, most agency files contain data from a number of different sources, collected for different reasons and with different instruments, updated in different ways and on different schedules. This makes them, almost by definition, in a continual state of flux and makes knowing how and when to release information extracted from them much more difficult than it would seem at first glance.

Some of its dimensions of Government information management problem are technical: the need for standard definitions, procedures, and formats and the need for "metadata" or information about information (How was it collected? When? How reliable is the source? How often is it updated?). Standard statistical series usually handle such questions well. Often releases are made several times a year presenting a snapshot "frozen" at a point in time. The main database, however, continues to be updated and an all-inclusive annual summary is later released covering the entire year. Moreover, definitions have been settled for some time and any changes are heralded by long notice periods and extensive explanation.

Different technical questions affects the vast stores of government-generated information that have already solved the data problems just described. Many of the issues related to dissemination of government information, however, are not technical ones. They are policy questions about the priority such activities receive, the resources allocated to accomplish them, and the performance standards applied to gauge their effectiveness. Today, we know that multiple sources of related information could help answer many questions about our society and our economy. Tying disparate data systems together toward that end is no small task. It also generates some tough questions: Should government simply ease access to the data it has? Should it be responsible for routine analysis and release of statistical series and summaries? Should it charge fees for information? Should it interpret its data and make its conclusions available? If so, would that effort preempt private sector initiatives or investment in better information resources for everyone?

Collecting and processing data is costly. Analysing, interpreting and publishing information is even more so. The degree to which a public agency, a state, or any other jurisdiction invests in these activities rests mostly on the value both leaders and constituents place on publicly available information resources as a legitimate function of government. There are no of information technology applications are available for different uses as well as fast, cheap and transparent citizen services, such as Gyandoot, Soochnalayas, Computer-aided Administration of Registration Department (CARD), Andhra Pradesh Development Monitoring System (APDMS), The Secretariat Knowledge Information Management System (SKIMS), VIDYUTNET, Simplified and Transparent Administration of Registration (STAR), Telemedicine, Gram-Sachivalaya and many more other IT based project and applications are making people very near to governance.

Therefore, we conclude here that information and communication technology is playing very vital role in all the spheres of the life of the people in the country.

12

PRACTICING E-COMMERCE FOR COMMUNITY ECONOMIC DEVELOPMENT

Pradeep Nair

Introduction

Electronic Commerce (E-Commerce) has almost overnight become the dominant on-line activity. Equally quickly it has become a significant element in commercial activities globally, both in the developed and developing countries where suitable infrastructure support is available or likely to be available. E-Commerce, of course, has no single definition, meaning only commercial activity which is somehow linked to or supported by electronic communications. It may be anything from a simple advertising presentation available on the World Wide Web, or an e-mail communication; all the way to an entire multi-million dollar transaction initiated and promulgated in electronic form up; to and in some cases including the actual delivery via the net of information intensive goods or services.[1] (E. Turban, J. Lee, D. King, and H. M. Chung, 2000: 49-65).

Estimates of the volume of E-Commerce activity vary as widely as do the definitions but figures in the trillions of dollars are being widely circulated.[2] *(http://www.ecommerce.gov)* The initial and still most visible E-Commerce activities involved commercial relationships between businesses and individual consumers (B2C) such as *Amazon.com, or Grocer.com* or between consumers and consumers (C2C) as for example sites such as *eBay* or similar auction sites. However, the major developments which are causing the huge ripples economically and which underlie the astronomical sums which are being quoted are the Business to Business (B2B) undertakings, many of which are known only to those within particular segments of the business community.[3] (Steinfield, Charles and Pamela Whitten., 1999).

Advantages of E-commerce

The advantages of E-Commerce from a commercial perspective are numerous:

1. Online and more or less *instantaneous searches* with an unlimited number of criteria such as description, category, subcategory, location, color, size, and price range-i.e. The use of computerized information management for a huge and rapidly expanding globally distributed knowledge/information base along with the availability of full color media including graphics, animation, sound and now video and no space or time limitations as to information delivery.
2. Full *two-way 24 hours/day, 7 days/week communications/information access* capability which allows for instantaneous response and feedback concerning product/services and related information.
3. Full *processing of transactions* (including delivery) for information intensive goods such as software, text, images, video, and music; downloadable directly to the consumer's computer at the time of purchase and including the opportunity for limitless product comparison. All of this leads directly to greatly intensified competition in these markets and lower margins, reducing costs to the end user.
4. *The elimination of the need for middlemen (disintermediation),* leading to lowered transaction costs (including marketing, sales, transaction processing),

reduced overhead, and reduced inventory and labor costs.

5. The *delivery of after-sales service and support* directly and low cost.

Components of E-commerce

The principal components of e-commerce include:

1. *Web Browser*– A software program that allows people to access the World Wide Web. Internet Explorer and Netscape Navigator are the two most popular Web browsers.
2. *Web Servers*– Computers that host the information that Internet users access via their Web browser. Web servers are special Internet computers that store and deliver (serve) Web pages. A Web page is a specially formatted document that you can view in your Web browser. A Web server can host one or more Web sites.
3. *Payment System/Transaction Manager*– Electronic money exchanges including via (primarily) credit cards, electronic checks, smart cards, digital cash, and electronic funds transfer (EFT).
4. *Standards (existing and emerging)*–Methods for facilitating e-commerce interactions include and are meant to ensure transaction security, reliability, Electronic Data Interchange, and privacy.
5. *E-Commerce Software*– To the end user, the most visible part of the e-commerce system is the software that puts it all together. The basic functions of e-commerce software include: customer registration and authentication, online catalog viewing, order capturing and processing, customer service (e.g. enable customers to check order status and order history), and reporting and analysis (tools to analyze the activity on the e-commerce site for customer tracking). Optional functions include order fulfillment and payment processing, to name a few.

6. *E-mail*– Electronic mail serves as a support E-commerce Web sites.
7. *Mailing List Server*– An optional component of E-commerce is a mailing list server which automates the management of mailing lists for groups of users.
8. Search, Intelligent Agent, and Knowledge Management technologies these include the variety of software tools for "managing" information on the Net-"spiders", "bots", "inference agents" and so on.
9. Multimedia and broadband access technologies.

E-Commerce and Community Economic Development

E-Commerce presents significant challenges to Community Economic Development (CED).[4] (CED-Net@sfu.ca) CED has for the most part been low technology, focusing on those sectors of the economy which traditionally have not been technology or knowledge intensive and with relatively low technical skill requirements such as real estate development or rehabilitation, food retailing, craft manufacture and sale, tourism and particularly eco-tourism and so on. Most regions and communities with a strong interest in CED have been low income, with low skill levels, and little technology or training infra-structure. They have been ill-equipped to take leading edge advantage of the development of technology opportunities and have been "implementers" not "innovators" in technology use.[5] (C.M. Gurstein (Eds.) 2000: 65-75).

In many cases the Internet has come to be a central element in certain areas of social development and particularly in social advocacy, with those involved in these activities having developed innovative Internet based approaches and even applications. However, overall there has until recently been a strong feeling among those with Internet interests that the Net, whose origin was non-commercial should in fact remain non-commercial. Those with a social activist perspective and highly developed technical skills such as many of those who have been involved in the Free Software Movement and Open Source developments such as Linux, have resisted and even opposed the application of their skills and outputs for commercial purposes even in support of social sector economic activity.

There have however, been a variety of efforts mostly from those already involved in CED to adapt or develop electronic based supports for their economic activities notably the work of the Public Web Market[6] *(http://development.civicnet.org/webmarket/index.html)*, the work of the Centre for Community and Enterprise Networking (CCEN) in Cape Breton, Nova Scotia[7] (M. Gurstein, 2000: 28-63) and a variety of developing country initiatives some linked to the World Bank and others to other agencies. What characterized these early efforts was a lack of sustained funding which translated into the inability to develop the capacity for the on-going research and experimentation required to find optimal strategies for Net based commerce.

Lacking the resources or in many cases the skills to explore opportunities, those with an interest, were unable to develop sustained approaches and when initial efforts were only partially successful, they were left to whither. The entrepreneurial zeal and creativity which has marked the progress of the Internet and particularly E-Commerce in the last few years has been notably absent from the not-for-profit sector, partially it might be assumed because the very individualism and entrepreneurialism which has been the basis for development and success in the for-profit (and small business) sectors are precisely what is generally not found in the not-for-profit sector where there appears to be much more concern for general (rather than personal) advancement and much less economic risk taking.

But all of these aside, the range and significance of E-Commerce is such that it can no longer be ignored by the CED sector as it is presenting too great a competitive threat to this sector as to others. The threat to local economic development from E-Commerce is several folds:

- E-Commerce tends to shift economic activity towards pools of skill or in otherwise advantaged locations (because of climate, geography and so on) and away from marginal or disadvantaged regions.

- The success of E-Commerce is often at the expense of local enterprises who now find themselves in direct competition with huge number very low cost suppliers who may be located anywhere.
- The range of goods available on the Net is very large and cannot be matched by any supplier let alone smaller local ones thus putting local enterprises at a significant disadvantage in certain sectors.
- The cost of developing an effective E-Commerce site has risen dramatically and is now out of the range of many local enterprises.
- There is an on-going migration of the variety of information intensive services to the Net and away from local delivery (and local employment) as local distribution or service agents are centralized and down-sized as for example banks, government information offices, the producers of local directories and so on.
- Disintermediation allows local purchasers to by-pass local suppliers or local wholesalers and buys directly from manufacturers thus eliminating whole strata of local intermediaries.

Those concerned with local development ignore the threat (and opportunities) presented by E-Commerce at their peril.

E-Commerce Opportunities for Community Economic Development (CED)

It is notable and interesting that one of the most active areas for business development in E-Commerce has been attempts to develop "community" E-Commerce web-sites or portals. There have been a number of attempts in this direction including failed attempts by Microsoft and a variety of start-ups which looked to create E-Commerce portals. These for example, attempted to provide substitutes for local newspapers with local news, sports and entertainment information, or in other cases civic and civic government information. In general, they are looking to "capture eyeballs" through these locally oriented web-sites, on the well known principle that individuals are mostly interested in things that are relatively close physically to themselves and their families.

Many of the free-standing commercial "community portal" sites have disappeared or are not being updated. They do not have sufficient advertising revenue to support the cost of the staff required to keep the sites up-to-date. A number of sites linked to local newspapers are still surviving since they can reuse information collected for other purposes, but even these do not appear to be independently profitable.

A second development of some interest is the current concern with developing "community networking" among a number of the major Internet supplier firms such as for example, Nortel and Newbridge. They are looking on this as a way of generating sufficient traffic in local communities to require the installation of their high band-width networks. All of the major bandwidth suppliers and their associated firms are moving extremely aggressively to provide ever greater amounts of digital delivery capacity without having a clear sense of how all of this bandwidth could be used (and thus paid for). Several of the firms are operating on the assumption that only the development of local applications and a sophisticated user community in local areas will generate the demand of the educational, health and other community based applications they require to justify their services.

The question then, is how local communities can or those concerned with CED adapt the technology and the methodology/business models developing to support E-Commerce applications to their requirements.

E-Commerce Business Models for Community Economic Development (CED)

A quite large number of business models have evolved in the short life span of E-Commerce to support the transactions and to take advantage of the unique capabilities which the Internet and the World Wide Web afford. A number of these models are being or could be adapted to support local and CED enterprises along with the enterprises at a distance for which they were originally developed. There are a number of E-Commerce business models and here the paper suggests how they are being or could be used in a Community Economic Development (CED) context.

The Web-Site as an On-Line Billboard

The first and still most common use for the WWW is as a substitute for conventional display advertising whether in paper, billboard or other format. The idea is that one does one's advertising copy and then finds someone to put it into HTML and onto a server and then waits for the traffic to flow. Of course, sometimes it does and there are anecdotes about rug weavers and hammock makers who have increased their sales by factors of 1000 or more but there are fewer stories about the hundreds and thousands of local business folk who have paid for display web-sites and found that no one visited them.

A variation on this are sites which attempt to consolidate information and links relating to a sector or region (also known as a "portal"). The advantage of a portal is that where one enterprise might have difficulty in generating traffic to the site, a site which gives access to a number of enterprises might generate much more traffic. This principle has proven partially true, but the problem has been that the proliferation of sites has now been matched by the proliferation of "portals" all competing for the same users and often in overlapping areas.

Those concerned with CED might consider developing local enterprise portals (a number of them already have done so). These portals would have the advantage over competing portals in that they might be in a position to start off with a relatively loyal band of local users with an interest in local information, local products and the promotion of local community interests. In some cases, the development of local portals of this kind can be scaled up to include regional portals through which local portals can be accessed and at some point, these web-sites and those who are using them to display and present their goods and services will have a sufficient breadth and depth to become of interest to the larger world. At this point of course, they begin to come into competition with commercial sites with large promotion and advertising budgets, but CED based portals have been successful by using word of mouth and informal lines of communication to bring attention to their sites (academic or religious groups, not-for-profit networks, newsletters and so on).

The Attention Business: Portals and Traffic-Builders

The first and still most common business model on the WWW is based on the initial function of the web-site as a place to display/present information or graphics and in this way capture "attention". Having captured the attention, the use to which that attention was put has been primarily to push advertising at the site user and then to charge the advertiser for having captured the users attention and used it in this way. The more "attention" captured and thus the more and more elaborate, eye-catching, knowledge and service rich the site/portal, the more the advertising on the site could be sold for.

Community groups equally of course, could create web-sites or portals of local or other interest and capture the attention of their own clientele. The attention of this clientele might be of less interest to commercial advertisers but might be of some interest to others who would be similarly willing to pay for the delivery of their information-public health, education, civic-to this clientele as well. It might also be of interest to other groups with a for example interest in selling CED produced goods or services who might be willing to pay or exchange services for this opportunity.[8] (Romm, T. Celia and Fay Sudweeks. 1999: 44-57).

Adding Value: A "Service" Model

A number of web-sites have been developed whose function is to grab attention by providing the user with one or another type of service-email, web hosting, rate calculations and so on. The notion here is again that by getting the user's attention this in turn can be re-sold. In the CED world it may be possible to see a different opportunity. Since the local users will be one's with a clearly specifiable range of interests and service requirements, it should be possible to develop a range of locally focused services including information, news, links, useful applets and so on which are of sufficient value to their local users that they may either be willing to pay a subscription fee, or give a contribution to support the site or alternatively it may be possible to find someone willing to sponsor the site simply to be associated with it. This kind of development serves two functions-developing a local E-Commerce activity (and employment) and also providing an otherwise unavailable or costly set of services to the local community.

One interesting example is the development by a local business of a web portal which substitutes for what used to be their or their suppliers catalogue (and part of their inventory) which allows customers to comparison shop through the Net, order through the local dealer's portal at the price offered through the Net. The local supplier receives a commission from the ultimate seller of the good, but also the local supplier will be in a preferred position to enter into after-sales service contracts both with the goods supplier and with the consumer. In this way the local supplier maintains their position in the commercial cycle. This model is very likely one that could be adopted by local consumer co-operatives for CED service enterprises as well.

A Community "E-Commerce Community" Model

A very "hot" area in commercial E-Commerce is the building of "virtual communities" in association with web-sites and linking these to their associated products or sponsors. The notion is being that if an individual comes to identify with a (in this case "virtual") community then they are more likely to accept the norms of that community and their behavior as a consumer will be influenced as a result, including and not incidentally overcoming the distrust which seems to accompany much on-line interaction. The business model here is based on the assumption that these "virtual communities" represent a set of consumer "loyalties" which have commercial value and thus these communities can have a commercial value (and can be bought and sold sometimes at very significant values!).

In the context of CED of course, the issue is not the creation of a "virtual" community but rather the creation of a linkage between a real physical community (Baker calls this a "proximal" community)[9] (Baker, Paul, 2000: 73-89) and the "virtual" world where this community may undertake certain of its activities. The availability of these proximal community linkages for transfer into the virtual domain provides an opportunity for community enterprise developers to use these community ties as a framework within which to construct economic and trade relationships. Thus for example, a proximal community may wish to act together to procure goods and services at more favourable rates than they would receive as individual consumers. This can much more easily be effected on-line than face to face and mirrors directly the types of E-Commerce activities which are being done for commercial purposes. Similarly a proximal community can use the Net to "sell" themselves either as a market or as a supplier of goods or services into the commercial E-Commerce sphere.

Brokering or Facilitating Transactions

One of the most active areas for development on the net has been the replacement of brokers or mediators in some areas and their redevelopment in others. The range of information access and the speed of communications allows for the development of a new brand of intermediaries who are in a position to negotiate "with the world" on behalf of the individual or the group as for example by putting together groups of unconnected consumers as units for negotiating best prices with suppliers.

Such a development would work well in the CED world as well where previously unconnected CED groups or activities regionally, nationally and even internationally could find their negotiating strength considerably amplified by creating a common cause for commercial activity or for the variety of lobbying efforts which would support their activities.

Another interesting possibility here would be the use of the forms and information management capability of the Web for handling scheduling and resource allocation as for example, in co-operative purchasing environments. An example of this would be a car co-op where a number of individuals would go together to purchase one or more cars for joint use.

A current problem with this is the book-keeping and scheduling involved and the cost of maintaining an office and a staff to manage this. In a web environment the scheduling could all be done in a web displayed interface where individuals could see dynamically updated scheduling and automobile availability and in real-time enter their own scheduling requirements into the system which in turn would be immediately available to everyone with suitable access (this would of course, be best done within a secure or password protected environment).

Auctions or Dynamic Pricing

A very familiar by now form of business activity on the Net is the "auction" as for example that undertaken by eBay. These are now also available for a very wide range of goods and services where previously auctions were unknown such as for airplane tickets, hotel rooms, industrial components and so on. The unique communication and information management features of the Net (not excluding the capacity of the net for facilitating and presenting feedback on suppliers and purchasers) have facilitated this development.

Apart from the conventional auctioning of goods and services by CED enterprises, a much wider range of auction activities have been suggested as being possible in the context of the Internet. Thus for example, the development of regional, national and even global markets with "dynamic (auction)" pricing for recyclable and waste materials-one person's waste is another person's raw material.

Also the use of this model to sell perishable food products produced by CED or co-op enterprises expands potential markets considerably and can assist in managing the problem of wastage and inventory control for small and local enterprises as easily as for larger businesses.

E-Money

An intriguing development is what is being called E-Money or money which only exists in the virtual domain. An example of this is "Beanz.com" which provides a facility for electronic payment in an on-line currency they call "Beanz" which can be used in the purchase of goods or services from co-operating sites or businesses. Individuals in this case, receive "Beanz" for visiting web-sites, for undertaking transactions on web-sites and so on. Importantly the management of the transaction and of individual client and supplier accounts is done electronically and for free to the user, through the "Beanz" site (and back office).

Conclusion

The future as they say in technology circles is wireless, mobile, multi-media (voice, video, 3D) and broadband. All of these technology changes are rapidly developing and being incorporated into on-line and E-Commerce activities. From a CED perspective they are also following the path of earlier on-line technologies with a very steep decline in entry cost and ease of use or the non-professional user. Thus while CED enterprises need not be "first" users they certainly need not be "last" users nor should they be. Commercial firms are discovering that at least one leg of the stool on which virtual commerce is resting and will continue to rest is face to face physically delimited communities and it is here, where the on-going and future strength and opportunities for growth and development of CED rests. By recognizing that E-Commerce and the opportunities it presents is no more technologically or dare it is better to say that they are ideologically daunting than credit cards or ATM machines and thus the possibility for E-Commerce to enhance the growth and local contribution of CED is significant.

Notes and References

1. E., Turban, J. Lee, D. King and H.M. Chung (2000), Electronic Commerce: A Managerial Perspective. New York, Prentice-Hal: 49–65.
2. U.S. Department of Commerce (2004), *The Emerging Digital Economy*. The Report is available *on http://www.ecommerce.gov.*
3. Steinfield, Charles and Pamela Whitten (1999). "Community Level Socio-Economic Impacts of Electronic Commerce", *Red Rock*

Eater News Service, Phil Agre. The Report is available on *pagre@alpha.oac.ucla.edu.*

4. E-Commerce and Community Economic Development. The discussion is available on CED-Net@sfu.ca.
5. C.M. Gurstein (Eds.) (2000), Community Informatics: Enabling Communities with Information and Communication Technologies. Hershey PA: Idea Group: 65–75.
6. *http://development.civicnet.org/webmarket/index.html.*
7. Gurstein, M. (2000), Burying Coal: The Centre for Community and Enterprise Networking and Local Economic Development. Vancouver: Collective Press: 28–63.
8. Romm, T. Celia and Fay Sudweeks (1999), Doing Business on the Internet: Opportunities and Pitfalls. Berlin: Springer Verlag, 44–57.
9. Baker, Paul (2000), "Community Informatics and the Virtual Metropolis" in Gurstein, M. (Eds.) Community Informatics: Enabling Communities with Information and Communication Technologies. Hershey PA: Idea Group: 73–89.

13

IMPACT OF GLOBALIZATION ON BRANDING SELF HELP GROUP PRODUCTS

T. Karthikeyan, V. Balakrishnan & R. Asokan

Introduction

The Indian marketing scenario has seen radical changes in the past decade. Entry of multinational brands, emergence of young professionals, growth of luxury and leisure markets, media impact, westernization, mobility of consumers, availability of global brands have forced the Indian companies to undergo different competitive strategies. Indian market consists of variety of products varying from low-involvement product categories to high-involvement product categories.

Hindustan lever limited has identified that the money available to spend on Fast Moving Consumer Goods (FMCG) products is Rs. 63,500 crores in rural India. National Council of Applied Economic Research (NCAER) report suggest that the number of middle and high income households in rural India is expected to grow from 80 million to 111 million by 2007, 40% of students graduating from colleges are from rural areas, they became the decision makers and are similar in education, exposure, attitudes and aspirations to their counter parts.

In an another angle, 70% of the population lives in 6,27,000 villages in rural areas. In that almost 90% of the population is concentrated in the villages with a population of less than 2000. These milestones clearly focus that emerging market in India is rural market. The micro enterprises started under self help groups have involved in lot of productive and marketing activities in rural market. Once these products are branded it becomes easy for identification and differentiation. The emergence of self help groups (products) not only opened up new market but also provides employment opportunities and improve informal micro enterprises. The self help groups as collective group effort emerges from each and every village of the country.

The women in the informal micro enterprises sector constitute a large section of the work force in developing countries. Official data base clearly pointed out that in developing countries the informal sector consists of 40% to 90% of the non-agricultural labour force and beyond 90% agriculture is also included. In addition the contribution to the national income varies between 25% and 70%. Thus there is no doubt that informal micro enterprise through self help groups play a vital role in national economy. Therefore branding is considered to be the critical issue for promoting and marketing self help groups products in this globalized environment.

Objectives

This paper revolves around the following objectives.

- To study the global brand strategies and their impact on self help group (products).
- To identify the different branding strategies adopted by self help groups.

Global Brand Strategies and Self Help Groups

International companies have traditionally followed two types of strategies to create their global brands. The first is to strategy has consisted of expand successful local brands on international markets. This strategy has been followed over decades by many multinational firms. For example, a brand like "Evian" was a first successful local brand in France before it was expanded on a worldwide basis. Evian has now become the leading global brand in the worldwide mineral water market.

The second strategy is to create global brands from the start. These brands are launched on a worldwide basis at the same time. This is the most recent strategy adopted by certain multinationals such as Procter and Gamble. The creation of global brands such as Pringles, Swiffer or Kangoo is good examples of this strategy. The key advantage is to rapidly build a world brand with the same name and positioning in every market and benefit from substantial economies of scale.

In this situation the globalization strategies adopted by many MNC's too concentrate on think and acting according to local conditions. Most of the self help group products are unbranded were, the consumers in the market are not aware of it because these products don't possess any brand identity and image. Factors like place of origin could be used as a strategy for marketing self help group products. The self help group products don't posses any brand image for which consumers are now looking for it. The multinational companies use self help groups as a channel for their distribution networks. But self help group products (SHG products) which are considered to be *Rural Local Jewels* (RLJ products) will loose its market share due to the emergence of global brands. New brand building, positioning, extending and equity creating strategies are to be devised. Branding strategies like umbrella branding, cult branding could also be used according to the situation. To highlight this factor few cases of branded self- help groups and their strategies are discussed below.

Branding Strategies among Self Help Groups

Banacraft

The Self Employed Women Association (SEWA) has worked as a NGO for a decade to assist women producers and it is involved in marketing of their products. The self employed women association (SEWA) introduced a brand name called 'Banacraft' which is a direct marketing outlet of several thousand crafts women of the Bana Skantha district of Gujarat State.[1]

Bana craft is a means of providing livelihood to desert families whose only source of income when rains and harvest fails is craft that feed them well. Banacraft is a brand for the poor women to reach the market through SEWA. Currently, 3000 women get work and income of around 500 rupees a month, with an annual turnover Rs. 50 lakhs. They consider that the brand name 'Banacraft' and SEWA's assistance has grown with their earnings.

Gramhaat

Gram haat is yet another brand of SEWA salt. Gramhaat through its website procured industrial and expert orders. The groups now sell 40,000 tonnes of salt annually with an increasing earning Rs. 200 per tonne per annum. The brand image of gram haat not only helped to up scale the production but also doubled the income. To promote the poor women products SEWA has taken holistic responsibility and introduced new brands for them.

Mayurbhanj

Mayurbhanj, a District Supply and Marketing Society (DSMS) established with a mandate to provide non-credit inputs like procurement/purchase of raw material and sale of IRDP/DWCRA/TRYSEM products was established and registered in the year 1994 which is a district unit of Orissa Rural Development And Marketing Society (ORMAS)[2]. At present DSMS is engaged in market promotion and facilitating marketing of SGSY and self help groups products like forest honey, Siali leaf plates and buffer plates, Sal leaf plates and cups, Dhokra (an antique expression), Sabai (threaded to perfection), Stone carving and sarees which are marketed by DSMS under the brand name of Mayurbhanj. This is a best example for marketing self help groups products through district supply and marketing societies.

Conclusion

National brands like Hindustan Lever Limited (HLL) too focusses on self help group for its distribution of products. Then why not these self help groups products be branded. The brand image for the self help groups products can be built either for a individual product or even all the products produced by self help groups can be branded under single name so that the consumer price perception of the products will be high. More over it is the scenario of flexible globalization which made global brands like coke to even react to local condition[3] (i.e., think local and act local) when global brands adopt a localization strategy then the rural local jewels (self help groups products) to be marketed where, When there is no proper brand positioning and brand image building strategies are not devised by the government. When you compare the number of self help groups in India very few self help groups are known to customer by their brand name as discussed earlier. Thus, this paper puts for the strong resolution that self help groups (products) are to be compulsorily branded so that they can improve the living standard of poor women who are below the poverty line (BPL).

Notes

1. Faculty Member in Management, Directorate of Distance Education, Annamalai University, Annamalainagar-608002
2. Professor and Head, Management wing of DDE, Annamalai University, Annamalainagar - 608002
3. Faculty Member in Economics, Directorate of Distance Education, Annamalai University, Annamalainagar-608002

References

Reema Namavaty, (2004), Making the Poor Women Ready Market: 'SEWA's Journey', SEWA Academy, SEWA, Ahamadabad, India.

file://p:/shgproduct/dsms.htm

Assaal Henry, (2001), "Consumer Behaviour and Marketing Action", 6th Edition, Thomson Learning, pp. 503-509.

Moorthi YLR, (2005), "Brand Management the Indian Context, Vikas Public House Pvt. Ltd.

14

COMPARATIVE STUDY OF THE CAPACITY ASSESSMENT TOOLS

B. Sripirabaa & R. Krishnaveni

Introduction

Globalization has augmented competition whereby, organizations need to meet the challenges—negative as well as positive. The globalized era demands a generation of future-oriented, anticipatory managers capable of developing visions, manage organizations, compete for resources, plan and design activities for successful accomplishment of organizational objectives (Farazmand 2004).

Capacity Building is one of the methodologies available for managers to assess and build the capabilities of organizations. World Bank in 1996 and UNDP in 1997, concentrated on how the capacities of individuals, institutions, organizations, societies and practices could be developed (Table 1).

Later, Wange (1997) expressed Capacity building as a "continuous and multidimensional process of nurturing the ability of individuals and institutions to undertake quality policy analysis and economic management."

Concept of Capacity Building

Capacity building refers to activities that improve an organizations ability to achieve its mission ("CapBuild GMI," n.d.).

It is the process that increases the capability of organizations and individuals to produce or perform. Capacity building could be carried out at the macro level focussing the organization as a whole and at micro level which focuses on the individuals.

Table 1
Views Regarding Capacity Building

World Bank	The combination of people, institutions and practices that permits countries to achieve their development goals
UNDP	The process by which individuals, organizations, institutions, and societies develop abilities (individually and collectively) to perform functions, solve problems and set and achieve objectives

Capacity building may relate to any aspect of the organizations work; improved governance, leadership, mission and strategy, administration, program development and implementation, fundraising and income generation, diversity, partnerships and collaboration, evaluation, advocacy skills, training/speaking abilities, technical skills, organizing skills and other areas of personal and professional development ("CapBuild GMI," n.d.). The idea of capacity building is limited to adding new functions and raising more money, buildings or technology.

When the focus of Capacity Building is at the micro level it involves giving individuals knowledge, providing opportunities for them to make decisions, empowering them to act and enabling them to carry out their tasks to the best of their ability. It is the process of building on the innate skills and abilities, which exist within the individuals.

The concept of Capacity Building is being used by organization development researchers and consultants to help small companies, non-profit organizations, non government organizations, civil society organizations and community development agencies to discover innovative ideas in management, effective disbursement and utilization of its limited resources. Majority of the Capacity Building activities in the past two decades were focused on Community development, environmental protection and empowerment of non-profit organizations (Baumqarten. 2004, Cosio, R. 1998, Farazmand. 2004, Northridge, Sidibe., Goehl., 2004, Orazeo, Lapointe 2004, Panagiotis, Despoina 2004, Richard 1995). Having gained the attention of Organization Development researchers and consultants, different tools were developed and applied to measure and enhance the capacity of organizations. An attempt has been made in this paper to compare and analyze such tools that were developed and used.

Objective

The focus of this paper is to identify and compare the various tools that are available in the literature in the last decade for measuring and building the capacity of organizations.

Methodology

Twelve tools that have been developed and used by small companies, non-profit organizations, non government organizations, civil society organizations, community development agencies, Philanthropists, funding agencies like UNDP, organizations involved in community based programs, facilitators providing capacity building support, partnership organizations etc., for capacity building, during the last ten years (1997 to 2006) were identified and included in this study.

Analysis

Table 2 gives in concise, the tools that have been taken up for the comparative analysis along with the organization/ individual who developed it and the purpose for which the tool was developed.

1. *Discussion Oriented Organizational Self Assessment–(DOSA):* This tool was developed by Beryl Levinger and Evan Bloom in 1997 with assistance from the United States Agency for International Development/Office of Private and Voluntary Cooperation (USAID/PVC) and numerous Private and Voluntary Organization (PVO) colleagues ("DOSA,"n.d.). This tool was used as:

- An organizational capacity assessment tool, to measure and profile organizational capacities and consensus

Table 2
Tools used for Capacity Building

Sl. No.	*Year*	*Tool*	*Developed by*	*Application*
1.	1997	Discussion Oriented Organizational Self Assessment–(DOSA)	Beryl Levinger and Evan Bloom	Organizational capacity assessment, Organizational development and service
2.	1998	Participatory Organizational Evaluation Tool (POET)	Beryl Levinger and Evan Bloom	Organizational capacity assessment and organizational development
3.	1998	Simple Capacity Assessment Tool (SCAT)	Beryl Levinger and Evan Bloom	Organizational capacity assessment
4.	2000	Participatory Capacity Assessment (PCA)	CARE and BEF	Organizational capacity assessment
5.	2001	McKinsey Capacity Assessment Grid	McKinsey & Company	Identify the areas of capacity that are strong and those that need improvement
6.	2001	Marguerite Casey Foundation Organizational Capacity Assessment Tool (MCF OCAT)	McKinsey and Company	Strengthen low-income families and mobilize their communities to achieve a more just and equitable society

Contd...

Sl. No.	Year	Tool	Developed by	Application
7.	2001	SVP Organizational Capacity Assessment Tool (SVP OCAT)	Social Venture Partners	Organizational capacity assessment
8.	2003	Self assessment tool (SAT)	Southern Minnesota Initiative foundation	Serve clients better
9.	2004	Benefits Planning, Assistance and Outreach Performance Excellence Instrument (BPA&O PEI)	Cornell University	Assess the efficacy of services and supports delivered and the effective management of Benefits Planning, Assistance and Outreach programs
10.	2004	Organizational Assessment Tool (OAT)	Marco Kirschbaum	Help organisations improve their performance
11.		Organizational Self Assessment Tool (OSAT)	Capacity Development Consultancies	Improve performance through Organization Development
12.		Cap Map	Organizational Development Initiative and LISC Operating Support Collaborative[7]	Map current capacity of an organization

levels in six critical areas. The tool helps to assess over time, the impact of these activities on organizational capacity (benchmarking).

- An organizational development process, to build capacity by bringing staff together in cross-functional, cross-hierarchical groups for open exchange. This helps to identify divergent viewpoints to foster growth, create consensus around future organizational capacity development activities and then select, implement and track organizational change and development strategies.
- A service, funded by the United States Agency for International Development/Office of Private and Voluntary Cooperation. They provide training and certification to volunteers in administering the tool. Later they receive the comprehensive analyses of capacities measured by the tcol and the capacity building efforts carried thereon.

Fourteen PVOs participated in the DOSA exercise as a cohort in 1997. A cohort is a group of organizations that wants to improve performance, engage in deep organizational learning, and are open to change. Table 3 gives the focus areas of DOSA.

Table 3
Focus areas of DOSA

Area	*Focus*
External relations	Constituency development, fundraising and communications
Financial resource management	Budgeting, forecasting and cash management
Human resource management	Staff training. supervision and personnel practices
Organizational learning	Teamwork and information-sharing
Strategic management	Planning, governance, mission, and partnering
Service delivery	Field-based program practices and sustainability issues

DOSA produces two kinds of measures, a capacity score, which indicates the perception of the organizations' strengths and weaknesses with respect to the capacity areas, and a consensus score, which indicates the degree to which assessment team members agree on their assessment of organizational capacity. The procedure for using the tool is:

- A 5 point Likert's scale indicating a lesser capacity for a lower average point and higher capacity for a higher average point is used
- Scoring is done by an assessment team with representatives from the organizations
- The raw capacity and consensus scores are calculated for all the six areas.
- The standardized capacity and consensus scores are calculated.
- The standardized capacity and consensus scores are converted to scaled capacity and consensus scores.
- GRID is plotted with the capacity scores on the horizontal axis and consensus scores on the vertical axis.
- The areas that need improvement are identified and consequently strategies are planned.

2. *Participatory Organizational Evaluation Tool (POET)* was developed in 1998 by Beryl Levinger of Education Development Center and Evan Bloom of Pact with assistance from the United Nations Development Program (UNDP) and numerous civil society organizations (CSO) colleagues.

POET has two concepts rolled into one-it is a tool, and a process. As an organizational capacity assessment tool, Civil Society Organizations (CSO) and their partners use POET to measure and profile organizational capacities and consensus levels in seven critical areas, and assess, over time, the impact of these activities on organizational capacity (benchmarking). As an organizational development process, CSOs and their partners use POET to build capacity by bringing staff together in cross-functional, cross-hierarchical groups for open exchange. This helps them to identify divergent viewpoints to foster growth and create consensus around future organizational capacity development activities and select, implement and track organizational change and development strategies ("POET," n.d.).

POET is based on a methodology called PROSE (Participatory, Results-Oriented Self-Evaluation) a methodology for assessing and enhancing organizational capacities ("POET Manual," n.d.). The POET Manual was designed for three different types of users;

- a CSO as part of a cohort,
- a cohort administrator,
- an independent CSO.

POET could be used by organizations that are part of a cohort to study their scores in comparison with peer organizations for benchmarking purposes and also by individual organizations. The concept underlying POET is similar to that of DOSA. (Table 4).

Table 4
Focus areas of POET

Sl. No.	*Area*	*Focus*
1.	Human Resource Management	Staff development, recruitment, compensation (salary and benefits), personnel evaluation, and grievance and conflict resolution.
2.	Financial Resource Management	Budgeting, forecasting, fundraising, and cash management.
3.	Equitable Participation	Field-based program practices related to project access and project benefit
4.	Sustainability of Program Benefits	The impact of environmental, economic, political, institutional, and cultural factors
5.	Partnering	Collaboration with other CSOS, donors policy makers, and private sector entities
6.	Organizational Learning	Teamwork, information-sharing and capacity for generating information that leads to improvement of current practice
7.	Strategic Management/ Governance	Board practices; planning practices; and, commitment to goals, mission and philosophy

The procedure for administering POET is similar to that of DOSA.

3. *A Simple Capacity Assessment Tool (SCAT):* This tool was developed by Beryl Levinger and Evan Bloom. The application of this organizational capacity assessment tool requires broad participation by the organization that wishes to employ it. The tool was developed to provide support organizations with procedures for assessing the organizational capacity of potential partners and to provide a process through which relevant and context specific indicators could be developed in a collaborative manner. A support organization working with the SCAT will identify appropriate indicators, develop an appropriate scoring nomenclature, and begin to develop a strategy for implementing a program of organizational capacity assessments ("SCAT," n.d.). Table 6 gives the focus areas of SCAT.

Table 5
Focus areas of Participatory Capacity Assessment

Area	*Focus*
Governance	Vision/Mission/Goal, Constituency Participation, Board/ Leadership, Legal Status
Management practice	Management Administration, Human Resource Financial Management, Planning, Monitoring and Evaluation
Program development and service delivery	Program Development and Service Delivery
External relationships and networking	External Relations and Networking
Sustainability	Sustainability
Education	Education

Scoring is done by an assessment team using a rating scale of 1 through 4 (1=nascent; 2=emerging; 3=expanding; 4=mature). The average score for each component is calculated.

4. *Participatory Capacity Assessment:* The Participatory Capacity Assessment (PCA) uses the POET and was developed by Cooperative for Assistance and Relief Everywhere (CARE)

and Benin Education Fund (BEF). The outcome of PCA is an objective measurement of the organisation's capacities and the degree of consensus about this level of capacity. Table 5 gives the focus areas of PCA.

Table 6
Focus areas of Simple Capacity Assessment Tool

Area	*Focus*
Governance	Board, Mission, Goals and Philosophy, Executive Leadership, Legal Status
Management practice	Organizational Structure, Information systems, Administrative Procedures, Planning, Program Development, Program Reporting
Human resources	Personnel Management, Diversity Issues, Supervisory Practices, Salary and Benefits
Financial resources	Accounting, Budgeting, Financial and Inventory Controls, Financial Reporting
Service delivery	Sectoral Expertise, Constituency Ownership, M&E Systems
External relations	Constituency relations, Government, Relations, Donor Relations, Public relations, Media relations
Partnering	Intra-sectoral partnering, Inter-sectoral partnering

PCA uses a 5 point Likert's scale and scoring is done by an assessment team with about twelve to fifteen representatives of the organizations. The assessment provides information about the capacity of their organization. Self-assessment has the advantage of organizational learning and building of ownership of the capacity building process ("CARE," n.d.). Each member of the assessment team "scores" the level of capacity, based on discussions and their own views and experiences. The average score in each area is calculated and associated with the organizational life cycle concept and the results are plotted on a graph.

5. *The McKinsey Capacity Assessment Grid:* This tool was created by McKinsey and Company and published in Effective Capacity Building for Non-profit organizations in 2001. This tool was developed to identify the areas of capacity that are

strongest and those that need improvement, to measure changes in an organization's capacity over time and to draw out different views within an organization regarding its capacity ("McKinsey," n.d.). The seven areas of the Capacity Assessment GRID are: Aspirations, Strategy, Organization skills, Human Resources, Systems and infrastructure, Organizational structure and Culture.

Assessment is done by nonprofit staff members, board members, or external parties who have a good knowledge of the organization. Scoring is done on a four point scale as 1=Clear need for increased capacity, 2=Basic level of capacity in place, 3=Moderate level of capacity in place, 4=High level of capacity in place. The average capacity dimension in each area is calculated and the values are plotted on a graph.

6. Marguerite Casey Foundation Organizational Capacity Assessment Tool: It is a derivative product of the Capacity Assessment Grid created by McKinsey and Company for Venture Philanthropy Partners and published in Effective Capacity Building in non-profit organizations in 2001. This tool was developed to help low-income families strengthen their voice and mobilize their communities in order to achieve a more just and equitable society for all ("Marguerite Casey," n.d.). The assessment is intended for self-guided use by nonprofit organizations to identify capacity strengths and challenges and establish capacity building goals. Table 7 gives the focus areas of the tool.

Table 7
Focus areas of Marguerite Casey Foundation Organizational Capacity Assessment Tool

Area	*Focus*
Leadership capacity	The ability of organizational leaders to inspire, prioritize, make decisions, provide direction, and innovate
Adaptive capacity	The ability of a nonprofit organization to monitor, assess, and respond to internal and external changes
Management capacity	The ability of a nonprofit organization to ensure the effective and efficient use of organizational resources
Operational capacity	The ability of a nonprofit organization to implement key organizational and programmatic functions

Assessment is done by the Executive Director/Chief Executive Officer and Board President, Staff, board members, and/or constituents individually. They then gather and discuss their ratings and reach consensus on one set of ratings that best represents the organization and submit it on behalf of their organization. Four levels from 1 to 4, carrying points 1 to 4 are assigned to each item and the average capacity dimension in each area is calculated. The values are plotted on a graph.

7. *SVP Organizational Capacity Assessment Tool:* This tool is used as a baseline assessment of capacity to measure improvements over time. It helps non-profits identify capacity strengths and challenges and establish capacity building goals ("SVP," n.d.). This tool was developed by Social Venture Partners to assess organizational capacity to provide cash grants, skilled volunteers, professional consultants, leadership development and management training opportunities. It was published in Effective Capacity Building for Non-profit organizations in 2001. The ten focus areas are; Mission/Vision Strategy and Planning, Program Design & Evaluation, Human Resources, CEO/ED/Senior Management Team Leadership, Information Technology, Financial Management, Fund Development, Board Leadership, Legal Affairs and Marketing Communications and External Relations.

Three to five persons form various levels of the organization viz. Board President, Executive Director, Staff complete the assessment individually. Upon completing the Assessment on an individual basis, participants gather to discuss their ratings and reach consensus on one set of ratings that best represents the organization and submit it on behalf of their organization. Scoring is done on a four point scale as 1=Clear need for increased capacity, 2=Basic level of capacity in place, 3=Moderate level of capacity in place, 4=High level of capacity in place. The average capacity dimension in each area is calculated and the values are plotted on a graph.

8. *Self assessment tool developed by Southern Minnesota Initiative Foundation:* This tool helps non profit leaders assess their organization performance enabling them to better serve their clients ("SMI," n.d.). The tool was developed by Southern

Minnesota Initiative foundation in 2003. The tool encompasses seven areas: Mission, Deep and broad leadership, Resilient organizational system, Access to sufficient and sustainable assets, Mission driven programming, Learning and self reflection and Integrity.

A diverse team of organizational employees, lead volunteers and board members are selected. Each team member completes the evaluation and the group analyses responses and come to a consensus. There are both status and change questions. Status questions describe the current practices and the change questions ties responses to time; past, present and future. For the status questions the scoring is 1=Disagree, 2=Tend to disagree, 4=Tend to agree, 5=Agree, X=Unsure. For the change questions the scoring is 1=Absent, 2=Declining, 3=Improving, 4=Regained, 5=Stable. The average of the status and Change scores in each section are calculated and plotted in the graph with the change scores on the X axes and status scores on the Y axes.

9. *Benefits Planning, Assistance and Outreach Performance Excellence Instrument:* This is a comprehensive assessment tool developed by Cornell University to assess the efficacy of services and supports delivered and extent to which Benefits Planning, Assistance and Outreach (BPA&O) programs are managed effectively ("BPA&O," n.d.) in 2004. This tool help BPA&O assessment teams to determine areas of improvement in their organization and to create action steps to improve targeted areas. The tool comprises six areas: Leadership, Strategic Planning, Customer Needs and Satisfaction, Work Organization and Flow, Human Resources and Organizational Performance and Results. Organizational assessment should be facilitated by an assessment team for the entire agency or individual projects. The indicators are rated as 1=strongly disagree, 2=disagree, 3=neutral, 4=agree, 5=strongly agree. The average score in each area is calculated.

10. *Organizational Assessment Tool (OAT):* OAT was developed by Marco Kirschbaum in 2004 to help organizations improve their performance. It helps to find out their strong and weak points ("OAT," n.d.). Table 8 gives the focus areas of the tool.

Table 8
Focus Areas of Organizational Assessment Tool

Area	*Focus*
Governing structure	Mission, Vision statements, Values, Statues and board
Management process	Process orientation, Organization chart and staff access to leader, Meetings, team work and knowledge management, Planning Implementation of work plan and monitoring of progress achieved, Reporting and information exchange
Human Resources	Human resources policy and development, Human resources unit, Staff numbers Promotions Salaries and other benefits, Incentives and rewards system, Performance appraisal Training, Complaints and performance problem, Staff representation
Financial Resources and Administration	Registration, Economic and Fiscal environment, Budgeting, Funding, Accounting, Cost efficiency, Accountability, Financial Reporting, Administrative procedures, Infrastructure
Relationships	Social and cultural environment, Stake holders engagement, Partnerships with other NGO's, networks, companies, government authorities, Media
Results	Results achievement, Stakeholders satisfaction, Financial Results, Human Resources Results, Impact on Society

Managers and staff participate in the assessment. An internal assessment manager or an external facilitator leads the assessment process. Structured or semi structured interviews, team-based discussions are used. A SWOT for each of the questions using the SWOT Brainstorming Sheet is done. Relevant actions to be taken based on the results of the SWOT analysis using the SWOT Action Plan Sheet are identified and the plan of action is presented using the summary sheet. Level of achievement is scored as A=not yet started, B=some progress, C=considerable progress, D=achieved. The level of Priority scored as Top/medium/ low. The SWOT analysis is done and the OAT summary sheet is prepared with Priorities 1-4 for implementation as 1=to be resolved in up to three months, 2=three to six months, 3=six months to one year, 4=more than one year.

11. *Organizational Self Assessment Tool developed by Capacity Development Consultancies (CADECO):* CADECO'S core business is helping organizations to improve their performance through Organization Development. They help clients become more conscious of their responsibility for the development of their organizations and the need to create both efficient and humane organizations. This is a Proverbs based tool that would enhance the communication of the organizational issues in a language people would easily understand ("CADECO," n.d.). and comprises six areas; Culture, Leadership and Vision, Strategy, Roles and Responsibilities, Policies and Sustainability. Rating (0–5) are used where 0 = we do not experience this in our organization, 5 = we strongly experience or observe this in our organization. The average score in each area is calculated.

12. *CapMap:* This diagnostic tool was created and designed by the Organizational Development Initiative and *Local Initiatives Support Corporation* (LISC) Operating Support Collaborative ("CapMap," n.d.). It assists LISC program staff in mapping the current capacity of an organization, working in partnership with Community Development Corporations (CDC) ("LISC," n.d.). It assists LISC staff and CDCs to:

- Map an organization's baseline performance in nine core competency areas.
- Identify intervention strategies that move an organization from one stage of measurable performance to the next.
- Assess and quantify an organization's internal growth along a spectrum of progressive measurements.
- Evaluate the need for and effectiveness of capacity building strategies.
- Enhance institutional knowledge around organizational development and contribute to our various research and development efforts in the field.

The focus areas are Board Governance, Community Connections, Executive director, Financial Management, Fund development, Human Resources and staff development, Management information systems, Real estate Asset Management and Real estate development.

Apart form these, capacity assessment tools were developed and used for specific programs like:

- The Communities Responding to the HIV/AIDS Epidemic (CORE), helps ensure that grantees and southern and strategic partners have the necessary skills and strategies they need to implement effective community-based HIV/AIDS programs in United States of America ("CORE," n.d.).
- The North Central Regional Technology in Education Consortium of United States of America developed a tool to compare the current instructional practices with a set of indicators for engaged learning and high-performance technology for educational institutions ("NCRTEC," n.d.).
- Tool to assess Program Capacity to Integrate Cervical Cancer Prevention into Reproductive Health Services to assess program capacity for adding cervical cancer screening and dysphasia treatment services to existing reproductive health services in United States of America ("Integrated Cervical Cancer," n.d.).
- Capacity and Performance Standards for Community Development Corporations is an evaluation tool designed to document the capacity of the Community Development Corporations (CDC), to assess the CDC's performance, and determine the CDC's development stage ("Standards for CDC," n.d.).
- Intervention Capacity Assessment Tool to understand Agency's Capacity to Implement an Evidence-Based Intervention ("Agency Capacity," n.d.).
- Organizational Assessment Tool designed to identify the level of Community Participation to Improve Adolescent Reproductive and Sexual Health in Burkina Faso ("Adolescent Health," n.d.).

- Land and Water Australia's (LWA) Capacity Assessment Tool for Riparian Rehabilitation ("Land and Water Australia," n.d.).

Individual organizations too have developed specific assessment sheets to assess their performance from time to time like:

- Organizational surveys to improve operations of the organization promote good employee relations and establish benchmarks for evaluating the progress of both ("Organization surveys," n.d.).
- Exploring the Conscious and Unconscious Mind of Organizations ("Conscious Mind," n.d.)
- Questionnaires for Satisfaction at the work place ("Questionnaire for Satisfaction," n.d.) fo measure the learning climate and profile of organization characteristics.
- Organization health surveys ("Organization health surveys," n.d.).
- Founder's syndrome to identify whether the organization operates primarily according to the personality of a prominent person in the organization ("Founders Syndrome," n.d.).
- Small Business owner/Operator Competency Guidelines to identify the knowledge, skills and best practices for individuals managing small businesses ("Small Business Owner Competency," n.d.).

Discussion

The review of the various tools that have been developed for assessing the capacity of non-profit organizations, non government organizations, civil society organizations, community development agencies, Philanthropists, funding agencies reveal that DOSA was the first tool designed for PVO's to assess their capacity. Other tool like the Organizational Assessment tool, Organizational Self assessment tool, Participatory Capacity Assessment, SVP Organizational

Table 9
Comparison of the Capacity Assessment Tools

Sl. No.	Dimensions of Assessment	DOSA	POET	SCAT	PCA	MCF OCAT	SVP OCAT	McKinsey Capacity Assessment Grid	SAT	BPA&O PEI	OAT	OSAT	CapMap
1.	Recruitment and Compensation	*	*	*	*	*	*	*	*	*	*		*
2.	Personnel Evaluation	*	*	*	*	*	*	*	*	*	*	*	*
3.	Staff Development	*	*	*	*	*	*	*	*	*	*		*
4.	Grievance and conflict resolution	*	*		*				*		*	*	
5.	Budgeting	*	*	*	*	*	*	*	*	*	*		*
6.	Forecasting	*	*	*	*	*	*	*	*	*	*		*
7.	Fundraising	*	*	*	*	*	*	*	*	*	*		*
8.	Cash Management	*	*	*	*	*	*	*	*	*	*		*
9.	Increased stakeholders participation	*	*	*	*	*	*	*		*	*		*
10.	Customized projects	*	*	*	*	*	*	*		*	*		*
11.	Programs built on local knowledge and best practices	*	*	*	*	*	*	*	*	*	*		*
12.	Impact of environmental, economic, political, institutional and cultural factors	*	*		*	*	*	*			*	*	

Contd..

Sl. No.	Dimensions of Assessment	DOSA	POET	SCAT	PCA	MCF OCAT	SVP OCAT	McKinsey Capacity Assessment Grid	SAT	BPA&O PEI	OAT	OSAT	CapMap
13.	Collaboration with policy makers, NGO's, donors, policy makers etc	*	*	*	*	*	*				*		
14.	Enhancement of financial benefits and technical skills through partnering	*	*	*									
15.	Result based indicators for project assessment	*	*	*	*	*	*	*	*	*	*		*
16.	Recognition of interdependence of organizations units in analyzing problems	*	*			*	*	*	*		*	*	
17.	Open information sharing	*	*	*	*	*	*	*	*	*	*	*	*
18.	Teamwork	*	*	*	*	*	*	*	*	*	*	*	*
19.	Leadership	*	*	*	*	*	*	*	*	*	*	*	
20.	Informative reports to donors	*	*	*					*				

Contd..

Sl. No.	Dimensions of Assessment	DOSA	POET	SCAT	PCA	MCF OCAT	SVP OCAT	McKinsey Capacity Assessment Grid	SAT	BPA&O PEI	OAT	OSAT	CapMap
21.	Competency of board members in their activities	*	*	*	*	*	*	*	*	*	*	*	*
22.	Initiatives consistent with strategic and operational plans	*	*	*	*	*	*	*	*	*	*	*	*
23.	Monitoring and Tracking progress	*	*	*	*	*	*	*	*	*	*	*	*
24.	Commitment to goals, mission and philosophy	*	*	*	*	*	*	*	*	*	*	*	*
25.	Strategic Planning	*	*	*	*	*	*	*	*	*	*	*	*
26.	Knowledge management		*		*	*	*	*	*		*		*
27.	Infrastructure					*		*	*		*		
28.	Telecommunications and Computers					*	*	*	*		*		*

Capacity Assessment tool, Simple Capacity Assessment tool, McKinsey Capacity Assessment Grid and CapMap were developed to help organizations measure their current capacity and henceforth develop strategies to augment their capacity. Marquerite Casey Foundation Organizational Capacity Assessment tool, Self assessment tool and Benefits Planning, assistance and Outreach Performance Excellence Instrument were developed to asses the effectiveness of their programs so that they could better serve their clients. POET is the improved version of the DOSA developed by the same authors an year after. The former encompass seven critical areas whereas the later only six areas. Though all other tools contain four, six, nine or ten critical areas, still could be fit within the seven areas of the POET and hence could be viewed as the modified version of the POET having developed for a specific purpose. Hence POET could be taken as base for all the tools that have been developed consequently. Therefore POET appears to be more comprehensive for assessing the capacity of organizations among the tools available. The comparative analysis of the tools taken for the study is depicted in Table 9.

Conclusion

The concept of Capacity Building has been used by non profit organizations, CSO's and CDC's to measure and improve their capacity over time or benchmark their capacity with the cohort. Organizations have either developed specific tools to assess their capacity and to identify their level of service to their clients or have used common tools like the POET. Therefore POET appears to be the baseline tool for assessing the capacity of organizations. Since globalization has offered extensive opportunities for worldwide development, there is scope for the concept of Capacity Building being extended to profit organizations also. These organizations could use POET to assess and enhance their organizational capacity or could modify it and apply to a single department or few of its critical functions.

References

Richard. K. Mulligan (1995), "Catalyst for Community Capacity-Building: A Role for Public Sector Practitioners", *Journal of Economic Development Review,* 13(4): 58-62.

Floden. Goertz and O'Day (1996), *http://www.ncrel.org/sdrs/areas/issues/content/currclum/cu3il24.htm*

Cosio, R. (1998), "Social Constructivism and Capacity Building for Environmental Governance", *Journal of International Planning Studies,* 3 (3): 367- 390.

Baumqarten.Liz (2004), Building Capacity for Public Advocacy, *http://www.clpi.org.*

Blumenthal. Barbara, Investing in Capacity Building: A Guide to High–Impact Approaches.

Farazmand. Ali (2004), "Innovation in Strategic Human Resource Management: Building Capacity in the Age of Globalization", *Journal of Public Organization Review,* 4: 3-24.

Northridge E. Mary, Sidibe. Saika, Goehl J. Thomas (2004), "Environment and Health: Capacity Building for the Future", *American Journal of Public Health,* 94 (11): 1849-1850.

Orazeo, Manuel, Lapointe Michelle (2004), "Mexican Hometown Associations and Development Opportunities", *Journal of International Affairs,* 57(2): 31-49.

Panagiotis. Getimis, Despoina. Grigoriadou (2004), "The Europeanization of Urban Governance in Greece: A Dynamic and Contradictory Process", *Journal of International Planning Studies,* 9 (1): 5–25.

DOSA *http://www.edc.org/GLC?CapDev/dosafile*

POET *http://www.comminit.com/planningmodels/pmodels/planningmodels*

POET *http://www.comminit.com/pdf/POET_UsersManual.pdf*

Marguerite Casey *http://www.caseygrants.org*

SVP *http://www.svpseattle.org/key_documents/OCAT.xls*

McKinsey *http://www.emcf.org/evaluation mckinsey_assessment_tool.htm*

CADECO *http://www.impactalliance.org/*

CapMap *http://www.lisc.org*

LISC *http://www.lisc.org/docs/odi/IIB_imagine.pdf*

CARE *http: //www.careinternational.org.uk/download.php*

BPA & O *http://www.ilr.cornell.edu/ped/benequal*

OAT *http://www.ngomanager.org/tools/OAT_July_2004.pdf*

SCAT *http://www.gdrc.org/ngo/bl-scat.htm*

SMI *http://www.smifoundation.org/NPAssessmentTool.pdf*

CORE *http://www.aidsalliance.org.*

NCRTEC *http://www.ncrtec.org/capacity/profile/profwww.htm*

Integrated Cervical Cancer *http://www.path.org/files/Tool-16-july.pdf*

Standards for CDC *http://www.dca.state.ga.us/housing/housingdevelopment/programs/downloads/SFY2004_COAP_CAT.pdf*

Agency Capacity *http://chipts.ucla.edu/interventions/resourcemats*

Adolescent Health *http://www.foodaid.org/worddocs/localcapacity/Organizational%20 Assessment%20Tool.doc*

Land and Water Australia *http://www.waterwatch.org.au/publications/2005conference/pubs/thomson.pdf*

Organization Survey *http://expertss.objects.net/*

Conscious Mind *http://www.change-management-toolbook.com/*

Questionnaire for Satisfaction *http://www.change-management-toolbook.com/*

Organization Health Survey *http://www.od-online.com*

Founders Syndrome *http://www.managementhelp.org/misc/founders.htm*

Small Business Owner Competency *http://www.councils.org/1small business/owner operator/index*

CapBuild GMI *http://www.gmi.org/research/capbuild.htm*

Capacity *http://www.gdrc.org/uem/capacity-define.html.*

http://www.imf.org/

http://www.oceansatlas.org/

15

FOREST POLICIES AND LEGISLATIONS IN INDIA AND NEPAL: A COMPARATIVE STUDY*

Yogesh Ranjit

Background

The terms 'Forest Policy' and 'Legislation' mean the programmes and actions of a government for protection, management, optimal use and sustainable development of forests and forest products in a given period of time. It is also defined as a set of principles or/and guidelines adopted by a government to attain fixed objectives and targets in forestry for the welfare of people and nation as a whole. In early days, there was no any specific forest policy and legislation. People at that time were much conscious about self belonging to the nature and importance of forests. The use of forests and forest products was undertaken on the basis of indigenous and traditional management system with the sufficient customary rights of people over the use of forest. Custom itself prohibited the cutting of certain trees like *Pipal, Bel,* and *Banyan* and protected certain patch of religious forests (*Dharmic Ban*). Similarly, there was very less or almost no problem in forests use and management due to the existence of vast tracts of forests, a small size of population and less demand for forest products. However, some rulers in those days had made some specific guidelines for better use and management of forests. After some time when forest degradation started widely due to it's over use and exploitation, the Governments of both India and Nepal have announced various forest policies and legislations which became tighter one after another over time period. But it did not produce anticipated results. So, ultimately, governments pursued people-oriented forest policy and legislation in mid of 1970's in Nepal and in late 1980's in India which are functioning till to date with increasing level of participation but facing with some problems like less effectiveness and socio-economic inclusion of real users.

Objectives and Methodology

The main objective of the paper is to critically examine various forest policies and legislations of India and Nepal along with comparison of them in general. So, the paper is fully based on the secondary source of information. Hence, it involves a review of various available forest policies and legislations of both countries. A deep consultation with experts in the field of joint forest management (JFM) in India and community forest management (CFM) in Nepal was also undertaken in order to explore more idea about the implementation of those forest policies and legislations. Besides, informal discussions with the members of forest related organizations like VFCs in India, FUGs in Nepal and forest officials were also held in order to have better understanding about the impacts of concerned policy and legislation in grass root level as well.

Historical Development in India

Pre-British Government (Before 1757)

Ancient India (up to 800)

Indian civilization, economy, culture, society and livelihoods are being closely associated with forests and forest products since the time immemorial. During Maurya rule, Chanakya (Kautilya), a renowned teacher and prime advisor to the King

Chandra Gupta Maurya in his book '*Arthasastra*' written during 325 to 273 B.C, mentioned some valuable guidelines related to forestry like classification of forests, plantation in boundaries among villages, separate forests for special trees like *chandan, ashok* and *palash,* proper exploitation and good marketing for forest products, appointment of superintendent of forest, specific fines for destroying or harming tress of different kinds etc. Although there were no any formal forest policy and legislation for using forests during the rulers of Maurya Dynasty, forests were found in the large tracts with a sound system of conservation.

Gupta Dynasty also followed almost similar system of forest management. But the conservation of forest might have been paid lesser attention in comparison to the Maurya period. After ending of Gupta dynasty in 673, the country was again divided in to small states that usually fought among themselves that caused destruction of forests. People destroyed forests for their settlement and extension of farm land. This was singular period in the history of India that forests were destroyed on the account of political instability (Lal, 1989). But during the period of Harshvardhan, a famous king of 7th century, forests had been in prosperous condition that remained till 800 A.D. Hence, it can be concluded that forestry had been maintaining to a large extent under the guidelines of Kautilya.

Medieval India (800-1526)

During Medieval India, forests had occupied a large percentage of geographical areas of the country through natural regeneration. Although the Sultans of Medieval India had deep interest in keeping sound forests, the exploitation of natural forests had gradually increased due to increase in demand for forest products with increasing both human and livestock population and pace of urbanization. They paid very less attention towards the promotion and better exploitation of forest (Jha, 1994). But, a few Sultans took keen interest towards the promotion of social forestry like Ala-ud-Din-khalji (1296-1316) and Firoz Tuglak (1351-1388). However, the Sultan's efforts towards promotion of Indian forestry deteriorated during

Medieval India in comparison to Ancient India though the coverage of forestlands had remained satisfactory during the rule of Sultans and forests had been meeting the requirements of the country.

Mughal India (1526–1757)

Mughal kings had shown favourable attitude towards forestry. They adopted various programmes of fuel-wood trees plantation, block plantation and shady trees in both sides of all-important roads like in social forestry (Mahajan, 1970). A few tree species were specified as 'Royal Trees' and a high fee were charged on their felling and removal. But there was no such a tight restriction policy on cutting of other trees (Lal, 1989). The condition and area of forest was satisfactory in general. Although the area of forests started decreasing on the account of settlement and cultivation, they were capable of producing as much as the requirement of people and government revenue. But, the pace of urbanization has notably hampered the balanced growth of forest. Besides, some factors adversely affected to the condition of forests due to occurrence of natural calamities, series of battles and weak administration after the death of Aurangzeb in 1707 (Jha, 1994).

Hence in pre-British Period, it can be concluded that forests in India were collectively managed and customarily used based on a set of cultural, religious and social norms, values and beliefs which ensured the protection, management, optimal use and sustainable development of forests and forest resources.

British Colonial Period (1757-1947)

Although Victory laid the foundation of British Empire in India in the battle of 'Plassey' in 1757, the British Administration remained indifferent towards the problems of Indian forestry up to nearly the first half of 19th century. So, when the British Administration realized the commercial value of forests, they started formally imposing a number of restrictions on the use of forests and forest products through various forest policies and legislations on the name of better forest protection and management (Chaudhari, 1989).

When Captain Watson was appointed as a 'Conservator of Forest' in November 1806, he started felling maximum quantities of timber for building the ships of the British Navy. So, he was regarded as a plunder rather than conservator. The first step taken by the British Government to improve forests in India was the teak plantation at Nilambu of Madras in 1842 undertaken by Chatter Memon, a sub-conservator of forest (Lal, 1989). However, no other steps were taken for central and north India. The situation continued up to the year 1858 when the Queen Victoria was declared as Emperor of India by Royal proclamation. The years started massive felling forests nearly all over the country to obtain timber for railway sleepers. Hence, the British administrators had only concerned to secure big supply of teak and other timber for the Royal Navy and railway sleepers. So, their attitudes towards forest till the mid of 19th century were to obtain large quantities of Indian timber for the use of local construction, ships, railway sleepers and export the scanted sandalwood to various European countries and free extension of farm land by clearing forests.

The First forest Memorandum (charter) 1855

The forest memorandum of 1855 was the first written step of British Government of India during the period of Lord Dalhousie, the Governor General that provided many guidelines restricting the rights of the different communities particularly the forest-dwellers and tribal on the name of forest conservation and promotion. This memorandum starts scientific forest management in India. According to this memorandum, state forests are administered for only national benefit not to the personal benefit. Although, the policy was never fully implemented, a successive forest acts put more and more restriction on people's rights over forests (Kulkarni, 1989). The charter was later modified in 1894 as the first forest policy of India.

However, the systematic management of forests in India began with the appointment of Dietrich Brandis, a trained German forester as the first Inspector General of Forest in 1864. Then, he changed the objectives of forests management from obtaining supply of timber for various purposes as above mentioned to protection and improvement for biological growing entity. The immediate task of the newly created Forest Department were exploration and demarcation of forests, protection of forest fire, control on shifting cultivation and assessment of growing stock in valuable forest etc. (Lal, 1989). At the same time, the British government of India also started treating forests as a state property and thereby abandoned individual rights over forests.

Indian Forest Act-1865, 1st, May

The first Forest Act of British Government of India, under the guidance of Dietrich Brandis in 1865, formulated various rules about tree growth, prohibition of forest fire, removals of natural products, shifting cultivation and grazing of cattle. The Act fully empowered the state governments to declare any land covered with trees or brushes as government forests without any objection of individuals or communities. Besides, the state governments were also empowered to prescribe punishments for the branch off against the Act. Basically, the major objective of the Act was to establish strong control of state government over forests on the name of effective protection and management of forests and to attain the standard of forest management on lines of Western Europe. However, this Act was not a comprehensive one.

Indian Forest Act-1878

Indian Forest Act-1878 was an amendment of Forest Act-1965. The new Act was more comprehensive and improved than the earlier one by providing classification of forests like 'Reserve', 'Protected' and 'Village' forests. The Act also empowered local governments and officers to record, ensure and notify the use of pasturelands, forests and forest products. Hence, the Indian Forest Act-1878 fully extended the government control over forests. However, this Act preferred to some extent the claims of people's traditional rights to forests and forest products in the proposed 'Reserve' and 'Protected' forests (Kulkarni, 1989).

Forest Policy-1894 (19th October)

The first Forest Policy of India was implemented in October 1894 under the initiation of Dr. Voolcker (Kulkarni, 1989) by emphasizing on productive function of forestry. The policy basically consisted on three elements like public benefit of forests, permanently conversion of forestlands to farm land and functional classification of forests into four types like 'Preserve', "Product', 'Minor' and 'Pasture Forests'. The policy also paved rights and privileges of forest-dwellers over forests and forest products to some extent (Jha, 1994). But the policy was fully failed to give any guidelines for forest protection, maintenance of ecological balance, environmental stability and biological diversity. It did not pay any attention to the problem of forest-based industries, sustained supply of forest products and tree plantation. The policy has also not conceived any definite proportion of forest area to geographical area (Jha, 1994). However, it is not difficult to say that the policy has provided base for conservation of forests and the foundation of forestry education and research in India even though many aspects of Indian forestry had been ignored in the policy.

Forest Act-1927

The Forest Act of 1878 was revised and replaced by the comprehensive Indian Forest Act-1927. The new Act highly focused on the control aspects of forest governance and regulation of felling trees under private ownership. However, the prime motive of the Act was to establish the ownership of the British Government of India over forests and forests resources of India in order to provide timbers to the British Navy (ship industry) and Indian Railways. However, the Act took place a representative of forest legislation of its Era so that it also served as the base of forest laws in Nepal up to 1970's and many other British colonies as well. At the end of Second World War, Sir. Herbert Howard framed a new post-war forest policy of India in 1944 (Jha, 1994). But at the same time, the national freedom movement against the British Government took place at the top most level and thereafter the fag of British administration end on 15th August, 1947. So, no action could be taken accordingly the Draft Forest Policy.

Hence, it can be concluded that the main thrust and objective of forest policy of British government of India was to create monopoly ownership over forests, land and other natural resources of India. It never gave any priority to forestry in the Indian economy so that there was much shifting (*Jhum*) cultivation to maximize the state revenue on the name of better protection and management of forests by giving only 'Lip Sympathy' to environmental stability, ecological balance and meeting the basic forest products to the people. The overall proportion of forests was also not satisfactory. At the end of the British rule, it handed over only about 14% of forest area of poor quality to the Independent India in 1941 (Joshi, 1992).

However, looking back once, British rulers made a huge change in the notion of importance of forest in India. Basically, they gave a good system of regular forest working to the country. It was no doubt that the British Administration started forestry education and research in India, but never put up it to the mark. So, it is not difficult to say that the British administration laid the foundation of efficient forest department and effective forest research institutions. Last, but not the least, we may conclude that the British ruler introduced some good notion of forestry in India with some mistakes in principle and practice and also left some important gapes among the objectives, targets and efforts.

After Independence (1947-1988)

The partition of the country in 1947 obviously disturbed the equilibrium of Indian physical, socio-economic, cultural, environmental and ecological balance of the country. Due to the partition, India shared 77.2% geographical area and 80.8% of population of the undivided country (Jha, 1994). So, after Independence, there was some rethinking on the issues of forests and forest management. After celebration of first and second '*Van Mahotsava*' in 1950 and 1951 respectively, people started realizing the importance of forest (Lal, 1989). In addition, the government also owns most of the forests through the

'Forest Nationalization and Land Reform Laws-1951'. So, to have uniformity in forest management activities among all the states, the Independent Government of India realized a new forest policy to be implemented and that was enunciated on the 12th May, 1952.

National Forest Policy-1952 (12th May)

The new National Forest Policy-1952 was announced under the initiation of Shri. K.M. Munshi, then Food and Agriculture Minister of the Union Government on 12th May, 1952. The policy emphasized ecological (protective function) and social (productive functions) aspects of forests and gave only the secondary importance to the needs of commerce, industry and government revenue (Kulkarni, 1989). The policy took four types of functional classification of forests like 'Protection', 'National', 'Village' forest and 'Tree Lands'.

But, the forest activities were highly based on increasing government revenue by supplying timber for industries, railways, urban markets, exports and for defense needs. The concept of forest protection, conservation, sustainability, maintaining biological diversity and botanical regeneration was put only on paper and almost forgotten in practice (Indurkar, 1992). The policy shifted the traditional diverse and mixed forest to single plantation of commercial species like Teak and *Eucalyptus*. Hence, after announcement of the forest policy, the foresters who were to be conserver the forest eco-system became the main agents of reducing the diversity of forest species (Saxena, 1993). Although the policy paid due attention to supply basic forest products to the rural people in regular basis through village forests, *Adivasis* living in and around the forests were discouraged from using it as if they were enemies of forests. So, in this regard the policy looked like an extension of the old policies British Administration.

But, despite above shortcomings, we find a several marked decisions and improvement of the policy over the policy of 1894. It stated not conversion of forestlands into farm land throughout the country, proper control over private forests, importance of forest research in silviculture, botany, wildlife, forestry education and training for forestry staff. But this policy was failed for providing adequate finance for the scientific research. At the top most, fixation of one-third geographical area of the country under forests was a landmark achievement in the development of the history of Indian forestry in which the Mountain and Hills regions where erosion was the serious problem must be covered by 60% of forests and 20% of forest for plain area of the country where erosion was not a serious problem (GoI, 1952). But it did not recommend any fixing time-bound programme for the attainment of that fixed geographical coverage of forests. However, despite such given shortcomings, there is no room for hesitation to say that this policy displayed a marked improvement and exhibited an importance over the previous policy.

Indian Forest Bill (Forest Conservation Act) 1980

As the 42nd Amendment of Indian Constitution-1976 shifted the subject of forests from 'State List 'to 'Concurrent List', the state governments can divert forestlands for non-forestry purposes (like road, dam, canal etc.) only with the permission of the Central Government. So, following the amendment of constitution, Indian Forest Bill of 1980 curtailed the powers of the state governments over forests. But, in the beginning, there were not many clear implications in this regard to the state governments so that in many cases, they did not take any permission from the Central Government for some years before diversion of forestlands to non-forestry purposes. The real restriction imposed by the Act in diversion of forestlands was felt only after 1985 (Saxena, 1995).

But, on the other hand, the Act made state governments more powerful in order to declare any lands as forestlands even without trees or shrubs just like in the forest act of 1865. Similarly, forest officers and government staff are given more power to arrest and safeguard. But, unfortunately, they could not use that power in sufficient degree. The Bill also emphasized on forest protection through the cooperation of local people. But, unfortunately, that forest was not for the people. Because, the Act denies the real worth of forests in being a source of livelihood for tribal, *Adivasi* and millions of the poor people who live in and around the forests. Thus, the Bill clearly showed the pro-rich, pro-urban and anti-rural people bias (Kulkarni, 1989). It will also lead towards flooding of unskilled rural labourers into urban markets by driving the forest dwellers out of the forests which will increase the mass poverty in rural area. But the Bill, yet to be enacted, has evoked a lot of controversy.

Hence, it can be concluded that the first thirty years of Independent India were primarily used the national forests for timber and industrial needs by ignoring the de-facto rights and needs of forest dependent communities. Similarly, the next twelve years from 1976-1988 continued commercial forestry for some years and then slightly shifted the notion to meet the basic forest products for rural people and forest based industries through plantation in non-forests and private lands under social forestry programme.

After 1988

New Forest Policy 1988

Following the strong recommendation of the National Agricultural commission-1976 for the formulation of new forest policy, the Government of India announced the New National Forest Policy in 1988. The Policy basically changed the traditional notion and objectives of forestry from productive to protective function for ensuring environmental stability and maintenance of ecological balance along with satisfying people's basic needs of forest products like fuel wood, fodder and grass. So, the policy made some specific guidelines for the preservation, maintenance, restoration, sustainable utilization and enhancement of natural environment by conserving of total biological diversity and genetic continuity, national parks, sanctuaries, biosphere reserves and other protected areas. After Independence of India, the policy of 1988 for the first time highly considered the customary rights and concessions of tribal and other poor people living in and around the forests by providing basic forest products on priority basis and carrying capacity of the forests. The policy gave higher priority to forest conservation rather than to earning government revenue.

The policy made some improvement over the previous policy accepting minimum 33% of geographical area under forests and tree cover along with 66 % for Mountain and Hill regions in order to prevent effectively erosion and land degradation and 20% area of plain area to ensure the stability of the fragile eco-system (GoI, 1988). But it did not make any separate policy for the Mountain/Hills and Plain area. The policy also paid a special attention towards the problems and importance of forest-based industries, private forests and social forestry including both farm and agro-forestry and tree plantation alongside of roads, rivers, railway lines, streams and canals. It also discourages monocultures plantation. The policy also provides guidelines to stop the century-old practice of forest encroachment and shifting cultivation. The policy also paid a special emphasis on promoting forest education, research, mass media, audio-visual aids through out the nation for sustainable scientific forest management and creating consciousness amongst people. But this policy was failed to lay guidelines for providing adequate finance for the scientific research and education in forestry. Thus, the forest policy of 1988 was radically different from the previous policies that removed the shortcomings of the forest policies of both 1894 and 1952. At the top most, the policy emphasized the imperatives of people's needs of forest products, preservation, maintenance, sustained utilization, enhancement of environmental stability and maintenance of ecological balance through active people's participation. Although the policy is highly people-centered, it lacks statutory force as forest administration is based on the Indian Forest Act-1927 that does not reflect the spirit of the new policy.

Joint Forest Management Order-1990 (1st June)

Following the forest policy of 1988, the MoEF has issued memorandum/guidelines (No. 6.21/89-FP) on 1st June, 1990 to all the state governments for the involvement of village committees as a partner and voluntary agencies as facilitators in the forest protection, management, optimal utilization and sustainable development of degraded forests. With in the few years of that, it spread to most of the states of the nation. However, in the first decade of implementation of JFM, the outcomes were largely influenced by some factors like the attitude and ethos of the forest bureaucracy, lack of understanding of social-economic and cultural value system of the locals, participation of women, poor, disadvantaged and marginalized people, inter and intra village conflicts, lack of statutory authority to local institutions and coverage of only degraded forests under JFM etc. So, the central government revised the JFM order in time to time.

Joint Forest Management Guideline-2000 (21st February)

The Government of India revised the JFM order on 21st February, 2000. This guidelines solved the problems of above mentioned to a large extent with the compulsory registration of all VFCs under the societies registration Act-1860, 50% women participation in general body, 33% in executive committee and at least one official person chosen from amongst the female members of the committee, extension of JFM in good forest areas as well, and preparation of micro-plan, conflict resolution, 25% contribution of forest benefits in the Village Development Fund for conservation and development of the forests, monitoring, evaluation and transparence etc. But, after few years, some practical problems emerged in smoothly functioning JFM.

JFM Strengthening Guildeline-2002 (24th December)

The Government of India again revised the guidelines to make more strengthen the JFM programme by incorporating various above issued in 2002 like memorandum of understanding for Forest Department and VFCs, non-political relationship between *Panchayats* and VFCs, institutional reforms, capacity building for the management of NTFPs, equity in distribution of forest-benefits among poor, women, disadvantaged and marginalized people etc. Thus, it shows that the government of India has been increasingly concerned about the conservation of the country's forests through people's participation by formulating various forest policies and legislation in different time period based on people's needs with out compromising the national interest.

Hence, it can be concluded that from 1988 onward, there was a radical and paradigm shift from the earlier revenue-oriented to conservation-oriented forestry through a decentralized forest policy by inviting local people with VFCs as partner and NGOs as facilitator in forest regeneration and management of degraded forestlands. But starting with 21st century, it was extended to good natural forests as well and social inclusion in the programme. The historical timeline pattern of forest policies and legislation in India can also be revealed with the help of given Box: 1.

Historical Development in Nepal

Pre-unification of Nepal (Before 1768)

Prior to 1768, Nepal was consisted of a number of small kingdom, principalities and tribal areas. So, before unification of the country by the Shah Dynasty, the nation was governed by different rulers of different dynasty like *Kirats, Lichivis, Devas* and *Mallas* for several centuries. All royal orders related to forestry at that time were taken as forest policy and legislation. Basically, the historical account of this period is mainly based on chronicles, inscriptions and travelogues by foreign travelers (Bhattarai and Khanal, 2005).

During the Lichhivi period, royal orders were normally issued for harvesting trees and other NTFPs for domestic purposes and other authorized local bodies like Panchalis (a committee of village elders) to settle the matters of the use of forest and forest products (Tiwari, 1989). States taxes known as *'Sinkar'* on the export of wood products and herbs were also levied during the Lichhivi period.

Similarly, during the Malla period royal orders were frequently issued to protect forests of different areas of Kathmandu Valley like Kritipur, Soyambhu, Balaju, Changu, Gokarna, Bajrajogini as *Ban Gadh* (forest moats) and people in

Box 1
Historical Timeline of
Forest Policies and Legislations in India

Policies and Legislations/Years	Main Thrust	Remarks
Charter of Indian Forestry , 1855	Restriction on the free use of forest and forest resources to private individuals.	First written document in forestry as a starting of scientific forest management but it is not for the benefits of local people, only to the state.
Indian Forest Act - 1865	Fully empowered the state governments in judicious use of forests and forest resources.	Starting objective-oriented forestry and fully State controlled over forests in the name of its protection and management.
Indian Forest Act - 1878	Extension of State control over forests with 3 types of classification of forests.	Giving very less local rights in the forests to fulfill only subsistence needs
First Forest Policy of India - 1894	Priority for conversion of forests to farm land, protection of forest for ecological balance, reclassification of forests by giving some rights to forest dwellers over forests.	Fail to give proper attention in ecological balance giving emphasis only on maximum revenue generation in practice
Indian Forest Act- 1927	Containing all major provision of the earlier Acts by providing regulation of felling in forests under private ownership.	A bold and comprehensive Act mainly to establish a strong ownership of the British over forests and lands of India.
Forest policy -1952	Emphasizing the ecological and social aspects of forestry, functional classification of forest and fixation of 33% geographical area of the country under forests.	Commercial use of forests highly dominated for increasing government revenue with out ensuring ecological balance and biological diversity.
Forest Conversation Act- 1980	State government can't divert forestlands for non forestry purpose without permission of the Central government of India.	Curtailed powers of State governments over the use of forests but that was effect in full-fledged only after 1985.
New Forest Policy- 1988	Giving top priority to forest protection not for government revenue by satisfying the minimum needs of forest products to the local people under people's participation.	Reestablished the customary rights of local people on using forests by clearly inviting people's participation in the protection and management of forests.
JFM Resolution- 1990 (1st June)	Legally invites local people as partner and NGOs as facilitator in forest protection and management and regeneration activities.	The first decade of JFM was largely influenced by the attitudes of forest bureaucracy and socio-economic factors.
JFM Guidelines - 2000 (21st February)	Extension of JFM to good forests, compulsory registration of all VFCs, preparation of micro plan, 50% women participation in General Body and 33% in Executive Body.	It solved the given problems to a large extent but not sufficient to go ahead.
JFM Strengthening Guildeline-2002 (24th December)	Strengthen of JFM programme through institutional reforms, non-political relationship between *Panchayat* and VFCs, capacity building, equity in distribution of forest benefits among all social groups etc.	The government of India has been increasingly concerned about the conservation of forest through people's participation.

those areas were prevented from cutting trees. Any violations of the royal order were immediately punished as per the given rules and regulation. The responsibilities of forest protection and other forest related activities were also assigned to some State functionaries like *Vaskaradhikarta* and *Basota* (in Lichhivi Period) and *Mahane* (in Malla Period). However, *Kipat* system was very common and popular land holding system in the Hills of Nepal before unification of Nepal which gradually changed with political changes. Moreover, there was a strength law relating to forest use and management in the royal orders of king Ram Shah of Gorkha (a small but powerful kingdom of Nepal) during 1606-1633. The similar type of policy of forest use and management was continued during the time of Prithivi Narayan Shah (a king of Gurkha who unfired the Kingdom of Nepal in 1768) and afterwards.

Hence, it could be concluded that the pre-unification period of Nepal was a time of abundance in forests and forest products and that was generally controlled and managed under traditional and indigenous system with out any formal forest policy and legislation.

Post-unification of Nepal (1768-1846)

After taking over the three small Kingdoms of the Kathmandu Valley in 1768 as the last conquest during the regime of Prithivi Narayan Shah, the unification process was further continued by the rest of Shah's descendants. Due to the lack of other natural resources, Prithivi Narayan Shah started a system of distributing a large area of land and forests as grants or reward to army officers and senior office holders/nobility in the forms of *Jagir* and *Birta* respectively in order to bring into cultivation (Mahat et. al., 1986a, 1986b). The system was also continued by other successive rulers as well. Besides, a number of indigenous ethnic groups origin of a particular area also owned lands and forests on a communal basis without any legal entitle like *Kipat* which is an ancient, traditional and communal land holding system in Nepal. Most of the indigenous hill tribes of Nepal held all their lands under a form of *Kipat* (Poffenberge, 2000). No doubt, the Kiratis (Limbu) of the eastern-hill region are the most important Kipat owning community in Nepal. Some other communities like Danuwar, Sunwar, Tamang, Sherpa, Kumales and Lepchay etc. also held lands and forests under such tenure system in both the eastern and western hill regions (Regmi, 1971). However, in most of the places, the *Kipat* system was abolished after the conquest by the Gorkhalies and also changed gradually with political changes. Moreover, another ancient type of indigenous forest management and land revenue collection system is *'Shingo Newa'* which was very popular among the Sherpas of the Khumbu region, an eastern-mountain part of Nepal in which *Sherpas* appoint forest guards for the protection of forests and forest products.

Basically, there was no any formal forest policy and particular forest management program after the unification of Nepal. It was generally believed that there was no need to regulate the forest as the forest resources were plenty and size of population was small. On the contrary, people were encouraged to convert the forestlands into farmlands in order to increase the land-tax revenue of the government. Therefore, in absence of state control and regulation of forests, the people live in and around the forests collected forest products as much as they need. But occasionally some royal orders were issued to regulate specified forest area for special purpose (Shrestha, 1999). Then gradually the government had started controlling over forests and forest products with the new order announced in 1799. By 1886, the Terai forests were classified with high commercial value (*Sira*), low commercial value (*Jhora*) and protected forest. The government staff carefully regulated the system of exports of forest products (Poffenberger, 2000). So, after unification of Nepal, much area of forestlands was distributed in the forms of *Jagir* and *Birta* grants to be converted into farm land. A very little interest was paid in forest protection and management process.

Hence, during post unification of Nepal, an active land reclamation policy was adopted which led to heavy clear of forests especially in the Hills.

Rana Regime (1846-1950)

For the period of 104 years (1846 to 1950), Nepal was ruled by a 'Hereditary Dynasty' of Rana Prime Ministers in which the position of Shah Kings was just figureheads as king only on name like a parrot in a prison There was no any formal forest policy and legislation in written form. In those days, what ever the thoughts emerged in the mind of Rana Priministers and what ever the words come out through the speech of them on any matter that became the national rules and regulation. In fact, during the period, there were some informal forest rules that were very strict so that cutting even a small tree without permission of the authority was prohibited. Any one found having cut a tree without permission might be jailed or heavy punished. One who cut a *Bijaya Sal* (Pterocarpus marsupium) tree could be punished death penalty. But, on the contrary, individuals were also encouraged to convert forestlands into farm land as a means of extending state control over the territory and increasing state revenue through land tax.

Along with some strict forest rules, forests of Nepal were exploited for the expansion of agriculture and government revenue generation (Hobley et. al. 1996) like in earlier period. It may be due to lack of proper and formal forest policy and legislation in that period. Basically, successive Rana Priministers took the policy of extending the cultivation in Terai plains by clear felling the forests for government revenue generation. Exploitation of forest was formulized through the legal judicial process under the rule of the first Rana Prime Minister, Jung Bahadur Rana during 1846-1877 (Hobley et. al. 1996). Besides, a large area of forests was also allotted as *Shorhana* in the Hills and *Birta* in Terai to the Rana family members (Rai, 1997). By the end of Rana Government in 1951, one-third of the countries farmland and forests were held under *Birta* land grants, out of which 75% belonged to members of the Rana family (Regmi, 1978). Those *Birta* forestlands also cleared after some time for cultivation that was tax free and heritable (Shrestha, 1999). In fact, there was a strong and significant British influence in the forest use and exploitation activities in Nepal. So at that time, massive exploitable of the national forest in Terai were carried out especially for excessive timber exports to British India. Although there was no any formal forest policy and legislation in Nepal, the forests were not much degraded as it did after 1950's that may be due to very tight informal forest rules in Rana Period (Rai, 1997).

Hence, it can be concluded that during Rana Regime the adopted policy was highly concentrated on rights over forests in the hands of ruling family and other courtesans, active reclamation of forestlands both in the Hills and Terai, commoditization of forest resources, indiscriminate felling of trees for timber exports to British Government of India for railway sleepers and Navy and encouragement of converting forestlands to farm land that promoted massive clearance of forests in many areas of the nation.

After Independence (1950-1988)

Following the democratic movement in 1951, many changes took place in political, socio-economic, cultural and forestry sector as well. The forestry sector of Nepal addresses all the sub-sectors including land use pattern, soil conservation, watershed management, national park and wildlife conservation etc. At the same time, the government was very knee to formulate a forest policy. So, a first draft forest policy was prepared in 1952 under the initiation of Mr. E .J. B. Rana (a forest officer) and E. Robbe (an expert of FAO) which made first time a clear provision for community forestry (Tiwari, 1989). But unfortunately, the then government did not approve the policy. On the contrary, the government felt a necessity to go for a radically centralized ides of nationalizing the private forests through the Private Forest Nationalization Act-1957. However, in Nepal, there were no any comprehensive forest policies and legislations before 1957.

Private Forest Nationalization Act (PFNA)-1957

Following the democratic movement in 1951, government of Nepal started taking officially full responsibility over forest control and management system all over the kingdom through the PFNA-1957. This was a first legislation as a bold step of the government in order to wrest private forests with out any compensation. The Act provided only 1.25 ha. of forests in the Hills and 3.25 ha. in the Terai to be held as private forests (Bhattarai and Khanal, 2005).

But, unfortunately, the Act let feudal landlords to large-scale feeling down of trees to prevent the land being classified as forestlands and therefore to become government-owned

(Hobley et. al., 1996). Similarly, villagers reacted negatively to the act because they feared that it would curtail their traditional and customary rights of forest uses. Likewise, communities had no any stake in the preservation of forests. As the result, the *de-facto* and *de-jure* responsibilities of forests disappeared so that gradually converted it into an open access and common property resource. Although the idea behind the act was ideal and noble, forests virtually became nobody's concern due to the increasing both human and livestock population and rapid migration from the Hills to Terai with the eradication of malaria in Terai that continued to put heavy and increasing pressure on Terai forests for new settlements and acquisitions of farm land. Similarly, there were no land records so that the land could be claimed as private property if forest was cleared and started cultivation. As a result of the act, there had been a widespread conversion of private forest into farmland especially in the Terai. At the same time, the government started resetting migrated people from the Hills in Terai and some Dun Valleys by clearing the forestlands. No efforts were made to control forest encroachments but people were rather encouraged to settle in the places as they chose. Basically, due to the lack of effective management and communication, limited infrastructure, limited forestry administration, technical expertise, trained manpower, public awareness, the de-facto owners took advantages and destroyed a large area of forests (Shrestha, 1999). In 1959, the first Ministry of Forest was established in order to control over the entire country. But, even after that Hill forests still were not brought under any management plan and the forest administration being understaffed and forests remained unmanaged in the true sense. Hence, unfortunately, state control over forests through the Act was failed to bring the anticipated results (Parajuli, 1997) or might be particularly successive (Hobley *et al.*, 1996).

In fact, the Act was implemented in the form of innovation. If the forest had not been nationalized, most of the accessible and important forests would have gone to the control of handful rich bureaucratic owners. Then at that time, rural poor would either not get permission to have access or have to pay a lot to use basic forests products (Joshi, 1990). But, unfortunately, people were confused with the Act and generally it was believed that the Act was not appropriate due to against the traditional system so that it produced further negative consequences. The process of deforestation was accelerated after 1960 and the rate was especially high during sixties and seventies (Dahal, 1994).

Forest Act-1961

Following the failure of the democratic movement and there by restoration of the power of monarchy in the early 1960's, a new party less system called *'Panchayat'* was introduced. And Thereby the Government of Nepal (GoN) enacted the Forest Act-1961 that sought to restore government administration, registration, demarcation and control over national forests. It also defined the duties of the Department of Forest (DoF), listed forest offences and prescribed penalties as well (Mahat et.al.1986a). Based on decentralization concepts, the act also made provisions for handing over forests to the newly formed *Panchayat,* a lower level of local political body which had far reaching consequences for local control of resources. Besides, private forests that were considered to be poorly managed could be taken over by the government for a period of 30 years and any income from such forest would be given to the owner with some deduction as management cost. Management decision also remained with the government (Hobley, 1996). Four types of forests were categorized by the Act like *Panchayat* Forest, *Panchayat* Protect Forest, Religious Forest and Contract Forest.

However, the act had little impact on those forests area which is situated in distant from Kathmandu (the capital city of Nepal) and inaccessible areas where local people continued to use the forests for subsistence needs regardless of their legal status and force legislation (Palit, 1996). Thus, the Act legitimized *Panchayat(s)* but not the 'Forest User's control over local forests. However the Act opened the way for later changes in legislation and provided the environment in which PFM could emerge (Hobley et. al. 1996).

Forest Protection Act-1967 (A special Arrangements)

The government of Nepal passed the Forest Protection Act-1967 that provided the forestry official judicial power. The local people in the accessible areas in the Hills overtime became apathetic towards government control of the forest, which they had been using for their daily needs. Alienation of people from resource use brought rampant destruction of the forests which was aggravated by the population growth, their need of more forest products and illegal conversion of more forestlands to agriculture. Similarly, a separate act of 'National Park and Wildlife Conservation Act of 1973' was also enacted with an aim to conserve the wild flora and fauna within the national parks, wildlife reserves and conservation area that gave more support to the Forest Protection Act of 1967.

But, the Act was designed in such a way that it facilitated the unhindered harvesting of trees located in the plains of Terai and not in the Hills (Bhattari and Khanal, 2005). In addition, it did not include any environmental consideration like carrying capacity and resource extraction patterns. It also did not respect the traditional individual and collective rights of local people over forest resources and created the forest bureaucracy as the monopolist landlord of forest like in India as the same ideology was imported into Nepal in designing forest laws during 1950s and 1960s. Ideologically, until early 1970s, the legal regime relating to forestry in Nepal was normally based on the Indian Forest Act of 1927 (Bhattari and Khanal, 2005). The Act, however, had little impact on forest protection in the remote areas in the Hills where local people continued to use the forest for their needs regardless of their legal status. In addition, the decision undertaken by the government in 1971 to legalize the encroached forest up to the date helped a large scale felling trees in order to settle there (Shrestha, 1989).

The National Forest Plan-1976

The GoN enacted the National Forest Plan-1976 based on the proceeding of 'Ninth Forestry Conference' held in Kathmandu in 1974. The plan showed a paradigm shift in the forest management by considering forests as inalienable social property (property of society) as against the prior stand it as national property. This plan also formally opened for the first time in the history of forestry of Nepal for involvement of local communities (people's participation) in protection, management and development of forest and forest products through elected local institutions called *'Gram Panchayat'*. The plan reinforced in allocating categories of forestlands to the *Panchayat* as mentioned in forest act of 1961 (Hobley, 1996). However, this plan laid a foundation for scientific forests management in the Hills and Terai. The major objectives of the plan were the restoration of the balance of nature, economic mobilization, development of technology and promotion of public cooperation and participation etc.

But, on the contrary, the local people were illegally using government forests to meet their basic needs of firewood, fodder, grasses and leaf litter. But, in many cases, access was regulated by local practice and not by the forest department staff. This situation has led to the current situation where only option for the sustained management of hill resources lies in a partnership between local people and forest department staff. It is because that the department of forest had neither been able to stop the destruction of the forest nor had been able to manage the remaining forests in successive years (Joshi, 1993). However, the scope of this Plan was limited to a few divisions of the Terai and Dang Forest Division in the Siwalik. It could not fulfill all the objectives specified in the plan and fully operational in all aspects due to various reasons (Parajuli, 1997). Actually, the Plan was the first official written document devoted to major policy guideline for forestry and also recognized past mistakes and emphasized the need to correct them.

In order to directly involve local people in forest protection and management activities, the HMG/N gradually amended the Forest Act of 1961 in 1977 and 1978 that classified the forests of Nepal into national, *Panchayat, Panchayat* protected, religious, leasehold and private forests. It also made a provision to handover village *Panchayats* much degraded natural forests to be planted and protected in the form of *Panchayat* forests and well natural forest as *Panchayat* Protect forests. This indicates that the government was not only interested to involve people in plantation in degraded forests but also in the management of good natural forests (Parajuli, 1997). Thus, we can see the commitment of the government gradually shifted the responsibility of forest resources management from government to local bodies that can be taken as an institution of a process of decentralization. However, to give legal authority for people's participation, the government promulgated the *Panchayat* Forest and *Panchayat* Protected Forest Rules in 1978.

The Panchayat Forest (PF) and Panchayat Protected Forest (PPF) Rules-1978

A serious and revolutionary wave was made in forestry policy by enacting of the PF and PPF Rules-1978. Under the supervision of District Forest Officer, this legislation provided handing over of any parts of accessible government forests to local people respective of concerned village *Panchayat* boundary in order to control and manage as a community forests. Each village *Panchayat* is eligible for 125 ha. of government degraded forestland for the creation of PF while 500 ha. of well natural forests can be handed over as PPF (HMG/N, 1978). Besides, the village *Panchayats* were prohibited to carry out some activities in the both types of forest like handing over, selling, mortgaging, cultivating fruits, orchard, constructing building and any other land use except allowed by the 'Working Plan'.

But, the success was very limited in management and handing over of forest area and much of them was further degraded. An enough interest for participation could not be generated among the real users who could protect the forest so that results were disappointed (Bhatia, 1999) due to the lack of a clear definition of user group and procedure for handing over the authority. There was an absent of 'Community Components' in 'Community Forestry' under the Rules. Basically, the responsibility of using forests and control of them should fall on the same group of people. But, the Rules provided only one way to participate where as forest resources were strictly controlled by the village Panchayats. Actually, the *Panchayat* is the lowest level of political body, not a user group (Kanel, 1993) so that politics and political affairs existed much in the village rather than the work of forest protection and management. In addition, due to the highly degraded forests and located them mostly too far to monitor, the elected village leaders of *Panchayats* did not show required incentives to control and manage them. So, lack of ownership on forests could not mobilize the grass root support from the real users of the forests.

Hence, from 1976 to 1987, only near about 2% area of forests (36,376 ha) out of targeted (18,35,000 ha.) was handed over to local communities (Bhattari and Khanal, 2005). Similarly, in the first fourteen years of implementing PP and PPF rules, only 2% of the potential community forest area of 61% of national forest (Tamrakar and Nelson, 1990) has come under management which indicates that the management of the remaining potential community forest area will take at least another 400 years, if the speed of activities remaining the same (Joshi, 1993). Hence, the failure of such 'local level' concern but '*Panchayat* level' application rule demonstrated decrease in forest area from 6.5 million ha. in 1965 to 5.5 million ha. in 1990 (Shrestha, 1996).

However, the legislation can be considered as bold with a major shift in forestry policy empowering local community in forest resource control and management in order to meet basic forest products. At the top most, on the one hand the Rules made some positive effects to mitigate the negative effects of the PFNA-1957 where as on the other, the year 1978 could be considered as a starting step for giving birth of community forestry programme in Nepal. The PF and PPF Rules were also fully supported by the Sixth Five-Year Plan (1981-1985), the Soil Conservation and Watershed Management Act-1982 and Decentralization Act-1982 and Regulation-1984. The PF and PPF Rules of 1978 were amended in 1988 for adopting the concept of 'FUGs' in forest management programme.

Hence, it can be concluded that after Independence, the forest policy was to export timbers to India, forest nationalization, conversion of forestlands to farm lands and settlement area through forest encroachment. But from mid

1970's, it is shifted to protection function of forestry with decentralized forest policy through community participation to meet their needs of basic forest products.

After 1988

Master Plan for the Forestry Sector (MPFS)-1988

The MPFS-1988 (approved by the GoN in 1989) provided a long term comprehensive and systematic development plan of the entire forestry sector by setting up medium and long term objectives for 22 years (1988-2010). The major objective of the Plan was to meet people's basic needs of timber, fuel-wood, dodder, grass and other forest products on a sustained basis and to promote people's participation in the forest protection and management (MPFS-1988). The MPFS also equally addresses the issue of poor and women participation by stipulating in its guidelines that one-third of any user committee's members should be women.

Hence, community forestry was given highest priority in the Plan with two major components like community plantation and management of degraded forests and management of natural forests as community forestry like in the PF and PPF Rules-1978. But now onward there is no ceiling on the area of forest handing over along with irrespective of residential and political boundary of village, ward and district. However, success was very limit by handing over only a small fraction of the total forest area more of which was further degraded or lost during these days. The major reason for disappointed results was the impractical nature of the rules which failed to create an environment for the full participation of all users. They did not provide a clear procedure for the transfer of authority for the protection, management and utilization of forests to the real users.

However, the policy highly supports the development and management of forest resources through the active participation of individuals and communities to meet their basic needs and embarks on the phased handing over of all accessible Hill forests to communities to the extent that they are able and willing to manage them. The Plan designated FUGs as the principal vehicle for local collective and stipulated the forest staff to adopt new roles as advisors and facilitator. Moreover, the weaknesses of PF and PPR Rules-1978 were removed by the policy advocated by the MPFS-1988 which recognized the concept of FUG. The Plan is also fully supported by the new Constitution of Nepal-1990 and other Plans related to environment like Environmental Impact Assessment (EIA) guidelines-1992 and Nepal Environmental Policy and Action Plan (NEPAP)-1993.

Forest Act-1993

Following the new national constitution-1990 and various environmental plans, the GoN implemented the Forest Act-1993 that is the latest and very revolutionary forest legislation with strengthening the MPFS policy-1988. The Act identified forests into two broad categories namely 'National Forests' and 'Private Forests'. The national forests also classified in to five sub-types like Government-managed Forests, Community Forests, Protected Forests, Leasehold Forests and Religious Forests (HMG/N, 1993). Basically the act highly emphasized on the concept of 'Community Forestry' and 'User Group' as an autonomous and self governing institution that assigned more responsibility to the people or communities to manage a part of government forests as community forests in accordance with the given 'Operational Plan'. It also recognized and legalized the process of handing over community forests to the 'User Groups. The Act also shifted the earlier objective of community forestry as to fulfill the subsistence needs of forest products to commercialization.

Forest Regulation-1995

In order to prescribe the procedural matters of the Forest Act-1993, GoN has enacted forest regulations-1995 by giving prime importance to community forestry and leasehold forests with more decentralized and people oriented than before. The regulation basically focused on the determination of forests on various types, preparation of 'Constitution' and 'Operational Plan' of user groups, their registration, procedure of handing over the forest, collection, pricing, selling and distribution of forest products, functions prohibited in the forests, transportation of forest products, maintenance of records, operation of users' group's fund etc. It also indirectly advocated a change in the role of forestry staff from policing job to a facilitator (HMG/N, 1995). The user groups can also legally cultivate various types of NTFPs and perennial cash crops for sale in the community forest if the activity does not decrease crown cover and productivity of the forest. But the Regulation did not define the name of cash crops. Both the natural and degraded forests could be handed over to user groups with 100% of the benefits which is one of the greatest strength of the community forestry program in Nepal. The price of forest products could be autonomously determined by the user groups but it should not be below the revenue rate fixed by the government or the cost price of the products. All income of the user group will go to the fund of user groups controlled by them that could be used for development of community forests and community development activities. But user groups are not allowed to sell or handed over forestlands to another user group or institution. The tenure rights of the forestlands still with the government.

However, both the Act-1993 and Regulation-1995 have many serious drawbacks as they did not contain even a single word or clause for balancing production and the distribution of forest products according to household needs and maximizing community income. Similarly, it is not clear whether a member of a user group can sell their share of forest products to another member of the same group or member of another group or to any other institutions. However, the Forest Act-1993 was amended in 1998 with making various provisions that included penalizing forest user committee members on the complaint of member of FUGs for acts committed against the 'Operational Plan' and 'Constitution' of FUG. Besides, following the commitments for the Earth Summit-1992, the first amendment of the Act in 1998 made FUG to spend a minimum 25% of their fund for the development of community forests for global carbon emission, mitigation and biodiversity conservation and only the rest 75% of the fund can be spent for rural development activities. But the Act does not mention whether the expenditure is in annual basis or not. Similarly, it does not explain about what activities can or can not be included under that headings of community forest development programme like study tour, skill development work, management training, salary to forest watchman etc. This has made some confusion among the user's group. Similarly, the first and second amendment of the regulation also took place on 6th September, 1999 and 12th August, 2002 respectively.

Community Forestry Directives-1995

The GoN has again implemented some community forestry directives on 17th September, 1995. The major directives are like determination of the community forests; formation and registration of user groups; preparation of 'Constitution' and 'Operation Plan' of user groups; procedure of handing over the community forests to them; transportation of the forest products; establishment of the forest based industries; inspection of the account and withdrawal of community forests and re-handover etc. The directives also initially included the names of cash crops like tea, coffee, cardamom, black cardamom and similar crops under this group. The directives was amended in 2000 (10th, February) which removed tea and coffee from the list of cash crops but nothing was mentioned about tea and coffee that had already been planted in community forests. Similarly, the amendment also made a provision for compulsorily inclusion of growing stock of community forestry and annual allowable cut in 'Operational Plan'. The directive helped a lot to implement both the Forest Act-1993 and Forest Regulation-1995 as well.

Forest Sector Policy-2000

The forest Sector Policy-2000 has again adopted community forestry programme with protection and conservation view point as it was initially taken in the beginning (Kanel, 2006). As the Terai accounts for 35 % of Nepal's total forest area and also being very rich in young *Sal* trees, the government may have some reluctance to lose control of the resources (Proffemberger, 2000). So, the Policy is especially prepared to handover the barren and isolated forest lands of the Terai, Inner Terai and Churia hills as community forests in which forest products will be used on the basis of annual increment. Under this policy, the government will collect 40% of the earnings from the sale of surplus timber of community forests of Terai, Inner Terai and Siwalik for the implementation of the programme. The large patch of forests in blocks in the Terai and inner-Terai will be managed by the collaborative solidarity of the local users, local political bodies (VDCs and DDCs) and the government but not to local communities as community forests. The users under collaborative solidarity will get only 25% of the income from the sale of surplus forest products and the rest 75% income will go the income of the government. The Churia Hill forests will not be handed over to the users but managed as protected forests for watershed conservation as they are important for recharging the underground water and conserving the soil of Terai. But the policy has created some antagonism between the Terai users and government. So, the Supreme Court annulled this decision. So, the government began to collect this revenue through the Financial Act (i.e. revised in 2003/04) and it is only 15% of the sale of surplus timber of only two commercial species in the Terai. However, we can say that the policy withdraws some of the rights of local users in the Terai and the outcome of the Pilot programme has yet to be seen in the field.

Community Forestry Development Guidelines-2001

The GoN again introduced 'Guidelines for Inventory of Community Forest-2000 that regulates the harvest of products from community forests. This policy restricts the user group to forest harvesting not exceeding 30% to 60% of mean annual allowable (MAI %) depending upon characteristics of species availability in the forests. The hardwood and slow-growing species have greater restrictions than softwood and fast-growing species such as 30 % for Sal, 40% for Sal-pine mixed, 50% for Pine, Khair, Sissoo and Oak, and 60% for Utish, Katus and Chilaune (HMG/N, 2000). The guidelines believed that it is likely to affect the ability of communities to meet their household needs. With the approval of District Forest Officer, the present forest law has allowed FUGs to mortgage community forest resources in order to get a loan from financial institution for the development of community forest like the construction of huts/ houses for security purpose but so far as no visible achievement has been made in this regard (Bhattari and Khanal, 2005). Moreover, as the settlement pattern of community and collection of forest products are not usually limited to single forest area, membership of multiple user groups is also allowed in primary, secondary and tertiary users.

Hence, after Independence, there was also continued commoditization and nationalization of forests to some extent up to mid 1970's. Then it went to fulfilling basic needs through people's participation with a political body '*Gram Panchayat*' up to 1988. From 1988 onward, the policy started real users participation with legally authorized and autonomous local body namely FUGs respecying social inclusion in decision making, equity in distribution of benefits etc. for poverty alleviation and rural development. Moreover, the policy adopted second generation issues of community forestry like good governance, livelihood promotion and sustainable development as a second generation issues in community forestry programme in the beginning of 21st century. The historical timeline pattern of forest policies and legislation in Nepal can also be revealed with the help of given Box: 2.

Similarities

Traditionally, people were much conscious about self-belonging to the nature and environmental importance of forests in both India and Nepal. In the virtual absence of formal and comprehensive forest policies and legislations, local people themselves normally controlled and managed the forests under traditional and indigenous systems and that practices were functioning well at that time. As their livelihood highly depends upon forest and forest products, the local community was much aware for the need of sustainable forest management by pursuing only the seasonal removal of forest products. The

Box 2
Historical Timeline of Forest Policies and Legislations in Nepal

Policies and Legislations/Years	Main Thrust	Remarks
Private Forest Nationalization Act-1957	Nationalized private forests giving only 1.25 ha. in the Hills and 3.25 ha. in Terai to be held as private forests but without any compensation.	First and bold forest legislation but the result is Indiscriminate cutting of forests and almost fully failed in implementation
Forest Act-1961	Protection, management and utilization of forests entrusted to the Dept. of Forest.	The government was unable to manage the forests effectively.
Forest Protection Act- 1967	Judicial Powers of DFO were strengthened further.	Ignoring ecological balance and de-facto rights of local people on use of forests.
The National Forest Plan -1976	Recognized the need for people's participation in forest management.	DOF was unable to stop destruction of forest and fail to fulfill all given objects
P Forest and PP Forest Rule-1978	Handing over only 125 ha. of degraded forests as P Forest and 500 ha. of good natural forests as PP Forest.	Birth of CFP but very limit success due to much existence of politics and lack of a clear definition of FUG.
Master Plan for the Forestry Sector- 1988	Long term comprehensive and systematic development plan strongly emphasizing community forestry through active participation of real FUGs as the principal vehicle in forest management.	The result was not very impressive due to the lack of clear procedure of transferring forest management authority to the real users. It removed some weaknesses of PF and PPF Rules-1978.
Forest Act-1993	Latest and very revolutionary forest legislation that highly emphasized on community forestry and FUGs as an autonomous and self governing body.	It legalized the process of handing over community forests with more responsibility of forest management to FUGs.
Forest Regulation-1995	FUGs can legally cultivate various types of NTFPs in CF and autonomously determine the price, sell and distribution of all forest products by holding 100% benefits to them.	More decentralized legislation but it did not mention about distribution of forest products according to household needs and maximizing FUGs incomes.
Community Forestry Directives-1995	Prescribing procedure for handing over, withdrawal and re-handover of CF with the names of cash crops to be cultivated in CF.	It helped a lot to implement both the Forest Act-1993 and Forest Regulation-1995.
Forestry Sector Policy-2000	Especially prepared to handover the barren and isolated forests of the Terai, inner Terai and Churia hills as CF.	The policy withdraws some of the rights of forest users in the Terai and the outcome has yet to be seen.
CF Development Guidelines-2001	It restricted the FUGs for forest harvesting not exceeding 30% to 60% of mean annual allowable (MAI%) depending upon features of species availability in the forests.	Hopefully, it will help the ability of communities to meet their household needs.

extraction of forests was less than the sustainable supply level of forest resources due to availability of a vast tract of forests, small size of population and less demand for forest resources. So, perhaps governments in both countries at that time did not feel essential of any formal forest policies and legislations.

But, as the time passes, the demand for forest products and the need of government revenue increased due to increase in population both human and livestock. The forest destruction activities also increased from both the sides of government and people as well. They used forests and forest products in such a way that they never considered the future of it. Then both governments started controlling use of forest and forest products through various policy and legislations. After Independence of national, both the governments of India and Nepal nationalized forests in 1950's in the name of controlling the quality and quantity of forest degradation. But the pace of destruction of forest was not stopped rather increased considerably. Besides, there were also no major differences of the process of forest use and exploitation in both countries due to significant influence of British India to Nepal. As the quality and quantity of forest went out of control, government of both nations implemented more and more tight forest policies and legislations. But it could not stop the pace of exploitation of forests and forest products. So, there was high pace of forest destruction took place during 1960 to 1980 in both countries.

Although the notion of forests for environmental protection and ecological balance started globally in 1960's, it was placed only on paper, speech in the programmes and lip sympathy of the government, not in practices in general in both countries. However, in mid of 1970's, as the need of people's participation in forest protection, management and sustainable development was highly felt all over the world, the forest policies and legislations also moved accordingly in many countries but particularly in India and Nepal. There was a parallel development of participatory forest policies and legislations in both countries through village *Panchayats* at the end of 1970's. But due to cancellation of *Panchayat* system in India in1984 (that was reinstalled in 1993 with 43rd amendment of Indian constitution) and in Nepal in 1990, there was a new paradigm shift of control and management of forests from centralized forest departments to decentralized people's institutions as participatory forestry. So, by the late 1980's, it was fully and strongly documented in forest policies and legislations about people's participation in protection and management of forests. But it received legal status and authority only in the beginning of 1990's through the local institution namely VFCs in India and FUGs in Nepal. Hence, the historical background and the legal basis of both the programmes are almost unique to each country. Besides, there are also broad similarities in both at the institutional and implementation level of forest policies and legislations. Though the communities' institutions are distinct, many of the problems and challenges of them are also similar.

Dissilarities

India has experience of 150 years of scientific forest management with the specific and formal forest legislation where as Nepal has only of about 50 years for specific forest legislation with out any scientific forest management practices. But the important policy level changes have been introduced in India only during the last six decades where as the similar changes in Nepal was occurred during the last three decades. The mass destruction of forests in India was especially for government revenue generation, industrial feeding and commercial use of timber. But the case of Nepal was especially for growing food and settlement, exporting timber to India for the British Navy industry and construction of railway lines and that destruction was also under the supervision of British-Indian foresters and Indian forest harvesters. The people of Nepal did not have to start a big movement in the name of '*Chipko Movement*' as did in India by the people of Uttarakhanda under the leadership of Chandi Prasad Bhatt in1973 and 2500 km. *Padyatra* (trek) under the leadership of Sundar Lal Bahuguna from Kashmir (Srinagar) to Kohima (capital city of Nagaland) in 1981 to have community control and manage over the forests for the benefit of the community and thereby save the national environment. However, Nepal is the last country in nationalization of forests but one of the first countries to empower local communities in protection and management of forests and forest resources.

Despite the parallel developments of participatory forestry in both India and Nepal in the form of JFM in1990 and CFM in 1978 respectively, the nature and extent of shifting control and management from government to community differ considerably. It is generally believed that the forest policy and legislations of Nepal is more decentralized and people-oriented as compared to India. So, JFM will be the first step towards CFM where the local community is wholly responsible for the protective, management, optimal use and sustainable development of forests and forest products. Besides, composition of general body and executive committee of user group, social inclusion, benefit distribution between the government and community, nature of community institutions and the given degree of rights, responsibility and liberty are also distinct in both countries considerably.

Conclusion and Recommendations

Historically, people pursue sustainable use and management of forests under full cooperation of local people with out any formal forest policy, legislation and intervention of the government. As the demand for food, forest products and land for settlement increases, the productive function of forest dominates its protective function. So, from both sides of government and people started over use and exploitation of forest and forest resources that ultimately led environmental degradation and ecological imbalance in local, regional and national level. So, government started controlling them through various forest policies and legislations and it became tighter one after another. But, it could not stop the process of forest degradation rather increased considerably. Consequently, the destruction of forests, environmental damage and ecological imbalance further went up seriously. However, in mid of 1970's, it was highly felt the need of people's participation in forest protection, management, optimal use and sustainable development all over the world so that the forest policies and legislations also moved accordingly in many countries but particularly in India and Nepal. In addition, as the notion of environmental protection and ecological balance globally increased in 1980's, the forest policy and legislation also highly moved towards protective function with less priority to productive function. Then, over the years, the policy became more open to decentralized, integrated and participatory in forest management in India and Nepal. So, both India and Nepal are today globally acknowledged as a pioneer in promoting PFM.

However, people's participation became the most effective vehicle for forest protection, management, sustainable use, environmental protection and socio-economic transformation of the rural community. The governments have been amending of forest policies and legislations time to time in favour of better people's participation focusing on social inclusion equity in benefit distribution which is till functioning at satisfactory level in general. But as the forest policy of both countries is becoming two decades matured, perhaps the time has come to revise with the demographic, socio-economic and cultural change along with proper combination of both protective and productive functions of forest. In addition, it should not be neglected some important factors like topography, growth of forests, its carrying capacity, sustainability and land use pattern etc. in formulation of new forest policy and legislation.

Now it is clear that there is no other option except people's participation in forest protection and management in the 21st century. So, the new forest policy and legislation, if any, should be more and more people-oriented and decentralized by giving more legal rights and authority to the people in decision making in forest protection and management activities. Moreover, it should be as simple as possible to make them better understanding and strengthening the programme. The role of forest department should not be custodial as a police like in those days but as partner, advisor, facilitator and more technical supporter in the days to come. In this regard, community forestry programme of Nepal is at a significant crossroads and also growing as a best model for natural resources management programme in the world.

No doubt, a creation of mass awareness about forestry and good environment is absolutely necessarily if the forestry sector is to be developed along with the objectives of the national policy. So, to create such an environment, the role of multi-stakeholders like NGOs, other government institutions, social organizations and civil society etc. should not be ignored in the process of better and effective people's participation, institutionalization, post-formation support and capacity building to forest users through policy advocating, facilitation, financial assisting, orientation and training programme etc. However, at the top most essential factor apart from these all is feelings of self belongingness of the people to forests and forest resources like 'Our Forests' or '*Hamara Ban*' in Hindi or '*Hamro Ban*' in Nepali language along with positive thoughts and views towards forests. Otherwise, any kind of people-oriented and fully decentralized forest policy and legislation do not work effectively to achieve anticipated results. Hence, all stakeholders should go hand in hand with the government for better people's participation irrespective of any class and caste which could help in protection, management, optimal use and sustainable development of forest and forest products and there by creating environmental stability, ecological balance and socio-economic transformation of rural economy.

Besides, with some twenty years experience of JFM in India and thirty years experience of CFM in Nepal, both countries should learn from each other that will provide some useful knowledge and guidelines in the process of ongoing practice of PFM in other to have better protection, management, optimal use and sustainable development of forests and forest products in the days to come.

Note

- This paper is based on my on-going Ph. D. research work entitled 'Participatory Forest Management and Environmental-Economic Impact: A Comparative Study of Four Himalayan Districts' Department of Economics, University of Jammu, Jammu, Jammu and Kashmir, India.

References

Bhatia, A. (1999), 'Participatory Forestry Management: Implications for Policy and Human Resources Development in the Hindu-Kush Himalayas, ICIMOD, Kathmandu, Nepal, Vol. V (Nepal).

Bhattari, A. M. and D. R. Khanal, (2005), Communities, Forests and Law of Nepal: Present Status and Challenges, FECOFUN, Kathmandu, Nepal.

Chaudhuri, B. (1989), Forest, Forest Dweller and Forest Development, in B. Chaudhari and A. K. Maiti (eds.), *Forest and Forest Development in India*, Inter- India Publication, Raja Garden Extn, New Delhi).

Dahal, D. R. (1994), *A Review of Forest User Groups: Case Studies of From Eastern Nepal*, ICIMOD, Kathmandu, Napal.

GoI, (1952), *National Forest Policy of India–1952*, Conservator of Forest, Soil Conservation Circle, New Delhi, India.

GoI, (1988), *National Forest Policy of India–1988*, MoEF, New Delhi, India.

Hobley, M., J. Y. Campbell and A. Bhatia (1996), *Community Forestry in India and Nepal: Learning from each Other*, a Discussion Paper, Series no. MNR 96/3, ICIMID, Kathmandu, Nepal.

HMG/N (1957), Private *Forest Nationalization Act–1957*, His Majesty's Government, Kathmandu, Nepal.

HMG/N (1978), Panchayat Forestry Rules and Panchayat Protected Forest Rule, Nepal *Rajpatra (Gazette)*, His Majesty's Government, Kathmandu, Nepal.

HMG/N (1988), *Master Plan for the Forestry Sector*, His Majesty's Government, Ministry of Forest and Soil Conservation, Kathmandu, Nepal.

HMG/N (1993), *Forest Act-1993*, His Majesty's Government, Ministry of Forest and Soil Conservation, Kathmandu, Nepal.

HMG/N (1995), *Forest Regulation-1995*, His Majesty's Government, Ministry of Forest and Soil Conservation, Kathmandu, Nepal.

HMG/N, (2000), Forest Sector Policy-2000, His Majesty's Government, Ministry of Forest and Soil Conservation, Kathmandu, Nepal.

HMG/N, (2000), Guidelines for Inventry of Community Forestry, His Majesty's Government, Ministry of Forest and Soil Conservation, Kathmandu, Nepal.

Indurkar, P. (1992), *Forest, Environment and Economic Development*, Ashish Publishing House, Punjabi Bagh, New Delhi.

Jha, L. K. (1994), India's Forest Policies: Analysis and Appraisal, Ashish Publishing House, Punjabi Bagh, New Delhi.

Joshi, A. (1992), Development of Forest Policy in India with a Focus on the Hill Region of Utter Pradesh, Giri Institute of Development Studies, Lucknow.

Joshi, A. L. (1990), *Literature Review on Resource Management in Community Forestry*, Centre for Economic Development and Administration (CEDA), Tribhuvan University, Kirtipur, Kathmandu.

Joshi, A. L. (1993), Effects on Administration of Changed Forest Policies, a Paper Presented at the Workshop on Policy and Legislation in Community Forestry, RECOFTC, Bangkok, Thailand.

Kanel, K. R. (1993), Community Forestry and the 1993 Forestry Legislations, Implications for Policy and Implementation in a journal of forestry information for Nepal *Banko Jankari*, , DoF, Kathmandu, 4: 1.

Kanel, K. R. (2006), Nepal's Forest Policies on Community Forestry Development: the Government Perspective, in P. Gyamtsho, B. K. Singh and G. Rasul (eds), *Capitalisation and Sharing of Experiences on the Interaction between Forest Policies and Land Use Pattern in Asia: Linking People with Resources,* Technical Papers, ECIMOD, Kathmandu, Nepal, Vol. 2.

Kulkarni, S. (1989), Towards A Social Forestry Policy, in *Forest and Forest Development in India* (eds.), B. Chaudhari and A. K. Maiti, Inter- India Publication, Raja Garden Extn, New Delhi.

Lal, J. B. (1989), *India's Forests: Myth and Reality,* Natraj Publication, Dehra Dun.

Mahajan, V. (1970), Muslim Kalin Bharat, S. Chand and Company, New Delhi.

Mahat, T. B. S., Griffin, D.M., and Shepherd, K. R. (1986a), Human Impact on Some Forests of the Middle Hills of Nepal: Forestry in the Context of the Traditional Resources of the State, in *Mountain Research and Development,* 6(3):223-334.

Mahat, T. B. S., Griffin, D.M., and Shepherd, K. R. (1986b), Human Impact on Some Forests of the Middle Hills of Nepal: Some Major Human Impacts before 1950 on the Forests of Sindhu Palchowk and Kabhre Palanchowk, in *Mountain Research and Development,* 6: 325-334.

Palit, S. (1996), Comparative Analysis of Policy and Institutional Dimension of Community Forestry in India and Nepal' a discussion paper, series No. MNR 96/4, ICIMOD, Kathmandu, Nepal.

Parajuli, D. P. (1997), Analysis of Forest Policy in Nepal, in S. Gyawali, K. Baral and C. Khatiwada (eds.), *Prabhat,* Annual Publication, Institute of Forestry, Pokhara, Nepal, Vol. 5 pp 9-16.

Poffenberger, M. (eds.), (2000), *Communities and Forest Management in South Asia,* WG-CIFM, DFID and IUCN.

Rai, S. N. (1997), Management of Tropical Forests in Nepal, in S. Gyawali, K. Baral and C. Khatiwada (eds.), *Prabhat,* Annual Publication, Institute of Forestry, Pokhara, Nepal, Vol. 5, pp. 25-31.

Regmi, M. C. (1971), *A Study in Nepali Economic History (1768-1845),* Manjushri Publishing House, New Delhi.

Regmi, M. C. (1978), *Land Tenure and taxation in Nepal,* 1(4), Ratna Pustak Bhandar, Kathmandu, Nepal.

Saxena, N. C. (1993), Sustainable Development of Forestland and Joint Forest Management in India, *Indian Journal of Public Administration,* 39 (3): 465-472.

Saxena, N. C. (1995), *Forests, People and Profit: New Equation for Sustainability,* Natraj Publication, Dehra Dun.

Shrestha, B. P. (1989), *Forest Plants of Nepal,* Educational Enterprises, Lalitpur, Nepal.

Shrestha, B. K. (1996), Decentralized Planning and People's participation in Decision making in Nepal, Paper Presented at the National Seminar on *Strengthening Participatory Democracy through Decentralization,* Political Science Association of Nepal, Kathmandu, Nepal, March, 14-15.).

Shrestha, K. P. (1999), *Community Forestry Evolution: Concept and Policy,* a Paper Presented in International Training Course, RECOFT, Kathmandu, Nepal, (18 Sep-10 Oct) 1999.

Tiwari, K. B. (1989), Nepalko Ban Byabasthako Aitihasik Simhalokan (A Historical Overview of Forest Management in Nepal), Abarta Press, Kathmandu.

16

OPENNESS, STOCK MARKET DEVELOPMENT, AND TOTAL FACTOR PRODUCTIVITY GROWTH IN PAKISTAN

Shaista Alam, Ambreen Fatima,
Muhammad S. Butt & Syed Ashfaq Ali

Introduction

Openness fosters open competition that drives innovation, greater resource allocation, efficiency, and technological advancement. Recent studies by Moreno (1993); Roubini and Sala-i-Martin (1991) and Gould, *et al.* (1993) have attributed the rapid growth of some developing countries, such as South Korea and Taiwan, to increased openness. Openness and the associated free flow of capital promote TFP growth and economic development [Park (1993), Roubini and Sala-i-Martin (1991)]. However, a more hotly debated issue is the role of external liberalisation (Liberlisation of trade and international capital flows) in economic development [Roubini and Sala-i-Martin (1991)]. The opponents of external liberalisation, or full openness to trade, agree that such policies remove barriers to trade and international capital flows, but argue that free cross-border capital flows may not enhance economic growth and welfare. This is because removal of capital controls (openness) may result in "capital flight", as capital is free to flow out in search of high rate of return. In the process of opening up, many developing countries have found themselves in serious internal and external imbalances [Bruno (1988); Edward (1985)]. These arguments suggest that liberalisation and its associated openness may in fact slow down economic growth. Thus, the theoretical literature is divided on issue of the growth effects of financial liberalisation, openness, and financial development.

At the theoretical level, there is yet little or no consensus among development economists regarding the macroeconomic impact of financial liberalization, openness, and financial development. Goldsmith (1969); Mckinnon (1973) and Shaw (1973) were the first to hypothesis that financial liberalisation and the associated openness and financial development would promote economic growth through their impacts on the growth rate of capital and the efficiency of capital allocation. However, while Goldsmith focuses on the relationship between financial development and the efficiency of investment, what is now called the Mckinnon Shaw model that emphasizes the strong positive effect of financial liberalisation on savings, investment, and therefore economic growth.

The empirical evidence on these issues is also largely mixed, or rather less conclusive. Some studies have found evidence that indicates strong positive correlation between financial liberalisation and economic growth [Gregorio and Guidotti (1995); King and Levine (1993)]. In particular, Dornbusch and Reynoso (1989) found that liberalisation and opening up of South Korean economy in the late 1970s and the early 1980s were largely responsible for the recorded high rate of real growth during the 1980s. but, surprisingly, a cross-country study by Dornbusch and Reynoso could not establish that financial liberalisation has any significant positive impact on economic growth. This later evidence is supported by a recent study by Park (1993) which suggests that financial liberalisation in South Korea and Taiwan in the 1980s could not have any significant positive effect on economic growth.

The argument of those proposing a positive link between financial sector performance and economic growth appears more convincing. Financial development spurs higher economic growth by mobilizing savings. Greenwood and Jovanogic (1990) and Khan (2000) show how a well-developed financial sector can enhance economic growth by pooling savings. In particular, a well-functioning stock market provides finance for long-term risky, but high-return, industrial projects rarely financed by other financial markets. This is because the stock market can pool together long-term funds needed for such projects; pooling of resources provide diversification, protects savers from idiosyncratic risk, and enables the stock market to fund lumpy and risky, though profitable, long-term industrial projects [Montiel (1995)]. Second, a well-developed stock market promotes efficient allocation of the accumulated savings. Becsi and Wang (1997) highlight the role of financial sector in channeling resources towards more profitable projects, or better investment opportunities. By allocating resources more efficiently to profitable long-term investments, the stock market increases productivity in the real sector.

The third role of a well-functioning stock market, or financial system as a whole, is its ability to guarantee adequate liquidity. That is, investment in long-term, high-return projects will be almost impossible without a liquid stock market or financial system. This is because savers may be unwilling to relinquish their funds if they are not assured of prompt and easy access to their savings when needed [Bencivenga, *et al.* (1996); Demirguc-Kunt and Levince (1996) and Levine (1991)]. The fourth role of a well-developed stock market is its ability to reduce investment risk by offering opportunities for portfolio diversification [Levine (1991)]. The availability of different investment opportunities with differing risk characteristics encourages savers to acquire diverse investment assets, as this ensures minimum risk exposure. Fifth, a well-functioning stock market improves corporate control, monitors managers, and stimulates information acquisition about firms. Recent studies by Kyle (1984) and Holmstrom and Tirole (1993) show that the incentives for investors to obtain information about firms and improve corporate governance can be substantially increased by developed highly liquid stock market. When a stock market is liquid, an investor can use information will further spur investors to embark on supervision and monitoring of firms.

The relationship between financial development and productivity growth is an issue that has also generated intense controversy; most theoretical expositions suggest that a well-functioning stock market can significantly influence TFP growth rate. But there are disagreements as to the direction of the effect on growth. While some development economists argue that financial development has little or no effect on growth, others predict a strongly positive link between economic growth and financial development. However, there is little disagreement that a well-functioning stock market guarantees liquidity, risk diversification, acquisition of information about firms, corporate control, and savings mobilization. Certainly, any changes in these factors will alter the rate of TFP growth.

Hasan and Schmiedel (2003) provide clear evidence that European stock exchanges have exhibited positive productivity growth over the period. The results indicate a small overall rise in pure technical efficiency and a more significant overall technological progress. The empirical findings of the study support the view that technological innovation plays a pivotal role in shaping trading service provision during the 1993-1999 period. Technological progress can be interpreted as a sign of the dynamic nature of the whole exchange industry where stock exchanges take extra-ordinary efforts to adopt new cost-effective technologies and to cope with a changing security market environment. As a result, stock exchanges were able to take advantage of an intense diffusion of new technologies and information systems to leverage themselves on a higher production frontier. Automation of trading, electronic trading platforms, remote trading facilities and creation of networks among exchanges represent important characteristics of this sector for the period and for the near future. Additionally, the results report higher Technological progress for exchanges that show characteristics of automation, equity and derivative trading, for-profit governance structure, large and mid-sized capitalized markets. This finding support the view that technological advances in stock exchanges has been an expensive exercise and that bigger and medium exchanges with larger capital backup and higher turnover of trades were more able to fund intense technological investments relative to their smaller counterparts.

Klaus and Kugler (1998) investigated the Schumpeterian conjecture that views the incremental flow of services by the financial sector as essential for funding investment in R&D and thus for economic growth. On this basis, the neo-Schumpeterian growth models predict that the evolution of manufacturing TFP and financial activity are intimately related in the long run. This interaction was interpreted as a cointegrating relation who was then estimated and tested in a time series context for 13 OECD countries. The null hypothesis of no cointegration between logged manufacturing GDP and logged financial sector GDP could not be rejected for half of the countries. This finding is more controversial for models in which the long-run link between the real and financial sides of the economy stems from externalities resulting from broad capital accumulation rather than the Schumpeterian process of creative destruction emphasized by King and Levine (1993b). Replacing manufacturing GDP by manufacturing TFP, the hypothesis of no co-integration was rejected more often. This evidence establishes a long-run relation between financial sector activity and technical progress, as measured by the evolution of TFP. Hence, the focus on endogenous cumulative productivity enhancement as the mechanism linking economic growth and financial development seems more appropriate. This interpretation is supported by panel cointegration tests. They also investigated whether there is a feedback from manufacturing GDP, respectively TFP, to financial intermediation activity. This seems indeed to be the case for several countries. As Goldsmith (1969) argued, it is hard to ascertain the originating direction of causality once the feedback process is under way. It is not possible to make a general statement encompassing the whole sample as to whether financial development is truly an engine of growth or just a sign of the evolution of the whole economy due to independent factors. Baier, Dwyer and Tamura (2002, 2003) have examined the effect of introducing stock exchanges on growth rates for twenty years after a stock exchange compared to twenty years before a stock exchange opens, they find that economic growth increases after a stock exchange opens in a country, primarily by increasing TFP growth. They are in the process of exploring whether other institutional changes and more general financial development and financial repression affect the growth of output, aggregate input, and TFP.

To resolve these issues requires further empirical investigations. As already indicated, the purpose of this paper is to provide further empirical evidence on the issue, using data on Pakistan and focusing on the effects of opening of the economy and stock market development on TFP growth. The relationship between openness to world trade and economic growth has remained a source of intense debate among development economists. Numerous studies have proposed that outward orientation and openness improve growth performance through its positive effects on capital flows, foreign direct and portfolio investments, and development of domestic financial markets. It is argued that foreign investment (direct and indirect) promotes competitiveness, efficiency in resource allocation, economies of scale, and technological knowledge or transfers. The scheme of the study is as follows: Section 2 specifies the empirical model and discusses the data series used to estimate the model. Section 3 presents the econometric methodology and estimation techniques employed for the study. Section 4 presents and analyses the empirical results. Section 5 contains the conclusions emerging from the study.

The Empirical Model

The primary objective of this study is to estimate the impact of openness to trade and stock market development on TFP growth in Pakistan, to ascertain whether openness and stock market development are important factors of TFP growth in Pakistan. To achieve this objective, we adopt a modified and extended version of the stock market and economic growth model formulated by Levine and Zervos (1997); Demiague-Kunt and Levine (1996) and Demingue-Kunt and Maksimovic (1996a,

1996b), is specified and estimated over the period 1970-2002. a functional from of the model is specified as:

$$tfp = f\,(gdp, inf, mxlr, mcp, nmex, opns, sse) \qquad (1)$$

Where tfp	is total factor productivity,
gdp	Gross Domestic Product
inf	Inflation Rate
mxlr	Maximum Lending Rate proxied by Govt. bond yield
nmex	Ratio of Non-Military Expenditure to GDP
mcp	Ratio of Stock Market Capitalization to GDP
opns	Openness to international trade
sse	Secondary School Enrolment

To examine the basic relationship a log-linear version of equation (1), is of the following from:

$$\begin{aligned} \ln tfp_t = \beta_0 + \beta_1 \ln gdp_t + \beta_2 \ln inf_t + \beta_3 \ln mxlr_t + \beta_4 \ln mcp_t \\ + \beta_5 \ln nmex_t + \beta_6 \ln opns_t + \beta_7 \ln sse_t + e_t \end{aligned} \qquad (2)$$

The fundamental proposition of this paper is that openness to trade and well-developed stock market, respectively, have a strong positive influence on productivity growth. We use market capitalization as the measure of stock market development because it is assumed that stock market size reflects to a considerable extent, the market liquidity and extent of integration. The greater the stock market liquidity and integration with stock market liquidity and integration with international capital market, the more it will encourage savings, investment, and economic growth. The proposition that increased openness accelerates economic growth is based on the fact that most developing countries have abundant raw materials to export in exchange for machinery and equipment, including technical skill for industrial development, and then economic growth.

Undoubtedly, public infrastructure investment is the major component of non-military expenditure: it is productive and complements private capital stock [Tatom (1991), (1993); Aschaucr (1990); Udegbunam (2000)]. A large number of studies have shown that inflation and high interest rates exert individually a significant negative impact on investment and output growth [Barro (1991, 1996); Clark (1993)]. The consumer price index (CPI), a proxy used for inflation and government bond yield is used as primed for maximum lending rate. A country grows faster if it begins each period with higher level of human capital. With a high level of education attainment, labour is better equipped to adapt to new technologies and management skills developed elsewhere. The secondary school enrolment rate is used as a proxy for human capital.

A large body of empirical literature, including Barro (1991), Lucas (1988); Levine and Zervos (1997), provides evidence of strong negative link between initial income measure by initial GDP and long-run productivity growth. This evidence is attributed to the convergence hypothesis, which posits that an economy grows faster the lower is its GDP. In other words, the rate of growth of an economy depends inversely on the gap between the economy's initial income and the economy's long-run on steady state GDP.

The Data

The data for this study have been compiled by collecting information from various published and electronic sources. The time series data (1970-2002) for gross domestic product (GDP), non-military expenditures, government bond yield (proxised by maximum lending rate) and consumer price index (CPI) (proxied by inflation) have been obtained from the International Monetary Fund's, International Financial Statistics (IFS) CD-Rom (2003). We used the ratio of non-military expenditure to GDP. The time series data (1970-2002) for stock market capitalization and secondary school enrolment have been collected from Federal Bureau of Statistics, Finance division's Economic Survey of Pakistan. We used the ratio of market capitalization to GDP (Market Capitalization/GDP). A large number of studies used school enrolment as a proxy for human capital input [Lucas (1988); Romer (1990); Stokey (1991); Barro (1991)]. In the case of openness to trade, we adopt the measure often suggested in the literature [Iyoha (1976); Wood (1997)]. This is the ratio of imports plus exports to GDP (Imports + Exports)/GDP]. The data on openness are obtained from Penn

World Table 1 compiled by Summers and Heston (1998). The time series of total factor productivity (TFP) is estimated by adopting the methodology given in Fatima *et. al.*, (2003)[1].

Econometric Methodology and Estimation Techniques

A Vector Error Correction Model (VECM)

Consider the vector autoregressive (VAR) model.

$$X_t = \Phi_1 X_{t-1} + \Phi_2 X_{t-2} + ... + \Phi_k X_{t-k} + \mu + \eta_t \qquad t = 1, ..., T \quad (3)$$

Where X_t is a 8 x 1 vector containing *tfp, gnp, inf, mxlr, mcp, nmex, opns* and *sse*. All these variables are measured by their natural logarithm so that their first differences approximate their growth rates. Suppose that these variables are *I(0)* after applying the differencing filter once. If we exploit the idea that there may exists co-movement of these variables and possibilities that they will trend together towards a long-run equilibrium state, then by the Granger representation theorem, we may posit the following testing relationships that constitute our Vector-Error-Correction Model (VECM).

$$\Delta X_t = \Gamma_1 \Delta X_{t-1} + \Gamma_1 \Delta X_{t-2} + ... + \Gamma_{k-1} \Delta X_{t-p+1} + \Pi X_{t-p} + \mu + \eta_t, \qquad t = 1, ..., T \qquad (4)$$

Where ΔX_t is the vector of the growth rates of the variables, the Γ's are estimable parameters, Δ is a difference operator, η_t is a vector of impulses which represent the unanticipated movements in X_t, with $\eta_t \sim niid(0,\Sigma)$ and Π is the long-run parameter matrix. With *r* cointegrating vectors. ($1 \leq r \leq 8$), Π has rank *r* and can be decomposed as $\Pi = \alpha\beta'$; with α and β both 8 x *r* matrices. $\beta s'$ are the parameters in the cointegrating relationships and α are the adjustment coefficients which measure the strength of the cointegrating vectors in the VEC model. The Johansen (1988, 1992) and Johansen and Juselius (1990) co integration techniques allow estimating the long-run or co integrating relationships between the nonstationary variables using a maximum likelihood procedure which tests for the cointegrating rank *r* and estimates the parameters β of these cointegrating relationships. As proved by Johansen (1991, 1992), the intercept terms in the VEC model should be associated with the existence of a deterministic linear time trend in the data. If, however, the data do not contain a time trend, the VEC model should include a restricted intercept term associated to the co integ-rating vector.

The cointegration[2] methodology illustrates well the conflict that exists between the equilibrium framework and the disequilibrium environment from which the data are collected. As formulated in the VECM model, this conflict can be easily resolved by extending the equilibrium framework into one that accounts for disequilibrium by including the adjustment mechanisms represented by the error-correction terms. Once the equilibrium conditions are imposed, the VEC model describes how the system is adjusting in each time period towards its long-run equilibrium state. Since the variables are supposed to be cointegrated, then in the short-run, deviations from this long-run equilibrium will feed back on the changes in the dependent variables in order to force their movements towards the long-run equilibrium state. Hence the co integrating vectors from which the error correction terms are derived are each indicating an independent direction where a stable, meaningful long-run equilibrium state exists. The coefficients of the error-correction terms, however, represent the proportion by which the long-run disequilibrium (or imbalance) in the dependent variables are corrected in each short-term period. If the adjustment coefficient of a dependent variable is not significant, it means that it is weakly exogenous, and the VEC model should be reformulated conditioning on this variable. In the reformulated model the weakly exogenous variable will have an equation that does not include the cointegrating vector and, hence, will behave as a random walk vari-able, with a drift term if the data contain a time component.

Empirical Analysis

Since the VECM requires that the variables are I (1), we herein, use the augmented Dickey Fuller (ADF) test to investigate the stationarity status of each variable. Tests for unit roots are performed on the level variables as well as on their first differences. The null hypothesis is that the variable under investigation has a unit root, against the alternative that it does not. Table 1 reports the ADF statistics for each variable. The results of Table 1 are consistent with the hypothesis that the level variables are each integrated of order one. Because data appear to be stationary in first differences, no further tests are performed.

Table 1
ADF Unit-Root Test

Variables	*Test Statistic at Level*		*Test Statistic at 1st Difference*	
	Intercept	*Intercept+ Trend*	*Intercept*	*Intercept+ Trend*
LGDP	-2.543044	-2.183396	-3.692652*	-5.627338*
LINF	-2.221395	-2.441701	-3.278061**	-4.164739*
LMXLR	0.784553	0.037155	-3.962913*	-4.169367*
LOPNES	-2.305555	-2.575637	-4.467537*	-4.366500*
LNMEXGDPRT	-1.476508	-1.015522	-5.452918*	-5.724453*
LMRKCPGDPRT	-1.050607	-2.001420	-3.367795**	-3.367795***
LSSENRL	-0.994546	-1.127874	-3.540401**	-3.609217**
LTFP	-0.813055	-2.727812	-6.425010*	-6.734763*

* Significant at 1%.
** Significant at 5%.
*** Significant at 10%.

Before undertaking the co-integration tests, first specify the relevant order of lags (p) of the VAR model. Given the fact that the sample size is relatively small as number of endogenous variable is large, we select p = 1 for the order of the VAR. On the basis of the above unit root tests, we apply the procedure of Johansen and Juselius (1990) to determine whether any combinations of the variables are co-integrated. Results reported in Table 2. Starting with the null hypothesis of no co-integration (r = o) among the variables, the trace statistics is above the 95% critical value. Hence it rejects the null hypothesis r = o, in favour of the general alternative r = 1. As is evident in Table 2 the null hypothesis of $r \leq 1$, $r \leq 2$, ..., $r \leq 6$ rejected at a 5% level of significance and $r \leq 7$ cannot be rejected at a 5% level of significance. Consequently, we conclude that there are seven co-integrating relationships among the eight variables. Turning to the maximal eigen value test, the null hypothesis of no co-integration (r = o) is rejected at 5% level of significance in favour of the general alternative, that there are seven co-integrating vectors. But the test fails to reject the null hypothesis of r ≤ 7. This confirms the conclusion that there are seven co-integrating relationships amongst the eight I (1) variables.

Table 2
Johanson's Cointegration Through VAR

Trace Statistics

Likelihood Ratio	*5 Per cent Critical Value*	*1 Per cent Critical Value*	*Hypothesized No. of CE(s)*
339.1802	182.82	196.08	None **
201.9287	146.76	158.49	At most 1 **
137.9813	114.90	124.75	At most 2 **
99.31384	87.31	96.58	At most 3 **
70.64701	62.99	70.05	At most 4 **
47.17489	42.44	48.45	At most 5 *
25.93210	25.32	30.45	At most 6 *
6.612110	12.25	16.26	At most 7

*(**) denotes rejection of the hypothesis at 5% (1%) significance level. L.R. test indicates 7 co-integrating equation(s) at 5% significance level.

Max. Statistics

Likelihood Ratio	*5 Per cent Critical Value*	*1 Per cent Critical Value*	*Hypothesized No. of CE(s)*
137.26	36.06	37.59	None **
63.95	31.86	33.74	At most 1 **
38.67	27.59	28.17	At most 2 **
28.67	24.32	26.53	At most 3 **
23.48	20.55	21.60	At most 4 **
21.24	17.12	18.00	At most 5 *
19.32	13.07	14.19	At most 6 *
6.61	12.25	16.26	At most 7

*(**) denotes rejection of the hypothesis at 5% (1%) significance level. L.R. test indicates 7 co-integrating equation(s) at 5% significance level.

Estimation of An Error-correction Model

Once a co-integrating relationship is established, then an VECM can be estimated to determined the short-run dynamic behaviour of the variables under investigation. Table 3 reports the results of VECM formulation. According to Engle and Granger (1987), co-integrated variables must have an ECM representation. The VECM strategy provides an answer to the problem of spurious correlation–the short-run dynamic relationship between openness, stock market development and TFP growth estimated from the VECM formulation. The error-correction term (ECT) reflects the long-run dynamics and appears in the set of regressors. Technically, the error-correction term measures the speed of adjustment back to the co-integration relationship. The ECM is posited to be a force causing the integrated variables to return their long-run relation when they deviate from it, and thus the larger the deviation, the greater would be the force tending to correct the deviation [Banerjee, Galbraith, and Henry (1994)]. The coefficients on the lagged values of the differenced variables are short-run parameters measuring the immediate impact the independent variables on the dependent variables.

Given, that, the set of variables are cointegrated, the VECM representation have the following form:

$$\Delta Y = \alpha_0 + \alpha_1 E_{t-1} + \sum_{i=1}^{n} \alpha_{2i} \Delta X_{t-i} + \sum_{j=1}^{m} \alpha_{3j} \Delta Z_{t-j} + \sum_{k=1}^{p} \alpha_{4k} \Delta W_{t-k} + ... + U_t$$

where E_{t-1} is the error-correction terms.

VECM analysis suggested that Δtfp did not caused by any variable under consideration in the short run. The F-Statistics of Δinf (change in inflation) is statistically significant at 1% suggested that Δgdp caused by Δinf (inflation) in the short-run. Analysis of VECM in the case of Δinf as a dependent variable indicated that inflation caused by tfp, gdp, maximum lending rate (mxlr), non-military expenditures (nmex) and openness (opns) in the short-run. Analysis of VECM indicated that non-military expenditure (nmex) has immediate impact on maximum lending rate (mxlr). In the VECM analysis (Δmcp as a dependent variable), market capitalization caused only by human capital (sse) in the short-run, whereas any other variable reveals no short-run impact on market capitalization. In the

Table 3
Temporal Causality Results Based on Vector Error-Correction Model (VECM)

Dependant	F-Statistics								t-Statistic
Variable	*Δtfp*	*Δgdp*	*Δinf*	*Δmxlr*	*Δmcp*	*Δnmex*	*Δopns*	*Δsse*	E_{t-1}
Δtfp	-	0.638	1.090	0.379	2.36	0.598	0.505	1.698	8.438*
Δgdp	0.595	-	3.006***	0.807	0.592	0.847	1.192	0.462	0.417
Δinf	7.879*	8.748*	-	7.580*	1.394	7.205*	23.354*	0.006	3.561*
Δmxlr	0.541	0.284	1.375	-	0.245	3.039***	0.312	0.418	2.914*
Δmcp	0.207	0.033	0.054	0.164	-	0.699	0.041	3.300***	3.033*
Δnmex	0.329	3.949**	1.858	0.675	0.141	-	2.373	0.303	-2.304**
Δopns	1.187	1.730	3.486**	1.111	1.208	1.171	-	0.459	3.004*
Δsse	0.501	0.205	0.319	0.266	0.012	0.396	0.706	-	2.994*

* Significant at 1% level.
** Significant at 5% level.
*** Significant at 10% level.

analysis of VECM (Δnmex as a dependent variable) non-military expenditures caused only by gross domestic product in the short-run, whereas the openness (opns) immediately caused by inflation rate.

The analysis of VECM also indicated that any variable did not have short run impact on human capital (sse). The t-statistics of error correction terms (ects) of all VECM equations except in the case of Dgdp as dependent variable indicating that there would be long-run dynamic impact from explanatory variables to dependent variable. The insignificance of t-statistics of ect of VECM Δgdp indicated that there would be no long-run dynamic effect from explanatory variables on gross domestic product (Δgdp).

Concluding Remarks

The question of whether openness and stock market development are important factors in productivity growth is empirically evaluated in this study using time series data for Pakistan. This effort is spurred by the raging debate on the relevance of free trade and financial development to economic growth in developing countries [Hetzel (1994); Gould, *et. al.* (1993); Roubini and Sala-i-Martin (1991)], and the fact that the empirical evidence, so far, is somewhat mixed and that there is none yet for Pakistan. Using a VAR model, the empirical evidence suggests that openness to trade and stock market development have a long run equilibrium relationship with total factor productivity growth. That is the empirical findings provides strong support for the proposition that openness and stock market development are among the key determinants of total factor productivity growth in Pakistan. The other key factors, as indicated by results, are human capital input provide by Secondary School Enrolment rate, non-military expenditure that largely reflects the level of infrastructure facilities, GDP that reflects the size of physical capital and level of aggregate demand and inflation rate.

Our results suggest that stock market development facilitate productivity growth by reducing the incremental cost of external capital rather than simply by lowering the overall cost of capital in the economy. This conclusion receives further support from the result that growth appears to occur through the creation of new establishments; which is more likely to require external funds; rather than through an expansion in the average size of existing establishments, which firms are more likely to finance with internal cash.

Notes

1. See also Kim and Lau (1994) and Eichengreen (2002).
2. To choose an adequate VAR order, resort is made to the Akaike Information Criterion (AIC) and the Schwartz Criterion (SC) (Judge *et al.* 1988, pp. 761-764). In the VAR context,

$$AIC(n) = \ln\det(\Omega_n) + (2M^2 n)/T, \text{ and}$$

$$SC(n) = \ln\det(\Omega_n) + M^2 n \ln T)/T$$

where M is the number of variables in the system; T is the sample size; n is the lag length taking values 0, 1, ..., N with N being a pre-specified upper bound for the VAR order; and Ω_n is an estimate of the residual covariance matrix obtained with a VAR(n) model. Since the multivariate error term is assumed to have a non-diagonal covariance matrix, it is better to apply Zellner's iterative method or the seemingly unrelated regression (SUR) in order to take account explicitly of the non-zero covariances of the error terms (Charemza and Deadman 1997, p. 183). The lag order for which either AIC or SC is minimum is the optimal order for the VAR model, and the model is therefore characterized as VAR (p).

References

Aschauer, David A. (1990), "Highway Capacity and Economic Growth", Federal Reserve Bank of Chicago, *Economic Perspective* 14, 17-24.

Baier, Scott L., Gerald P. Dwyer, Jr., and Robert Tamura. (2002), "How Important are Capital and Total Factor Productivity for Economic Growth?" Unpublished Paper, Federal Reserve Bank of Atlanta.

Baier, Scott L., Gerald P. Dwyer, Jr., and Robert Tamura. (2003), "Modern Economic Growth and Stagnation." Federal Reserve Bank of Atlanta *Economic Review,* 88 (Third Quarter), 45-62.

Banerjee, AJD, Galbraith J.W. and Henry D.F. (1994), "Cointegration, Error-correction and the Econometric Analysis of Non-stationary Data, pp. 48-49, 52-53 Oxford, Oxford University Press.

Barro, Robert J. (1991), Economic Growth in a Cross-section of Countries, *Quarterly Journal of Economics,* May, 407-443.

Barro, Robert J. (1996), Inflation and Growth. Federal Reserve Bank of St. Louis *Review,* 78:3, 153-169.

Becsi, Zsolt, and Ping Wang (1997), Financial Development and Growth, Federal Reserve Bank of Atlanta, *Economic Review,* Fourth Quarter, 46-62.

Bencivenga, *et al.* (1996), Equity Markets, Transaction Costs, and Capital Accumulation, An Illustration, *The World Bank Economic Review,* 10:2, 241-265.

Bruno, Michael (1988), Opening UP, Liberalisation with Stabilisation. In R. Dornbusch and C. H. L. Helmers (ed). *The Open Economy, Tools for Policy Makers in Developing Countries.* EDI Series in Economic Development.

Charemza, Wojciech W. and Deadman, D.F. (1997), New Directions in Econometric Practice: General to Specific Modeling, Cointegration and Vector Auto regression. Cheltenham: Edward Elgar, 2nd edition.

Clark, T.E. (1993), Cross-country Evidence on Long-run Growth and Inflation, Federal Reserve Bank of Kansas City, (Research Working Paper, (RWP 93-05).

Demirgüç-Kunt, A. and R. Levine, (1996), Stock Market Development, Corporate Finance, and Economic Growth, *World Bank Economic Review,* 10, 223-239.

Demirgue-Kunt, Ash, and V. Maksimovic (1996a), Stock Market Development and Financing Choices of Firms, *The World Bank Economic Review,* 10:2, 341-369.

Demirgue-Kunt, Ash, and V. Maksimovic (1996b), Stock Market Development and Financial Intermediaries: Stylised Facts, *The World Bank Economic Review,* 10:2, 291-321.

Dorbusch, Rudiger, and A. Reynoso (1989), Financial Factors in Economic Development, *American Economic Review,* Papers and Proceedings 79, May 204-209.

Edwards, Sebastian (1985), Stabilisation with Liberalisation: An Evaluation of Ten Years of Chile's Experience with Free Market Policies, 1973-1983. *Economic Development and Cultural Change* 32, 223-254.

Eichengreen, Barry (2002), "Capitalizing on Globalization", *Asian Development Review*, Vol. 19, No. 1, pp. 14-66.

Fatima, A., S. Alam and Butt (2003), "International Trade and Total Factor Productivity growth in Pakistan: A Multivariate Cointegration Analysis", *Indian Journal of Quantitative Economics;* 18 (1&2), pp. 31-54.

Goldsmith, Raymond W. (1969), Financial Structure and Development. New Haven, CT: Yale University Press.

Gould, David, *et al.* (1993), Theory and Practice of Free Trade. Federal Reserve Bank of Dallas, *Economic Review,* Fourth Quarter, pp. 3-15.

Greenwood, Jeremy, and H. Jovanovic (1990), Financial Development, Growth, and the Distribution of Income, *Journal of Political Economy,* 98, 1076-1107.

Gregorio De Jose, and Pablo E. Guidotti (1995), Financial Development and Economic Growth, *World Development,* 23:3, 433-448.

Hassan, I. and Schmiedel, H. (2003), "Do Markets in the Stock Exchange Industry Pay off? Euopean Evidence", Bank of Finland Discussion Papers.

Hetzel, Robert L. (1994), The Free Trade Debate: The Illusion of Security versus Growth. Federal Reserve Bank of Richmond, *Economic Review,* Quarterly, 80:2, Spring, 39-58.

Holmstrom, Bengt, and J. Tirole (1993), Market Liquidity and Performance Monitoring, *Journal of Political Economy,* 10:14, 678-709.

IMF (2003), "International Financial Statistics (IFS)" CD-Rom, International Monetary Fund.

Iyoha, Milton A. (1976), Demand for International Reserves in Less Developed Countries: A Distributed Lag Specification, *The Review of Economics and Statistics,* 53:3, 351-355.

Johansen, S. (1988), "Statistical Analysis of Cointegration Vectors", *Journal of Economic Dynamics and Control,* 12: 231 54.

Johansen, S. (1991), "Estimation and Hypothesis Testing of Cointegrating Vectors in the Presence of a Linear Trend", Econometrica, 59, 1551-1580.

Johansen, S. (1992), "Determination of the Cointegration ranks in the presence of Linear Trend", Oxford Bulletin of Economics and Statistics, 54(1), pp. 383-397.

Johanson S. and Juselies, K. (1990), "Maximum Likelihood Estimation and Inference on Cointegration with Applications for the Demand forMoney", *Oxford Bulletin of Economic and Statistics*, Vol. 52, pp. 169-210.

Judge, P. A. Nixon, V. J. Cahill, B. Tangney, and S. Weber, "Overview of distributed shared memory", Department of Computer Science, Trinity College, Dublin, Ireland, Tech. Rep. TCD-CS-1998. *http://citeseer.csail.mit.edu/judge98overview.html*

Khan, Aubhik (2000), "The Finance and Growth Nexus", Federal Reserve Bank of Philadelphia *Business Review*, January/February, pp. 3-14.

Kim, J., and L. J. Lau, (1994), "The Sources Economic Growth of the East Asian Newly Industrialized Countries", *Journal of the Japanese and International Economy*, 8: 235-71.

King, Robert G., and R. Levine (1993), Finance Entrepreneurship, and Growth: Theory and Evidence, *Journal of Monetary Economics*, 32:3, 513-542.

Kyle, Albert (1984), Market Structure, Information, Futures Market, and Price Formation. In G. Storey, *et al.* (eds.) *International Agricultural Trade: Advanced Readings in Price Formation.* Boulder CO. Westview.

Levine, R., and S. Zervos (1997), "Stock Markets, Banks, and Economic Growth," *American Economic Review*, 88(3), 537–558.

Levine, Ross (1991), Stock Market, Growth, and Tax Policy, *Journal of Finance* 46, September. 1445-65.

Lucas, Robert E. Jr. (1988), On the Mechanics of Economic Development, *Journal of Monetary Economics*, 22:1.

Mckinnon, Ronald I. (1973), Money and Capital in Economic Development. Washington, D.C.: Brookings Institution.

Montiel, Peter (1995), Financial Policies and Economic Growth: Theory, Evidence and Country– Specific Experience from Sub-Saharan Africa, (AERC Research Paper No. 18.)

Moreno, Ramon (1993), "Are World Incomes Converging? Federal Reserve Bank of San Francisco, Weekly Letter 26.

Neusser, Klaus and Maurice Kugler (1998), "Manufacturing Growth and Financial Development: Evidence from OECD Countries," *Review of Economics and Statistics*. 80: 638-46.

Park, Yung C. (1993), "The Role of Finance in Economic Development in South Korea and Taiwan", In *Finance and Development: Issues and Experience*. Cambridge University Press.

Robert F. Engle and Clivew Granger (1987), "Co-integration and Error correction: Representation, Estimation and Testing". *Econometrica* Vol. 55, pp. 251-76.

Romer, D (1990), 'Endogenous Technical Change' *Journal of Political Economy*, 98, 5, pages 71-102.

Roubini, Nouriel, and X. Sala-i-Martin (1991), Finaicla Development, the Trade Regime, and Economic Growth, National Bureau for Economic Research, Cambridge, Mass. (Working Paper, 3876).

Shaw, Edward S. (1973), *"Financial Deepening in Economic Development"*, New York, Oxford University Press.

Stokey l. Nancy (1991), "The Volume and Composition of Trade Between Rich and Poor Countries", *RES*. Credible Public Policy," *Journal of Economic Dynamics and Control*, 15 (October 1991), pp. 627-656.

Summers, Robert, and Alan Heston. (1998), "Penn World Tables 5.6." *http://datacenter.chass.utoronto.ca/pwt/ on February 8, 2000.*

Tatom, S.A. (1991), Public Capital and Private Sector Performance. Federal Reserve Bank of St. Louis *Economic Review*, May/June, pp. 3-15.

Tatom, S.A. (1993), "Is an Infrastructure Crises Lowering the Nation's Productivity?", Federal Reserve Bank of St. Louis *Review*, November/December, pp.3-21.

Udegbunam, Ralph I. (2000), Public Infrastructure Investment and Economic Growth in Nigeria. *The Indian Journal of Economics*, 81: 320, July, 1-13.

Wood, Adrian (1997) Openness and Wage Inequality in Developing Countries: The Latin American Challenge to East Asian Conventional Wisdom. *The World Bank Economic Review*, 11:1, January, 33-37.

17

DEVELOPMENT OF AFRICAN COUNTRIES: GLIMPSES ON ISSUES AND PRIORITIES

Shankar Chatterjee & K. Jayasree

Africa continent is second largest continent in area in the world in area with 53 countries. In many of the countries of Africa are rich in mineral resources but due to different types of problems poor more in Africa. Some of the problems about the Africa continent vis-à-vis with respect to some countries are analyzed here. Different secondary sources have been consulted for writing the article. According to Deputy Country Director Abnezer Ngowi 842 million persons in the world are undernourished of which 26 per cent are in Africa (UNMEE Newsletter). The newsletter of 'Africa Renewal' (January 2005) has stated more than 40 per cent of Africa's 600 million people live below the internationally recognized poverty line of $1 a day. The publication further states that except South Africa and Egypt, in many African countries not more than 20 per cent people (some countries even 5%) has direct access to electricity. The figure hovers around 2 per cent in rural areas.

Water is an important ingredient for human life. Although Africa is endowed with 17 large rivers and more than 160 big lakes but it uses around 4 per cent of its total annual renewable water resources for agriculture, industry and domestic purposes (Africa Renewal, July 2004).

The publication further states that "out of 55 countries in the world with domestic water use below 50 liters/person/day (minimum requirement set by the W.H.O) 35 are in Africa. Almost half of all Africans suffer from one of six main water related diseases". Nigerian Water Minister Mukhtari Shehu Shagari in 12th session of the Commission of Sustainable Development (CSD) held in New York, April 14-30, 2004 may be quoted, "water problems in Africa are acute and complex". Water bodies in Africa are shrinking. The size of Lakechad (as an example) has reduced from 25,000 square kilometers presently, affecting more than 20 million people (Africa Renewal, July 2004).

Slum is another problem in African countries. In some Afiican urban areas, growing slum is a great problem. This problem is due to neglecting housing issue of the people, which inter alia, include poor accountability and lack of capacity that hinder effective urban management. According to Ms. Rosemary Rop, a leading NGO activist of Kenya, the weakness of central government and municipalities gives rise to a situation, "where nobody is taking charge, nobody is providing guidance". She further stated that governments do not commit sufficient resources to address the problems of existing slums, further reducing them to wastelands of overcrowding, poverty and social exclusion. In her language, "Governments simply label these informal settlements as illegal and do not provide services to them". Altogether 60 per cent of the total population of Nairobi lives in slums which shares only 5 per cent of city's land. This is not a isolated case rather it prevails in most large African cities where in between 40 and 70 per cent urban dwellers live in slums. (African Renewal, July 2004). Mention may be made here that world leaders have pledged to improve the lives of 100 million slum dwellers by 2020, but the number of persons living in informal settlements is expected to be doubled i.e. 2 billion in the next 30 years. This is a shuddering picture for the world community.

A few of the issues based on some countries are discussed here.

Democratic Republic of Congo (DR Congo)

The country is having an area of 23.45 lakh sq. km. with an estimated population of about 5 crores. Two cases one on exploitation of child labour and other one on killing of hippopotamus are presented.

In eastern province of AR Congo viz., Katanga about 800 children in the age group of 5 years to 15 years is employed for digging of copper and cobalt. The children are employed as they can be paid fewer wages than a grown up man. Most of the children are from poor families. These children have never been to school, al beit, they are interested for playing and attending school. There are no safety standards. No one wears a hard hat even some children work with bare hands and bare feet. "There are vast mineral deposits beneath the soil here, but this treasure has always benefited the leaders not the people", (Eritrea Profile, 14 June, 2006).

Case-II

Virunga National Park is famous for hippopotamus, buffalo, elephant etc., It is reported that a militant group known as Mai Mai military has set up camp in Virnaga National Park. They kill the animals for meat and ivory. Within a period of two weeks in October 2006, hundreds of hippopotamus were killed as a result their number has come down to less than 400. Although twenty years ago there were about 22,000 hippopotamus in the National Park, but civil war has drastically reduced the hippopotamus population. The researchers from Zoological Society of London (ZSL) warned that, "The entire population may disappear before the end of the year without urgent action". (Eritrea Profile, 21st October, 2006).

Election in Gambia

Gambia is small country located in extreme west of Africa. Total geographical area is 10,689 square kilometers with an estimated population of 13.64 lakh. Illiteracy rate in the country is very high as a result instead of ballot papers marbles are used to elect the people's representatives. There are three parties in the country. These are (i) Alliance for Patriotic Reorientation and

Construction (APRC), (ii) United Democratic Party (UDP) and (iii) National Alliance for Democracy and Development (Nadd).

In the Presidential election held in September 2006, voters used marbles (three different colours). The process is like this, "A marble is inserted into the drum representing the candidate" (Eritrea Profile, September 2006).

Impact of Civil War in Somalia

Somalia located in the horn of Africa. It is spread over to an area of 6.38 square. kilometers with an estimated population of 1 crore.

Somalia is the only country in the world without a central government. The country has been suffering from civil war for last 15 years. During 1980s per capita income was 300 US Dollar which ahs come down to 30 US Dollar a year in recent times. "Besides inflicting heavy human losses, the civil war in Somalia had completely destroyed infrastructure, social services and economic activities. The complete chaos and destruction that had encumbered Somalia for the past 15 years is a sad historical reality the international community had failed to assure moral responsibility for which it should be ashamed". (Eritrea Profile, 5 August 2006).

Corruption in Nigeria

Nigeria is located in west of Africa is spread over to an area of 9.24 square kilometers. Its population was estimated as 11 crore. Although the country is having huge oil reserve but high corruption vis-à-vis poverty is also high in the country. It is Africa's highest oil exporter but most people are poor. According to Nuhu Ribadu, an activist against the corruption, "More than 380 billion US Dollar either has been stolen or wasted by Nigerian Governments since independence in 1960". "The country is regularly ranked as one of the most corrupt by graft watch dog Transparency International". (Eritrea Profile, 21.10.2006).

Value of women in Southern Part of Sudan

Sudan is a largest country in Africa continent with an area of 25.06 lakh square kilometers. Its population was estimated as little more than 3 crore. In Southern part of Sudan women is considered as a commodity as its value (price) is measured in terms of cows. In one community of Southern Sudan if "a man kills his wife will have to make restitution with a fine of 26 cows. Then his debt to society is considered paid".

Almost all parts of Southern Sudan men can have many wives as long as he is having cows to pay for getting wives. It is almost common to have 2/3 wives for every man in this part of Sudan. The richer the man, more wives likely to have. It is also a practice in Southern Sudan that if a girl is uneducated, isolated and closed at have fetches more cows for her father. The reason is that a girl is less exposed to the community is considered as fresher, innocent, a greater prize for a husband. The girls who go attend schools are considered as more independent thus may be disobedient and defiant Slowly the perception is being changed. According to Abu Maknai Makuei, head of Malikon Women's Association her own daughter is a perfect example. "She is going to marry a man who already has the wife. The man paid 13 cows for that wife, who is uneducated. My daughter can read and write. He will pay 50 cows for her (Eritrea Profile, 20.9.2006).

South Africa and Zambia Grapple with HIV/AIDS

Zambia is located in southern part of Africa with an area of 7.53 lakh square kilometers having population of little more than 1 crore. HIV/AIDS is a great problem in the country. In this country one out of five persons is the age group of 15-49 years is suffering from HIV/AIDS. As a result an increasing number of employees are doping which include skilled, experienced and productive persons. It is reported that unless effective policies to combat HIV/AIDS are initiated one day work forces may be wiped out. "Since he epidemic tends to claim the most skilled and productive sections of the population, it seriously impedes the Zambian economy's broader efforts to build up its human capital base and increase overall productivity". (Africa Renewal, July 2004).

South Africa: Problems of AIDS

South Africa is spread to an area of 12.19 lakh square kilometers with a total population of 4.5 crores. After many years of racial tensions with the first democratic election held in 1994 the same has come to an end. With the objective of Reconstruction and Development Programme (RDP) for the impoverished black majority, African National Congress (ANC) came to power in 1994. ANC could do some development works which inter alia, include construction of houses for the poor, establishment of schools, health centers, safe drinking water to the people etc. But the major problem the country is facing today is HIV/AIDS. Prevalence rate of HIV/AIDS in South Africa is very high. Out of every five adult one is infected with the disease (2001) thus 47 lakh people are directly affected. Another quarter million children are having HIV positive. In 2001, "some 360,000 (360,000) South African died that year alone and the number of AIDS orphans rose to 660,000. By 2005, average life expectancy will have fallen to 47 years from 60 years a decade ago (African Renewal, July 2004).

Sierra Leone: Sexual Violence

Sierra Leone is spread over to an area of 71740 square kilometers with an estimated population of 40 lakh. The Sierra Leone Civil War was internationally known for severe atrocities. Atrocity was committed on villagers by severing their limbs. Besides, violence against women was a routine affairs not casual phenomenon.

In 1991 civil war which lasted for 10 years started in Sierra Leone. To get an idea about the real picture of atrocities committed on civilians during and after the war Truth and Reconciliation Commission (TRC) was set up. The Report of TRC was released in October 2004. The 1500-page report throws light about atrocities carried out in the war. It is sated in the Report that, "All armed groups carried out human rights violations against women and girls. These included killing, rape and other sexual violence, sexual slavery, slave labour, abduction, assault, amputation, forced pregnancy, disembowelment of pregnant women, torture, trafficking, mutilation, theft and the destruction of poverty. The Report further mentioned that, "Because rape and sexual violence were so rife during the war, the country is now seeing a sharp rise in case of HIV/AIDS and other sexually transmitted infections (Africa Renewal, January 2005).

Conclusion

Africa is rich in various mineral resources vis-à-vis its natural beauty is a 'diamond in the crown'. There are lots of scopes for development in Africa from various angles. Its human resource is another asset. Every year huge number of qualified persons leave Africa. In this context Eritrea Profile, 18 January, 2005 may be referred, "according to a study by the Geneva based inter governmental body, the International Organization for Migration (IOM) and the UN's Economic Commission for Africa (ECA) between 1960 and 1975 an estimated 27,000 highly qualified Africans left the continent for the West. This number increased to approximately 40,000 between 1975 and 1984 and then almost doubled by 1987, representing 30 per cent of the highly skilled man power stock. In general, Africa lost 60,000 professionals (doctors, university lecturers, engineers etc) between 1985 and 1990 and has been losing an average of 20,000 annually ever since."

Thus it is estimated that Africa is rich in many respects, in spite of this it is poor? The problems are many; a few of them are analyzed in this article. So there is urgent need to address the problems. My personal opinion includes all good governance in all the countries, food for all, education for all, providing health facilities to all, awareness against HIV/AIDS, creation of employment (both self and wage), eradication of corruption (as it is very high), status to women, control of ethnic clash (lakh and lakh people died) and strict measures against militias.

References

Africa Renewal (July 2004), United Nations, Department of Public Information, New York, USA.

Africa Renewal (January 2005), United Nations, Department of Public Information, New York, USA.

Eritrea Profile, 14 June (2006), Asmara, Eritrea.

Eritrea Profile, 5 August 2006, Asmara, Eritrea.

Eritrea Profile, 20 September 2006, Asmara, Eritrea.

Eritrea Profile, 21 October 2006, Asmara, Eritrea.

United Nations Mission for Ethiopia and Eritrea, Newsletter, July–August 2005.

18

CHALLENGES FOR RESEARCH DEVELOPMENT IN ERITREA SOME OBSERVATIONS

Ravinder Rena

Introduction

Research is defined as a scientific and systematic search for pertinent information on a specific topic. It comprises defining and redefining problems, formulating hypothesis or suggested solutions; collecting, organizing and evaluating data; making deductions and reaching conclusions; and at last carefully testing the conclusions to determine whether they fit the formulating hypothesis.

Research is an original contribution to the existing stock of knowledge making for its advancement (Allen T., 1978). It is the pursuit of truth with the help of study, observation, comparison and experiment. In brief, the search for knowledge through objective and systematic method of finding solution to a problem is research.

A survey of geographical distribution of research capacity indicates very high correlation between a nation's research capacity and its economic development level. According to the survey, for example in Africa, there are only 71 researchers per one million people compared to almost 4000 researchers per million people in North America, Japan etc., Today research, in most of the African universities, is very poorly supported by the governments. Similarly, the African universities do not get enough local support. It is not due to lack of financial resources, because the governments have been spending enormous amounts of funds on foreign consultants albeit. However, local experts of equivalent qualification are available at much lower cost. The management of various organizations (government and private) should understand that the research is not to criticize any one but to present the facts. Research provides better opportunity to work more intelligently and efficiently. Therefore, the organizations can learn from their impediments and adopt better measures for capacity building.

It is observed that Eritrea, like many other developing countries, has allocated substantial resources to its tertiary sector of education. It hopes to produce the required manpower essential for rapid economic development. However, the allocation of resources has not been matched with the researches conducted in the country. It is imperative to determine effectively how such resources have been used for the research development.

Profile of Eritrea

Eritrea is one of the youngest nations in the world, which became officially independent from Ethiopia in 1993 after a debilitating war that lasted more than thirty years. It is located in the North Eastern of Africa with a total area of 124,432 km^2 and a coastline on the Red Sea of almost 1000km. Eritrea, bordered in the North and West by Sudan, in the South by Ethiopia and Djibouti, and in the East by the Red Sea. It has an estimated population of about 3.9 million with a population growth per annum is estimated (1999 est.) to be 2.9 per cent. It has nine ethnic groups and six *zobas* (provinces/regions) [1].

The country is a land of varied topography, climate and rainfall. It is an arid and semi-arid region consisting of a high plateau and coastal plains. Climate varies according to the different topographical regions, mostly hot and dry along the low lands and Red Sea coast and cooler and more humid on the inland plateau. Average temperature range from 35^0c in the low lands to 20^{0}c in the highlands. The highlands have a moderate climate with minimal seasonal temperature variation. Temperature variations in the lowlands are much greater than in the highlands. During the hot and dry season maximum temperature can reach 45^{0}c in the low lands and 29^{0}c in the central highlands. Red Sea coastal plain, particularly in the Dalul depression in the Southeast that falls 100 meters below sea level is notable for having some of the highest temperatures recorded on earth. It can reach an extreme high temperature in the summer, with occasional highs up to 60^{0}c.

The main economic stay of the people is agriculture of which crop production followed by livestock herding are the core economic activities. The agricultural sector employs about 70 per cent of the working population, but its contribution to GDP is less than 22 per cent.

This research paper is composed of five parts. The first part is introductory in nature. The second part deals with the Research Development in Eritrea with a special focus on agricultural research followed by the third part, challenges for research in the country. The fourth part provides some implications for research development in Eritrea. The fifth and final part of this paper provides concluding remarks of the study.

Development of Research in Eritrea

About a year ago, an International Symposium was conducted on the topic "The Role of Research in National Building" This symposium was organized by the University of Asmara during 15 - 18 June, 2002 at Inter-Continental Hotel, Asmara, Eritrea. There as many as 40 papers pertinent to different fields had been presented. The research papers presented were mainly related with agriculture, social and management sciences, education, technology, health care and other development related issues. Scholars from inside and outside of Eritrea presented these papers at the symposium. The University of Asmara is striving hard to develop the research in the country. It is trying to develop research as "transdisciplinary, collaborative, cross national, and socially accountable"

Research is a powerful tool for knowledge generation. As a newly born nation, Eritrea has to find its own ways and its own solutions to the challenge of applying knowledge to work in the economy. Whatever solutions the government or the related institutions propose, we have to understand the research plays a central role and can generate new ideas and innovative techniques. These ideas give birth to new industries, and stimulate the productivity, that would increase the standard of life for the people of Eritrea. The experience of other countries reveal that, during the last five decades, the role of universities evolved into a mere cause-and -effect relationship with society, technology and the economy. The president of University of Asmara, recently outlined that, "the university is reached a stage where it must pay a greater attention to building its research infrastructure and research capacity in order to create better conditions to retain its staff that it has developed a very high cost and to transform itself from a mere teaching to full-fledged research university".

Agricultural Research in Eritrea

The basis of indigenous research has been weak. It has been characterized by a limited number of researchers, high cost, and dispersion over many research stations, and activities coupled with high turnover and unproductively (Ravinder Rena, 2003:10). It is observed that, Eritrea has focused on basic research. However, shortage of finance has undoubtedly plagued research institutes in the country. And there are severe problems in formulating and obtaining data in making any accurate estimates of the levels of output, employment consumption and distribution activities in Eritrea.

It is to be noted that the national agricultural research institution in Eritrea is in its infancy and it needs time and resources to be fully developed. It has, indeed made an impressive progress. At present, it is focusing mainly to prepare the foundations such as human and material capacity building. It has also released some improved crop varieties selected through adaptive research. They include staple crops such as sorghum vulgaris and many more are under study. It has established a germplasm bank on plants, three research stations and contacts with the international research institutions. Applied research on plant pests, livestock, forestry and horticulture are in progress. The laboratories are also under preparation. The main constraints include shortage of research scientists, high-level technicians, facilities and equipment and an overall syndrome of being young institution (FAO, 1998:18).

Eritrea, however, has been attempting to implement modern technology in specific areas in the country such as *Eloborate, Halhale, Aligidher, Hagaz, Amalmalo, etc.*, from the mid nineties onwards. Besides, three agricultural sites in Eritrea namely; Golluj in the Gash Barka, Shi'ib in the Northern Red Sea and Hazomo in Zoba Debub are considered three "breadbasket" areas[2] of the nation (Ravinder Rena, 2004[a]:120).

Indeed, until recently, very little research addressed efficient use of inputs and balancing the external input use and internal sources of nutrients. Thus, from the policy perspective, there is case for public and private initiative on several fronts to reverse degradation–increased investment in crop and resource management research and extension, research to develop diversified and more sustainable cropping patterns and rotations.

Participating Agencies in Research and Development: Most of the international organizations, some bilateral and few NGOs are operating in Eritrea as partners in, inter-alia, research and agricultural development. Since recent times, participation of NGOs has been on the decline. The partners are either directly involved in research and development of agriculture and fisheries or indirectly in rural infrastructure or institutional strengthening. Within the UN-system, they include FOA, United Nations Development Program (UNDP), United Nations International Children's Emergency Fund (UNICEF), World Health Organization (WHO), World Food Program (WFP), United Nations High Commissioner for Refugees (UNHCR) and Danish Development Agency (DANIDA). Among the multilaterals and financing institutions the EU, the World Bank, International Fund for Agricultural Development (IFAD) and African Development Bank (ADB) are actively supporting the research and a wide range of sectors to create an enabling environment to achieve the food security and rural development (Ravinder Rena, 2004[a]: 121). Farm among bi-laterals, Denmark, Norway, and United States Agency for International Development (USAID), the Netherlands and Italy are the major partners. Among the NGOs, Africare, the Lutheran World Federation and the local churches are the main participating in the Eritrea agriculture development.

Other Special Initiatives include Sasakawa Global (SG2000) project, whose objectives are to assist small farmers to improve productivity and welfare technology transfer and to strengthen national extension services in technology dissemination. SG 2000 has started in zoba Maekel and zoba Debub. It distributes improved seed; fertilizer and pesticides to selected farmers, and gives them management and extension advice. SG 2000 provides group training in farmers fields complemented by field days, workshops and study tours. However, the system or the role of intensification also has been advocated earlier through the SG 2000 and FSP (FAO) programme operating in Eritrea since some years (MoA, 2002: 20).

It is observed that the analysis of agricultural, industrial production in Eritrea suffers from a lack of data and sharp variations in the information available from different sources. The data related to many sectors of the economy is seems to be non-existent or less reliable. The information is also subject to considerable controversy.

As stated earlier, there is a controversy over data on production in relation to the use of different sources, including National Statistical Office (NSO), Ministry of Agriculture, Food and Agricultural Organization (FAO) etc. For instance, in agriculture, the main trend, which emerges, is either stagnation or slow pace of growth in aggregate food crop production during the period 1998-2002. However, the trends need to be treated with caution because of the problems of obtaining accurate data in Eritrea.

Research Centers in Eritrea

In Eritrea, there are some research-centered institutions such as Research and Documentation Center (RDC), National

Statistical Office, etc., In addition every Ministry has its own research libraries and/or departments. Particularly, Research and Documentation Center is a de facto National Archives and Record Management of Eritrea. It is located in Asmara. The author had the privilege of visiting it many times for the purpose of collecting data for research. So author can vouch without doubt that RDC is a rich source for research. It can be considered as a repository of Eritrean history, culture and valued documents. It consists of written records, audio /visual records, cartographic, photographic records etc., It has the collection of Federation Period (1952-62) including daily minutes, biographies and security issues, the armed struggle, Eritrean Liberation Front (ELF) and Eritrean People's Liberation Front (EPLF) conference proceedings, Italian, the British and Ethiopian periods. It also comprises complete records of Referendum (1993), and Constitution Commission's records are some of its important collections. All these documents are found in Tigrigna, Arabic, Italian and English. It is reported that, Eritrea is the only country in Africa, which has preserved the comprehensive and systematic historical records after South Africa. It should be mentioned that, the Fourth Eritrean National Book Fair conducted recently in Expo Exhibition, Asmara, Eritrea from 14-20 March 2005 also stimulates the researchers and supplies some source knowledge to conduct research in the country.

Research Challenges in Eritrea

The Researchers in Eritrea, particularly those engaged in empirical research, are facing several challenges. Some of the important problems identified and discussed below.

1. *Lack of a scientific training in the methodology of research:* It is found to be a great impediment for researchers in Eritrea. There is paucity of competent researchers in Eritrea. Many researchers take a leap in the dark without knowing research methods. It is observed that most of the work, which goes in the name of research is not methodologically sound. Research to many researchers and even to their supervisors/

guides, is mostly a scissors and paste job without any insight shed on the collated materials. The consequence is obvious i.e. the research results, quite often, do not reflect the realities. Therefore, a systematic study of research methodology is imperative. Before undertaking research projects, researchers should be well equipped with all methodological aspects. Thus, efforts should be made by the concerned organizations to provide short-duration intensive research courses for meeting this requirement.

2. *Lack of Interaction between University research departments:* There is a lack of coordination between the university research department on one-side business establishments, government departments and research institutions on the other side. A great deal of primary data of non-confidential nature remains untouched by the researchers in Eritrea. Therefore, efforts should be made to develop satisfactory relationship among all concerned for better and realistic researchers. Hence, there is a need to develop some mechanisms by university-industry interaction programme so that academics can get ideas from practitioners on what needs to be researched and practitioners can apply the research done by academics.

3. *Lack of Confidence in Researchers in disclosing Data:* It is noticed that, most of the business units in Eritrea, do not have the confidence that the material supplied by them to researchers will not be misused and such as they are often reluctant in supplying the required information to researchers in Eritrea. The concept of secrecy seems to be blessed to business organizations in Eritrea. However, it proves an impenetrable barrier to the researchers in Eritrea. Thus, there is a need for generating the confidence that the information obtained from business unit/government office will be used purely for research purpose alone.

4. *Research Studies in Eritrea are Overlapping one another:* This results in duplication and fritters away resources. This problem can be solved by proper compilation and revision, at regular intervals, of a list of subjects on which and the places where the research is going on. Due attention should be given toward identification of research problems in different disciplines of applied science, engineering, information technology and social sciences etc. which are immediate concern to the economy of the country.
5. *Lack of Code of Conduct:* There is no code of conduct for researchers in Eritrea. Hence, there is a need for developing a code of conduct for researchers, which, if adhered sincerely, can win over this problem.
6. *Lack of Secretarial Assistance:* It is also observed that, many researchers in Eritrea face the difficulty of adequate and timely secretarial assistance, including computer assistance. This indeed causes unnecessary delays in the completion of research studies. All possible efforts are made in this direction so that efficient secretarial assistance is made available to researchers in Eritrea. The Government of Eritrea should play a dynamic role to establish a competent organization in solving this problem.
7. *Unsatisfactory Mode of Functioning Libraries:* Library management and functioning is not satisfactory at many places in the country and much of the time and energy of researchers are of course spent in tracing out the books, journal and reports, etc., rather than in tracing out relevant material from them. However, the libraries are expected to be research friendly.
8. *Lack of Related Documents:* There is another important problem that many of Eritrean libraries are not able to get the old and new copies of the Proclamations, reports, statistical bulletins and other government publications in time. Besides, it is very difficult to get the current issues of some important journals. If

problem is felt in libraries, which are in Asmara, think about the position of Zoba level and sub-zoba level libraries in Eritrea. Thus, efforts should be made for the regular and speedy supply of all governmental publications and important journals to reach the important libraries and other research centers.

9. *Delay in Publishing Documents:* There is also the difficulty of timely availability of published data from various government and other agencies in Eritrea. Researcher also faces the problem on account of the fact that the published data vary quite significantly because of differences in coverage by the concerned agencies.
10. *Problem of Conceptualization:* There may at times, occur the problem of conceptualization and problems relating to the data collection and related things.

Implications

(i) Encourage the need based research suitable to Eritrea; (ii) Open the Post Graduate courses in the University of Asmara and/or Eritrean Institute of Technology thereby create a basis for research development courses; (iii) There must be a collaboration between the University and industry in research; it is observed that different ministries have Research and Development Departments, but they have to be activated to conduct research on contemporary economic and social issues; make available the research results masses for their social and economic development; (iv) Apply the research outcome that leads to sustainable growth of the nation; (v) Build the information network and encourage the publishing industry which can induce the research development in Eritrea.

Conclusions

Research is a careful investigation or inquiry especially through search for new facts in any branch of knowledge. Further, research is a systematized effort to gain new knowledge. On the other hand, research as the manipulation of things, concepts or symbols for the purpose of generalizing to extend, correct or verify knowledge whether that knowledge aids in construction of theory or in the practice of an art.

In a rapidly globalizing world, the awareness of the global problems and threats are rapidly developing, resulting in greater commitments to global issues such as ecology, climatic changes, gender issues, poverty, illiteracy etc., which usually but not always overlap the national priorities. Since more resources are available for research on the global issues and research priorities on global issues are more clearly defined, albeit in the developed world, maintaining a focus on national and/or regional research priorities and integrating them global issues may be a challenging. However, the research wing is lagging behind Africa in general and Eritrea in particular.

Notes

1. The Nine Ethnic groups of Eritrea are: Tigirgna, Tigre, Sahoo, Afar, Bilen, Hidareb, Kunama, Nara, and Rashaida. Where as the six Administrative zobas or provinces are: Maakel, Anseba, Debub, Gash Barka, Northern Red Sea, and Southern Red Sea.
2. These areas are chosen as work sites where deep agricultural research is proposed.

References

Allen T. Harrel (1978), *New Methods in Social Science Research.* New York: Praeger Publishers.

FAO. (1998), *Strengthening the Agricultural Research and Extension in Eritrea.* GCP/ERI/001/ITA, Asmara: Food and Agriculture Organization of the United Nations in Eritrea.

Freedman, P. (1960), *The Principles of Scientific Research.* New York: Pergamon Press.

Kothari, C.R. (1998), *Research Methodology: Methods and Techniques.* Hyderabad: Wishwa Prakashan.

Krishnaswami, O.R. (1999), *Methodology of Research in Social Sciences.* New Delhi: Himalaya Publishing House.

Ministry of Agriculture (2002), *Agricultural Sector Policy and Strategy Framework: Background and Context Development and*

Management. Asmara: Ministry of Agriculture, The Government of State of Eritrea (November).

Ravinder Rena (2003), "Challenges of Research in Eritrea". Asmara (Eritrea) *Eritrea Profile (A Weekly Bulletin of News and Views) Ministry of Information and Culture, 10 (15), (31st May,) p.10.*

Ravinder Rena (2004[a]), "Green Revolution: Indian Agricultural Experience–A Paradigm for Eritrea". New Jersey, USA: *Eritrean Studies Review, Vol. 4, No.1 (A Biannual Journal Published by the Red Sea Press) pp.103-130.*

Ravinder Rena (2004[b]), "Fundamentals of Research Methods". Asmara: Asmara Commercial College, Unpublished manuscript.

Sharma, H.D. and Mukherji, S.P. (1976), *Research in Economics and Commerce: Methodology and Surveys.* Varanasi: Indian Biographic Center.

19

POVERTY ALLEVIATION MEASURES IN ERITREA: A COUNTRY LOCATED IN NORTH EAST AFRICA

Shankar Chatterjee

Introduction

Poverty is a major problem of the developing countries. African countries are particularly affected with this problem. Rampant starvation death was worldwide news during 2005 in Niger. Poverty issue was and agenda in G-8 Summit held in July 6-8, 2005 in Scotland where the slogan was that "make Poverty History", particularly in Africa (UNMEE News July/August 2005).

Eritrea a new independent country (independence in 1991) with 1,25,000 squares Kilometers area is having 4 million populations. The country is also not free from the problem of poverty as its huge population is living "Below the Poverty Line" (BPL). As per the survey carried out by National Statistics & Evaluation Office (NSEO) of Eritrea, 66.40 per cent of its population was Below of the Poverty line in the year 2003.

National Statistics & Evaluation Office (NSEO) conducted a survey under the title of "Household Living Standard Measurement Survey" in the year 2003, with a view to get through idea about the nature, extent and causes of poverty in Eritrea. During the same time there other studies on poverty were also conducted in Eritrea. These studies are

(i) Participatory Poverty Assessment Study (ii) Second Demographic and Health Survey and (iii) Rural Livelihood Security Assessment Study. Based on all these studies, NSEO produced a Report under the title of "Dimensions of Poverty in Eritrea". Revealing point of the Report is that poverty ratio in Eritrea is 66.40 per cent with rural and urban ratios of 64.64 and 70.30 per cent respectively. Again out of 66.40 per cent BPL categories, 36.97 per cent population has been identified as "Extreme Poor Category". Like other countries basis of determination of poverty is money income. The person is considered as poor, if his/her income per month is 240 Nakfa or less and 150 Nakfa per capita per month is for extreme poor category. The BPL data are shown in Table 1.

Table 1
Incidence of Poverty (Head count) in Eritrea

Rural/Urban	*Percentage of Poor*	*Percentage of Extreme Poor (out of total poor)*
Rural	64.64	38.90
Urban	70.30	32.65
Total	66.40	36.97

Source: Dimensions of Poverty in Eritrea 2002.

The Government of Eritrea is also serious to alleviate poverty from the country. Establishment of Savings and Micro Credit Program popularly known as SMCP is the first step in this direction. The Savings and Micro credit Program (SMCP) is an autonomous government micro finance institution operating under the Ministry of National Development, Government of Eritrea. It was established in July 1996 with the objective of providing credit to marginalized people including women who lacks access to the formal financial institutions. Its beneficiaries also include demobilized soldiers, returning refugees, deportees from Ethiopia, and internally displaced persons (IDPs). The program has four operational objectives:

(i) to extend credit who are presently outside the orbit of the formal banking network,

(ii) to strengthen community representative structures from village to higher levels, especially in the economic domain

(iii) to build institutional capacity and capability at the local level

(iv) to establish a legal base so that the SMCP could become an independent financial institution which is organizationally and financially sustainable.

A National Steering Committee (NSC) representing the ministries of National Development, Agriculture, Trade and Industry, and the Eritrea Development and Investment Bank (EDIB), and the National Union of Eritrea Women (NUEW) is the highest governing body overseeing its activities. A Program Manager assisted by different units (Administration, Finance, Internal Audit and Research and Training) oversees the day-to-day activities of the program. SMCP extends poor beneficiaries two types of loan–First tier and Second tier.

First Tier Loan: First tier loan is extended to those persons who are in the category of poor/very poor. As a primary step a minimum of 35 persons (in SMCP language it is known as clients, hence forth client word will be used) should come forward to form a group, which is termed, as village bank. Again sub-groups comprising of 3 to 7 members (SMCP's language solidarity group) are formed from the members of village bank. Thus all members of village bank are split into sub groups ranging from 3 to 7. Group members guarantee each other's loan. Loans are sanctioned on short–term basis.

The clients under first tier program can access loan ranging from 3000 to 40,000 Nakfa which is disbursed in ten progressive loan cycles (loan cycle means once one loan is repaid another loan is sanctioned). It is pertinent to mention here that 1 US dollar is equal to 15 (approx) Eritrea currency, which is known as Nakfa. For the first four cycles, the loan terms ranges from 3 to 12 months, while loans in the next six cycles can be paid within 24 months. Clients are required to pay in installments (mostly monthly). If loan repayment in four consecutive cycles is within the stipulated time in that case as an incentive, clients are extended individual loan. This type of borrowing is known as first tier B–category client.

Second Tier Loan: The second tier loan is extended to individual person. Clients eligible under this loan program can access loans ranging from 40,000 to 150,000 Nakfa, which is disbursed in six different loan cycles. Each loan is extended based on best performance and full repayment of prior loan. Loan term under this program ranges from 3 to 36 months. Most loans under this program are given to people owing small enterprises. Unlike in the group loan (1st Tier), for any one to be eligible under this program, a feasibility study is conducted and collateral/cosigners are a requirement.

Under both the tiers, there is a mandatory requirement of savings. First tier clients are required to deposit 10 per cent of the loan amount before accessing the loan and an additional 6 per cent is deposited over the course of the loan. This brings the total savings requirement for this group of clients to 16 per cent. For second tier clients, the total savings requirement is 11 per cent. Client savings are deposited in a nearest commercial bank branch. A loan fee of 0.5 per cent paid during each disbursement is also common to both categories of clients. The clients of both first & second tiers have to repay loan on the basis of simple rate of interest, which is 16 per cent and is calculated on the declining balance method. However, clients of second tier with perfect records of loan repayment, a 2 per cent rebate is given as an incentive.

The SMCP presently operates in all six regions (regions are known as Zoba synonymous to Province) and 48 sub regions out of 59 sub regions. As of December 31st 2004 it had 16,487 (42.6% women) active clients under the first tier loan program spread over to 207 village banks and another 1, 671 (42.4% women) active clients under the second tier loan program (individual loan). From its inception in July 1996 to December 2004, the SMCP has disbursed a total of 26.99 million Nakfa.

The Government of Eritrea and the World Bank fund the SMCP. Lately, other organizations (UNDP, NGOs like A.So.C, Manittese, and Concern Worldwide) have shown interest to collaborate with the SMCP. The performance of SMCP from July 1, 1996 to 31st December 2004 is presented in Table 2.

A few salient features of the table are:

Table 2
Performances of Savings and Micro Credit Program (July 1, 1996 to 31st December 2004)

Items	*1996*	*1997*	*1998*	*1999*	*2000*	*2001*	*2002*	*2003*	*2004*
Total No. of village banks	25	39	76	85	88	146	162	191	207
Total No. of new village banks	25	14	37	9	3	58	16	29	16
No of Active clients (I Tier)	1470	2373	5477	5779	5942	10304	11492	13765	15602
No of Active clients (II Tier)	—	7	27	36	245	925	1469	16311	1665
% of Women Beneficiaries (I Tier)	30.0	30.3	27.6	29.6	30.2	37.0	40.0	40.0	42.6
% of Women Beneficiaries (II Tier)	—	14.30	6.5	14.3	29.0	36.0	36.0	39.0	42.0
Loan Disbursed (Million Nakfa) I Tier	1.37	6.36	13.89	9.43	7.02	19.80	32.62	43.80	45.57
Loan Disbursed (Million Nakfa) I Tier	—	0.07	0.63	0.30	2.68	14.69	27.40	23.20	20.69
Total loan Disbursed (Million Nakfa)	1.37	6.43	14.52	9.73	9.70	34.49	60.02	67.00	66.26

Source: SMCP Report

(i) Within eight years (1996 to 2004), number of active members has increased more than 10 times in first tier.

(ii) Increase in active member in second tier, is more than 200 times within 7 years.

(iii) Amount of loan disbursement has also gone up several folds in both the tiers.

It is evident from the above table that SMCP's performance is praiseworthy. However, declining trend was observed in 1999 and 2000 as the country had war with Ethiopia during this period.

Economic activity wise loan disbursement shows that agriculture got maximum importance in case of first tier clients and in case of second tier, trade got importance. One can assume here that first tier clients hail from agriculture community while second tier clients are having trade and business. Economic activity-wise distribution of loan is presented in Table 3.

Table 3
Sector wise loan disbursed (From 1, July 1996 to 31st December 2004)

(In Per cent)

Economic Activity	*First Tier*	*Second Tier*
Agriculture	42.95	20.47
Service	15.92	31.51
Trade	40.25	41.23
Manufacturing	0.88	6.79
Total	100	100

Source: SMCP 2004, Annual Report, March 2005.

Field Study

Study Area and Period of Study

To get an idea about the implementation of its program, field study was carried out a Himbirty village of Maakel Zoba and Maiduma village of Debub Zoba. Himbirty village was visited during October 2005 and study was conducted at Maiduma in November 2005.

Methodology

The study includes both primary and secondary data. The clients of First tier and Second tier were contacted and discussions were held with them for which a checklist was prepared. Secondary data were collected from various reports, documents etc.

Field Study

The village Himbirty is 34 Kms away from Asmara city (capital of Eritrea). As reported, it is largest village of Eritrea in terms of population. It is well connected by surface transport with Asmara due to its proximity to capital. On the other hand, Maidama is located about 115 Kms from Asmara and around 60 Kms road is fair – weather rather some portions of road are so bad vehicles face problem for smooth movement in winter also and in rainy days vehicle ply with great difficulty. The village Maiduma was badly damaged by Ethiopian soldiers in May 2000 during the time of conflict between Ethiopia and Eritrea. The villagers revealed this problem many a time during the time of study. The basic facilities of both the villages are presented in Table 4.

Table 4
Basic Facilities Available at Himbirty and Maiduma villages

Name of the Facility	*Number*	
	Himbirty	*Maiduma*
Total households	2295	1357
Total Population	8788	4822
Kindergarten School	2	—
Elementary School (5th)	1	1
Junior School (6 to 8)	1	1
Clinic	1 (No doctor but 5 paramedical staff)	1 (No doctor but 5 paramedical staff)
Pipe water Supply	7 (common distribution points)	Nil (people bring water from nearby wells by donkeys)
Electricity	Available	No (But through private generators electricity is supplied)
Bank	No formal bank	No formal bank

Source: Field Survey.

As mentioned already villagers have to form group under the banner of "Village Bank". The study reveals that there two village banks at Himbirty village. One consists of 60 clients and other consists of 58 clients. Besides, there are 13 clients in Second Tier. So altogether 131 villagers have been benefited under SMCP.

Cases from Himbirty Village

Mrs. Rigbe, a middle aged woman with nine members family had lot of hardship to manage her family before getting credit from SMCP. She had inclination towards business but minimum availability of fund was her hindrance. In the year 2001, she came to know about SMCP credits and accordingly approached. She was extended an amount of 20,000 Nakfa under second tier client as credit by SMCP in 2001. With this she started ready-made garments business in the front side of her house. She fully devoted in the business which was yielding desired result as could she earn a net profit of 2000 Nakfa per month. She refunded entire amount principal as well as interest by the end of 2003. She took second dose of loan (30,000 Nakfa) in March 2004 for expanding her business. She revealed that by investing the amount she could able to earn more income. It was reported that second tier clients should have some knowledge about business vis-à-vis before getting loan as second tier client they should have some business.

Mrs. Meaza Berhe is also a middle-aged woman but she is widow. Mrs. Berhe is having 6 members family with little agricultural land (half an acre). She struggled like anything for survival up to 1996. In the year 1996, she came to know about SMCP credit and immediately joined in village bank. She was extended an amount of 750 Nakfa by SMCP initially as a member of solidarity group (first tier) in the year 1996. With this amount, she started shoe-repairing business. Although amount was meager but her effort was great as a result she could earn minimum amount for maintaining her family. Motivated with the activity, she not only repaid loan within the stipulated time but she borrowed money from SMCP in 9 occasions. And every time, he repaid with in the stipulated time.

Her last borrowing was in May 2005 (13000 Nakfa), which she invested in expanding her business–utensils and vegetables business. Every loan helped her to earn more income, although she was unable to tell her net monthly profit as she has been earning and spending which is her day-to-day affairs.

The clients who were studied randomly reveal that they cámp up from their economic hardship after SMCP credit. In fact, it was observed that the village due to its proximity to capital city is having both favorable "Backward and Forward Linkages".

Cases from Maiduma Village

Maiduma is located 115 Kms away from Asmara more than half of 115 Kms road is fair weather. Naturally one can imagine the location of the village. More over, infrastructure of the village has been badly damaged by Ethiopian soldiers during May 2000. Altogether three village banks have been formed in the village with total clients of 480 persons under first tier. Besides there are 135 clients have been benefited under second tier. Besides there are 135 clients have been benefited under second tier. A few of the SMCP clients who were studied randomly are presented below.

Emanuel, male person of about 55 years age having no agricultural land is carpenters by profession. He has a large family–10 members including 7 children. Since he had carpentry business (in a small way) so he wanted to expand it, as a sequel he applied for SMCP loan as second tier client. Accordingly, in the year 2001 an amount of 40,000 Nakfa was sanctioned. He expanded his carpentry business but faced severe problem of raw materials, as a result he could not repay full amount of loan. Only 50 per cent of his loan was repaid within the stipulated time. In view of this he applied to diverse his business to hotel business. SMCP thoroughly reviewed his case and permitted him to shift his business from carpentry to hotel business and extended his loan repayment period also. Diversification has helped him to earn more; as a result he could repay every month at the rate of 2500 Nakfa besides earning a net profit of 2000 Nakfa per month. According to him, a few more installments are required to fully repay his loan SMCP.

Hadish, is also a male person of about 55 years age having no agricultural land. He was tailor by profession and as a part time activity he is priest. He is having 8 members family. In the year, 2000 (June), he wanted to start his business because his business was severely affected by war. Accordingly requested SMCP for loan as second tier client. An amount of 10,000 Nakfa was sanctioned to him. With this amount, he started ready-made garments business. Due to his hard labour, he could reap the benefit from the business and within a year he repaid the entire amount with interest. Subsequently he took loan and repaid the same as shown below.

(a) Second dose of loan of 15,000 Nakfa from SMCP was sanctioned in 2001, which he repaid within 1 year.

(b) Third dose of loan (20,000 Nakfa) was sanctioned in 2002, which he repaid within 1 year.

(c) Fourth dose of loan from SMCP was 40,000 Nakfa in 2003; repayment period of this is 2 years, which he has been repaying.

To a query about earning of profit, he informed that after repaying loan amount of 2000 (approx.) per month, his net profit ranges in between 1300 and 1500 per month. He admitted that SMCP loan has greatly helped him to improve his economic condition.

Mrs Rezan, a widow (64 years age) is having 3 members family (self, daughter and grandson). She is having five children but except one daughter all are staying seperatelly. She has little more than 2 hectare of agriculture land but cultivation is done through sharecropper. Only in rainy season land is cultivated and she is given one-fourth to total production, which include sorghum and wheat. She was unable to tell quantity of crops received by him. However, quantity of crop is very meager for the sustenance of the family. In view of this, she joined solidarity group to get loan as first tier client. In the year 2001, she was given an amount of 2000 Nakfa with which she started grain business. Since she could repay the loan within the stipulated time, she was given further an amount of 3000 Nakfa in 2002, further 5000 Nakfa in 2003 and 7000 Nakfa in 2004. She was getting loan, as she was repayig within the stipulated time. Impressed with her performance, she was included as first tier client of B category. It has already mention that if loan repayment is within the stipulated time then under first tier a person can get individual loan which is categorized as First Tier – B category. So her loan amount of 7000 is an individual loan. She happily informed that with the increase in loan amount, she could expand her business and besides repaying little more than 500 Nakfa per month she has been earning net profit in between 1500 and 1700 Nakfa per month.

Mrs. Ethiiopia (40 years), Mrs. Ziman (35 years) and Mrs Salamawit (24 years) formed solidarity group in the year 2003. Ethiopia is divorced woman but having three members in the family. Zamin and Salamawit are living with their husband but Ziman is having 6 members family (self, husband and four children). Her husband is daily labourer. Salamawit is having one child and her husband is in army. Each of the members was extended at the rate of 3000 Nakfa for doing business. Ethiopia started sheep business (purchasing baby sheep and sell when it becomes adult). Ziman and Salamawit started poultry business (buying poultry bird from interior villages and selling the same in the local market). But all of them could not succeed in business as a result they became defaulter. Each of the clients has to repay in between 2000 and 2300 Nakfa. In other words, out of 3000 Nakfa (per person) only 700 to 1000 Nakfa has been repaid. However, Ethiopia instead of sheep business started "Local beer selling" business.

Issue of non-repayment was discussed with SCMP officials. It was reported that severe drought in 2004 badly hampered their business activities. According to SMCP officials since first tier clients are poor so they are given some more time to repay at the amount particularly if they face any natural calamity. Even if they are unable to repay at the last stage and after doings thorough study, the loan is written–off. But for second tier clients no such relaxation is given. They have to repay loan. Sometimes time is extended even refinance is also done to divert the activities. Even if all these don't work then as a last resort case may be referred to the court.

Conclusion

It is evident from the above that SMCP has been doing well to eradicate poverty from Eritrea. But failure of three cases in Maiduma reveal that arrangement may be made for proper backward and forward linkages, and if any problem occurs in this regard, steps should be taken to address it. Otherwise simply pumping of loan will not serve the purpose.

Reference

UNMEE–United Nations Mission for Ethiopia and Eritrea, July–August 2005.

20

INDUSTRIAL DEVELOPMENT IN ERITREA DURING POST-LIBERATION ERA: A STUDY

D.V. Madhusudan Rao & Shankar Chatterjee

Introduction

Eritrea, a young nation (1991 independence), is located in the extreme North East of Africa. Its north east side is surrounded by beautiful Red Sea (1000 Kms coastal line approx.). In the absence of population census, actual data on population are not available. Different estimations have been made by different organizations like Government of Eritrea and World Bank etc. According to World Bank's publication of "World Development Indicators" 2005, the population of Eritrea was 4 million in 2003 with a surface area of 118,000 square kilometers. Eritrea got its' independence in 1991. In fact it was a colony of Italy from 1887 to 1941. The country consists of six regions (provinces), locally known as Zoba. Capital of Eritrea is known as Asmara. Its currency is known as Nakfa, which in US Dollar value is equal to 15 Nakfa. (1 US $ = 15 Nakfa approx.).

Some basic particulars on Eritrea

To get an idea about the socio-economic conditions of the people of Eritrea, a few particulars are presented in Table 1.

Table 1
Eritrea: Basic Information

Particulars	*Statistics (2003)*
Population	4 millions
Surface area	118 thousand Sq. Kms
Population density	43 people per Sq. Km
GNP	0.9 $ Billions (Rank 175)
GNI per capita	190 $ (Rank 198)
PPP Gross National Income	$ 4 billions
PPP Gross National Income per capita	$1,020 (Rank 190)
GDP - % growth (2002-03)	3.0
GDP - per capita % growth (2002-03)	0.8
Female population (% of total)	50.4
Life expectancy at birth	Male (50) Female (52)

Source: World Development Indicators 2005, World Bank, 2005.

Manufacturing Units in Eritrea before Liberation: An Overview

Modern manufacturing establishments in Eritrea began with the advent of Italian colonialism. Before the Italian rule (1887) the traditional mode of production was the mainstay of the Economy in Eritrea. The majority of the people were dependent on pastoralism and caravan and other forms of petty trade. Of course various cottage industries such as blacksmith, pottery, weaving, and wood working co-existed with the traditional mode of production.

Italian colonization brought both exploitation and modernization into Eritrea. The Italians generally organised the Eritrean economy according to their own needs. They (Italians) established a number of manufacturing units in between 1887 and 1930. These manufacturing establishments were classified in fifteen groups, namely pasta making (food), button making, flour milling, salt works etc. This industrial growth led to the development of infrastructure.

There was a substantial growth in public investment between 1913 and 1937 of which a significant portion was invested in industries as flour mills, pasta factories, tanneries, textile mills and electrical workshops. During Second World War British occupied Eritrea in April 1941. Industrial firms started operation within five months. From 1941 to 1943 a continuous mushrooming of new manufacturing establishments were witnessed. After 1943, industrial production started falling due to the closure of some industries. In 1946 the British began to dismantle and transfer many industries and projects by selling off and scraping important infrastructure installed by Italians. (Census of Manufacturing Establishments, 2004).

The end of British rule in Eritrea was followed by ten years of federal rule under Ethiopia (1952-1962). During this period manufacturing units established by the British and Italian continued to function. For example cotton manufacturing, brewing, meat packing, glass manufacturing, button making, match producing and agro-industrial estates were exploited optimally.

Ethiopia annexed Eritrea in 1962. They "followed policies that were hostile to Eritrea's economic growth. An economic policy of slowing down the economic activities inside Eritrea was implemented, and as a result, the expansion of existing enterprises and investing in new ones was totally discouraged. Subsequently, the relocation of Eritrean firms into Ethiopia was carefully executed, while skilled Eritrean labour was exiled to Ethiopia and other parts of the world."

During Ethiopian communist regime (1975-91), a deliberate policy of destroying the economic foundation of Eritrea was pursued by Ethiopia government. All major industrial establishments were put under state ownership and their planning and marketing activities were subjected to centralized direction and control.

Manufacturing Units after Liberation

On 24th May 1991, the Eritrea was liberated and a Provisional Government was installed. All the public enterprises were made the property of the Provisional Government of Eritrea.

After independence in 1991, Eritrea inherited 42 public and 645 private manufacturing units which were almost in a non-operating condition. However, many of these units were later on revived. According to Business Licensing Office (BPO) of Eritrea, total number of licensed industrial manufacturing establishments was 2241 in 2004. Presently there are 276

Medium and Large Scale Manufacturing Establishments (MLSMEs) in Eritrea. Henceforth in this article the word MLSMEs will be used. Based on UNIDO's recommendation if employment size in any establishment is 10 persons and above, it is considered as MLSMEs. The number of MLSMEs based on type of ownership is presented in Table 2.

Table 2
Number of MLSMEs based on Type of Ownership 2004

Legal Formation	*Individual (Sole Proprietor-ship)*	*Partner-ship*	*Private Limited Co*	*Share Company*	*Others*	*Total*
No. of Establishments	110	13	110	21	22	276
Percentage	39.9	4.6	39.9	7.6	8.0	100.00

Source: Eritrea Industrial Statistics 2004, Ministry of Trade & Industry, 6 Statistical Bulletins, Nov, 2005, Asmara, Eritrea

The above table shows that out of total MLSMEs, lion share goes to sole proprietorship and private limited companies.

Region wise (Province) MLSMEs

As mentioned already there are six regions in Eritrea. Number of Medium and Large Scale Manufacturing Establishments (MLSMEs) are presented in the following Table 3.

Table 3
Distribution of MLSMEs by Regions, 2004

Administrative Region	*No of Establishments*	*Percentage of Distribution*
Anseba	11	4.0
Debub	43	15.6
Gash Barka	7	2.5
Maekel	204	73.9
Northern Red Sea	11	4.0
Southern Red Sea	0	0
Total	276	100.00

Source: Eritrea Industrial Statistics 2004, Ministry of Trade & Industry, 6 Statistical Bulletins, Nov, 2005, Asmara, Eritrea.

It is evident from the above table that region wise distribution of MLSMEs is not only un-balanced but also un-even as around 74 per cent of total establishments are located in Maekel Zoba region against nil MLSMEs in Southern Red Sea region.

Statistics show number of MLSMEs is increasing in recent years. For example in 2002 total number of MLSMEs was 250, went up to 252 in 2003 and 276 in 2004. This has helped to enhance employment also. A detailed picture may be seen in Table 4.

Table 4
Major Economic Indicators of MLSMEs (2002-2004)

Major Economic Indicators	*2002*	*2003*	*2004*
Number of Persons Engaged	13,413	13,842	14,818
Eritrean Male	6,983	7,176	7,732
Eritrean Female	6,243	6,486	6,857
Non-Eritrean Male	152	148	196
Non-Eritrean Female	35	32	33
Number of Persons Engaged by Occupation	13,413	13,842	14,818
Administration employees	721	774	817
Technical employees	843	921	884
Production workers	9,892	10,067	10.956
Clerical	770	834	883
Other office workers	858	932	945
Unpaid workers (working proprietor, family workers, etc.)	329	314	333
Total Number of Employees by Nationality	13,413	13,842	14,818
Eritrean Male	6,983	7,176	7,732
Eritrean Female	6,243	6,486	6,857
Non-Eritrean Male	152	148	196
Major Economic Indicators	2002	2003	2004
Non-Eritrean Female	35	32	33
Unpaid workers (working proprietor, family workers, etc.)	329	314	333
Eritrean Male	225	216	254
Eritrean Female	86	85	73
Non-Eritrean Male	12	8	3
Non-Eritrean Female	6	5	3
Annual wages and salaries ('000 Nakfa) (A)	127,021	146,240	170,768
Administration employees	15,858	17,495	21,189
Technical employees	12,349	14,580	15,935
Production workers	82,630	96,109	112,788
Clerical	9,334	10,207	12,810
Other office workers	6,846	7,844	8,046
Total Annual Benefits ('000 Nakfa) (B)	5,471	7,989	17,128
Total Annual Compensation ('000 Nakfa) (A+B)	132,492	154,229	187,896

Source: Eritrea Industrial Statistics 2004, Ministry of Trade & Industry, Nov, 2005, Asmara, Eritrea

A few important points derived from the above are:

(i) Over a period of three years employment for both male and female of Eritrean population has increased.

(ii) Besides Eritreans, non-Eritreans have also been engaged.

(iii) Increase of production workers (directly associated with production) is more than administration, technical and clerical staff.

(iv) Workers are paid both as compensation (wage and salaries) and in the form of benefits like bonus etc.

Compensation (wages) of Employees

Wage paid to workers is an important indicator of living standard. In this case, compensation paid to employees of different industrial groups is discussed. Total compensation paid to employees in 2004 was about 188 million Nakfa, of which about 171 million Nakfa was paid as wages and salaries, and remaining 17 million Nakfa consists of other benefits such as commission, bonus, professional hardship, allowances etc. Besides, employees are paid pension, life and causality insurance also.

Annual compensation of employees varies in different industrial groups; data for the compensation per employee is presented in the Table 5.

Number of employees is more in Textile followed by Food and Non-Metallic mineral products. Annual compensation of employees in 2004 ranges from the lowest ratio 8.89 Nakfa per employee in Textile Industry and the highest is 46.93 Nakfa per worker in Tobacco Industry. Compensation per worker in 2004 has increased in all industrial groups (except in Textile Industry) in comparison to 2003. The compensation in Tobacco industry is higher than any other industrial groups due to higher salary scales of administration and technical employees. The compensation per employee in the manufacturing of Beverage and Alcoholic drinks and Furniture stands in the second and third ranks respectively.

Table 5
Employees Compensation–Industry Groups

(In '000 Nakfa)

Industry Group	*2003*			*2004*		
	No. of employees	*Compensation (wages)*	*Compensation per employee*	*No. of employees*	*Compensation (wages)*	*Compensation per employee*
Food	2,472	24,180	9.782	2,627	28,860	10.986
Beverages & Alcoholic Drinks	1,083	17,147	15.833	1,321	25,645	19.413
Tobacco	49	2,065	42.143	44	2,065	46.932
Textile	2,924	28,130	9.620	2,991	26,596	8.892
Leather & Shoe	974	10,104	10.374	934	10,087	10.800
Paper and Printing	517	6,326	12.236	556	8,897	16.002
Chemical Products	542	7,315	13.496	585	9,284	15.870
Rubber& Plastic Products	578	4,414	7.637	582	5,689	9.775
Non-Metallic Mineral Products	1,952	21,011	10.764	2,233	27,202	12.182
Metal Products	1,083	12,788	11.808	1,088	15,754	14.480
Furniture	1,354	20,749	15.324	1,524	27,817	18.253
Total	13,528	154,230	11.401	14,485	187,896	12.972

Source: Eritrea Industrial Statistics 2004, Ministry of Trade & Industry, 6 Statistical Bulletins, Nov, 2005, Asmara, Eritrea

Productivity

Analysis of gross input and gross out put of each industrial group show that in the case of some industries ratio is not favourable, but in some cases favourable ratio is observed. Gross input and gross output in absolute term vis-à-vis in ratio may be seen in Table 6. It may be mentioned that relative growth of both output and input has shown a substantial increase of 26 and 31 per cents respectively from 2003 to 2004.

The above table 6 reveals that the gross input of MLSMEs was 1.39 billion Nakfa in 2003 increased to 1.82 billion Nakfa in 2004. On the other hand the gross output increased from 2.19 billion Nakfa in 2003 to 2.77 billion Nakfa in 2004. Food and Beverage and Alcoholic drinks contributed the highest percentage to the total gross input in both years.

To get an idea about the workers working in MLSMEs, an in-depth study was conducted among the workers of a tea packaging unit. This is the only tea packaging unit in entire Eritrea. The tea is distributed and sold only for domestic consumption. This unit is popularly known as ERTEPA. The unit imports tea from Kenya and then packaging is done in Eritrea. The unit has been established in 1998, (near Asmara capital of Eritrea), ie. after liberation.

Study Period and Methodology

The study was conducted in June, 2006. Of the total workers, about 25 per cent of workers numbering 23 were contacted randomly for which structured schedule was prepared. Both male and female workers were contacted, however 19 women workers were interviewed against 4 male workers. Besides the workers, some basic information was collected from the management.

Findings of the Study

The tea packaging unit ERTEPA is a MLSME under private sector. It was established in the year 1998. Altogether 90 workers work in the unit. Out of the total workers, 81 are female and 9 are male. Again skilled and unskilled distribution of workers reveal that 5 are skilled against 85 unskilled. The unit is basically

Table 6
Gross Output to Gross Input (Returns on Input) by Industrial Groups

(In '000 Nakfa)

Industry Group	*2003*			*2004*		
	Gross Output (A)	*Gross Input (B)*	*Gross O/p to Gross I/p (A÷B)*	*Gross Output (A)*	*Gross Input (B)*	*Gross O/p to Gross I/p(A÷B)*
Food	461,570	550,323	0.84	532,607	597,178	0.89
Beverages & Alcoholic Drinks	591,839	226,545	2.61	877,549	450,225	1.95
Tobacco	163,491	42,962	3.81	185,685	81,439	2.28
Textile	92,913	45,605	2.04	115,816	59,136	1.96
Leather & Shoe	82,671	55,189	1.50	98,329	60,857	1.62
Paper and Printing	57,179	27,171	2.10	75,917	36,053	2.11
Chemical Products	151,565	90,022	1.68	176,648	109,423	1.69
Rubber& Plastic Products	55,424	34,866	1.59	86,077	57,834	1.49
Non-Metallic Mineral Products	178,534	115,369	1.55	226,076	142,784	1.58
Metal Products	138,640	83,502	1.66	181,386	113,588	1.60
Furniture	220,635	121,922	1.81	210,522	115,962	1.82
Total	2,194,459	1,393,476	1.57	2,766,612	1,824,479	1.52

Source: Eritrea Industrial Statistics 2004, Ministry of Trade & Industry, 6 Statistical Bulletins, Nov, 2005, Asmara, Eritrea.

using labour intensive technology as a result more unskilled persons are employed.

The women workers are in the age group of 18 to 29 years. On the other hand age of male workers ranges from 18 to 65. The unit provides dress to the workers, which is blue in colour. According to the management this brings sporting attitude and feeling for oneness among the workers. All the unskilled workers interviewed are educated-schooling to junior college level. The wages of women unskilled worker per month ranges in between 500 and 800 Nakfa, depending upon their nature of job and experience. For skilled women workers the same is 1500 to 2000 Nakfa per month. On the day of study only one woman was working as skilled worker. For male unskilled and skilled workers minimum and maximum wages are 1000 and 1300 Nakfa per month respectively. It has been reported that, work of skilled workers is occasionally required. On the other hand, unskilled work is regular and full time. Moreover unskilled workers have to do heavy works like lifting of heavy tea cartons etc. So wages for male skilled and unskilled workers are almost same. With respect to wages and poverty (based on income) mention may be made that the poverty in Eritrea, as per Government report, is 240 Nakfa per person/month. That is anyone earning less than 240 Nakfa per month is considered as living Below the Poverty Line (BPL). In view of this it can be said that workers are paid wages which is above the poverty line category. Moreover most of the workers interviewed revealed that either husband or father/mother or both parents work in different institutions-Government/Private etc. So minimum of two earning members exist in each family (whom interviewed). Apart from wages, workers are paid bonus three times in a year. Total amount of bonus ranges in between 600 and 2000 Nakfa per year. Besides bonus, everyday the workers are provided tea and bread (two times) and monthly 200 grams of tea at free of cost.

It was reported that there is no trade union among the workers. The workers are not unhappy also for this. In fact the authors did a study in textile manufacturing unit in Asmara in May 2006 where more than 200 workers are engaged and it was observed that no trade union operates among the workers.

In spite of this, workers in both cases had no grievances against management. It is heartening to note that in both units (where authors did the study) workers reported that if unit is closed down then they have to beg for survival. According to them running of a manufacturing unit means earning of bread for the workers. No worker has been terminated till the day of study. Regarding the problems, the workers revealed that due to high price of vegetables, and food articles they find it difficult to manage their families, otherwise with management they have no problem. Query was made with the management about their problem in running of the industry. It was reported that non-availability of electricity hinders production otherwise the management is having no offer major problem. Both the labourers and management are in good relation. They are not having any logger-heads.

Conclusion

This study reveals that after liberation of Eritrea industrial scenario has been changed in the country. More and more MLSMEs are being established in every year. As a result many persons are getting employment. This helps for eradication of poverty also. The country with 66 per cent of its total population living below the poverty line is surely a not good indicator. So such employment opportunity definitely is helping to eradicate poverty from the country.

References

(The authors are thankful to the officials of Ministry of Education, Ministry of Trade and Industry and employees of Surveyed Units for their co-operation in carrying out the study).

Ministry of Trade and Industry, Government of Eritrea, "Eritrea: Report on Census of Manufacturing Establishments 2004", Statistical Report, Nov, 2005, Asmara.

Ministry of Trade and Industry, Government of Eritrea, "Eritrea Industrial Statistics 2004", Nov., 2005, Asmara, Eritrea.

Ministry of Trade & Industry, "Eritrea Industrial Statistics 2004", 6 Statistical Bulletins, 6 Nov, 2005, Asmara, Eritrea.

World Development Indicators 2005, World Bank.

21

DROUGHT IN SUB SAHARAN ERITREA: SOCIO-ECONOMIC CONSEQUENCES

Md. Arshad & Saidur Rahman

Introduction

Climate change is both and environment and development issue. Any human induced change in climate condition will affect not just ecosystems and biodiversity, but will also affect agricultural productivity, water quantity and quality, human health, and human settlement patterns. All this has direct and potentially damaging implications for developing countries as it can, ultimately, undermine their aspirations of sustainable development.

Currently, the issue of drought has become a big concern around the world and its social and economic consequences demand greater attention. Drought is phenomenon that arises out of the poor constitutions of rainfall. The negative effect of water shortage in terms of human sufferings is colossal. According to Oram (1989), many people around the globe are being reported to suffer from water shortage. Such a prolonged water shortage will lead to a complete crop failure and wide spread starvation of population and decimination of livestock in the drought stricken areas. The direct connection of drought with water, which is an essential element to produce goods and services, has called for more attention. Oram further argues that the sensitivity of agriculture to drought is another factor that makes drought important to address, although its characteristics vary significantly from place to place. Alexander (1993) mentioned that drought is one of the main natural hazards that cause food shortage in developing regions.

Nowhere is this more critical than Eritrea, where the poor are the most at risk from the increased variability and volatility in weather patterns. One of the key climate related vulnerabilities of Eritrea's economy is its heavy dependents on the monsoons. Monsoons analysis reveals that various regions of Eritrea have been hit by recurring drought. The Sub-Saharan area, which Eritrea forms a part, is one of the worlds that are prone to recurring drought. Eritrea lies in the Sahelian rainfall zone of Africa where the land is mostly arid and semi-arid and is characterized by erratic rainfall-usually unevenly distributed. Due to its geographical location in the arid and semi-arid zone of the Sahel belt, Eritrea lacks adequate rainfall and its underground resources are deteriorating from time to time. Thus, the agricultural activities in the country have been affected adversely.

The disastrous effect of feeble or failed monsoons has been particularly acute in Eritrea, where more than 80 per cent of the people depend on agriculture for their livelihood. As reported in the Eritrea Profile (2003), the agricultural output of 2003 was the lowest recorded in last 20 years. The Eritrean Relief and Refugees Commission (ERREC) and the Ministry of Agriculture reported that only 54 thousand metric tones of cereals had been harvested in 2002 which constitute only 11 per cent of the normal of the annual green production and only 9 per cent of the total food consumption in Eritrea. It is evident that 90 per cent of the food demand of the country had to be covered either from aid donations or from international market through purchase. The recurrent drought affects almost the entire population in Eritrea. UNICEF has repeatedly warned that the drought and consequent famine in Eritrea could have devastating consequences unless immediate measures taken to save lives.

During the past years, it was estimated that hundreds of thousand were affected by Eritrea. As a result of recurring drought people were either starved to death or malnourished and many other were displaced. According to the UN (2004), the recent drought in Eritrea is estimated to have had a critical effect in the living conditions of the population resulting a decreased a rural income by 18 per cent. And 65 of the Eritrean continue to live with income as less as one US Dollar a day. Generally, the scarcity of rainfall followed by its uneven distribution and a short rainy season led to drought. Drought reduces the crop yield, which caused human starvation and livestock dissemination. As a result of recurring drought, people have devised various traditional coping mechanisms to ensure their survival. However, drought continues to affect their lives adversely.

Definitions of Drought: Drought is normal, recurring climatic feature. It occurs in almost all climatic zones, but its characteristics vary significantly from one region to another. Drought is temporary aberration. It differs from aridity, which is restricted to low rainfall regions and is a permanent climatic feature.

Drought results from a deficiency in precipitation that persists long enough to produce a serious hydrological imbalance. It should be considered relative to long term average condition of balance between precipitation and evapotranspiration in a particular area. Drought differs in three essential characteristics: intensity, duration, and spatial coverage. Intensity is the degree of shortfall in precipitation and/or the severity of impacts associated with the shortfalls. It is generally measured by the departure from normal of a climatic index and is closely linked to duration in the determination of impact. Impact relates to timing and effectiveness of rainfall. Other climatic factors such as temperature, wind and humidity can significantly aggravate it severity.

Different scholars define drought differently. According to Bryant (1997), drought is defined simply as an extended period of rainfall deficit during which agricultural biomass is severely curtailed. Besides, the declaration of drought occurrence varies in different countries depending on their geographic locations, social and economic structures (CIDA, 2002).

The problem of drought has global dimension. Drought problem extends to most of the continents of the world. It occurs in Northeast United States, Southern Europe, Australia, Latin America, Asia and Africa which have a drier climate (Bryant, 1997, Mohammad Salih, 1994 and CIDA, 2000). Although drought is controlled by a natural process of cloud formation ij the atmosphere, the event is exacerbated by combined effect of human utilization of natural resources in non-sustainable ways and climatic changes taking place as a result of global warming (Bryant, 1997, GTZ, 1996). Hence, the catastrophe such as food and water shortages, and accompanying mal-nutrition, degeneration human health, and resulting conflict and mass migration that are associated with drought, are the ever pressing issues facing the modern societies (UN, 2004).

Drought and the Sub-Saharan African Region: The sub-Saharan Africa is characterized by arid and semi-arid climate. Starting from the early 20th century, some places around the fringes of the Sahara desert witnessed decrease in rain fall by almost 50 per cent (Bryant, 1997). Hence, drought has caused serious implications on the social economic situations of sub-Saharan African countries. The drought situation further deteriorated in the 1970s and 1980s (CIDA, 2002).

The people of Sub-Saharan Africa are severely affected by shortage of food and mal-nutrition. Poverty being seen here in these zones, often forces their inhabitants to utilize resources in non-sustainable ways in order to survive. The unsustainable use of natural resources exacerbates the process of desertification which is already a problem in these regions. Desertification which is the process of deterioration of dry lands reinforces the occurrence of drought (GTZ, 1996). In addition, the sub-Saharan African countries have high population growth rate (3-4 per cent annually). The increasing pressure of population and poverty has put a immense pressure in the natural environment conservation (GTZ, 1996, CIDA, 2002).

The poor soil management practices, increasing soil erosion, deforestation and desertification and/drought are decreasing the productive capacity of land that is already overused by high density of population in these societies. Further, the vulnerability to drought is felt differently by different section of the population. At local level, women and children often bear the burnt of land degradation. These groups are more vulnerable as they fail to take up opportunities that may increase their chances of pulling out of poverty. Women are obliged to become bread winners in addition to their domestic roles, particularly in response to male out migration (CIDA, 2002).

In the Sub-Saharan Africa, agricultural is marginal nomadic in character and highly dependent on monsoons. During the 1970s when the climatic condition over the Sahel switched to drought, world fuel price sourced, people shifted to forest resources as source of energy. The increasing population increased pressure on land to supply food. To aggravate the situation, in improved techniques of ploughing and other modern techniques to improve farming proved inappropriate in these regions. All these events have enhanced the negative feedback mechanisms to the atmosphere cloud formation process, facilitating the occurrence of drought and desertification (Norton & Alwang, 1993, Mohammed Saleh, 1994, Bryant, 1997).

Drought in Relation to Eritrea

Since independence of Eritrea in 1991, one of the serious challenges facing the new country was the repetitive occurrence of drought. During 1999–2002, Eritrea suffered its worst drought in many years (MOA, 2002). The situation was aggravated because of rampant poverty. The drought exacerbated by the conflict of border war with Ethiopia from 1998–2000. The severe drought created a situation of mass displacement of people from their villages. It posed a great challenge for the government of Eritrea (GOA, 2003). In the post war Eritrea, an estimated 38–52 per cent of the households are female headed, have higher dependency ration and large family size. They have limited access to basic social services and have; lower literacy rates. There shortage of basic inputs such as seeds, labor, oxen and irrigation facility etc. The majority of the farmers are under high debts. As consequences, there are large number of children in the streets and commercial sex workers in every nook and corner of cities and towns.

The government of Eritrea has shown a sense of commitment to address the underlying factors of food insecurity and poverty and making efforts to provide assistance to the people using its all resources (GOE, 2003). Hence, the basic challenge for Eritrea is mitigating the impact of drought on vulnerable section of the population and strengthening their coping mechanisms. This is in fact a very difficult task as according to the UN (2004) report, even in good harvesting years the country produces only 50– 60 per cent of its food requirements.

Climatic Variations in Eritrea

Eritrea has six administrative zones. All six administrative zones of Eritrea are dry to a greater or lesser extent, the main cause of drought being variation in the climate. To regions of Eritrea (Maechal and Debub) are grouped as dry sub-humid, three (Gash Barka, Anseba and Semenawi Kehih Bahri) as semi-arid and the Debubawi Keyih Bahri as arid (Table 1).

Observation of long-term climatic data for Eritrea indicates three important factors affecting agricultural and natural resource degradation (MOA, 2002). They are:

1. Eritrea's water balance: the gap between potential evapo-transpiration and rainfall has been steadily worsening over the past century. In fact, rainfall exceeds evapo-transpiration during only two months of the years, namely July and August.
2. The country has experienced a decline in rainfall over the past century. The data available from 1905-1995 suggest that rainfall has been declining, on average, by circa 0.4 mm/year.
3. The period between onset and cessation of the rainy season has been getting shorter over the past century.

Table 1
Aridity Indices for Eritrea by Zone

Zones	*Aridity* Index	*Length of growing* period (days)	*Typical Crops*
Maekel	0.50-0.65	120-179	Maize, Beans, Barley, Wheat, Teff etc.
Debub	0.50-0.65	120-179	Maize, Beans, Barley, Wheat, Teff etc
Gash-Barka	0.20-0.50	60-119	Baloush-millet, Sorghum, Sesame
Anseba	0.20-0.65	60-119	Baloush-millet, Sorghum, Sesame
SemenawiKeyih-Bahri	0.20-0.65	60-119	Baloush-millet, Sorghum, Sesame
DebubawiKeyih-Bahri	0.05-0.20	1-59	No crops, marginal, pasture

Source: Ministry of Agriculture, 2002.

It is important to note that in Eritrea, the incidence of drought and resulting famine has not been properly documented. Hence, much is learned from indirect sources of information (MOA, 20020. However, it has been observed that the vicious cycle of grain failures in Eritrea occurs in circa of years, such periods being closely co-related with years of poor crop production.

Research Methodology

Justification of the Study: Eritrea is a newly independent country in Northeast Africa. It forms a part of the Sub-Saharan area, which is prone to recurring drought. With more than 80 per cent of the population dependent on agriculture, the livelihood of Eritrean remains vulnerable due to crop failure, livestock loss and asset depletion. As Eritrea is exposed to recurrent drought, there is a serious need for a great effort to fight it. It is important that people are aware of and are knowledgeable about the social and economic effects of drought. Therefore, it is convincing to make a proper study of the socio-economic effects of drought in this Sub-Saharan region.

Objective of the Study

The main objectives of this study are:

1. To study the socio-economic consequences of drought in Eritrea.
2. To study the coping mechanisms employed by the people of Eritrea against drought.

Background of the Area of Study

Eritrea was overwhelmingly affected by drought in 2000-2003. However, the degree of vulnerability to drought differed from place to place. Himbirti Village was selected as the site for this study for the various reasons:

- Effects of drought were clearly seen in this village.
- Himbirti is only 34 Km from Asmara. It is easily accessible by transportation.

- It was interesting to study if this proximity of Himbirti village to Asmara, the capital city of Eritrea, has any effect on the adaptive mechanism of the drought affected area.

The area of study is in the Zoba Maekel. Himbirti is located in the southwest of Asmara and is 34 Km in distance. Himbirti is relatively bigger in size and is densely populated than its surrounding villages. The altitude of Himbirti is about 2080 meters above the sea level and is sloppy on the top, steep slop in the middle and flat in the bottom. The main farm land lies down the slope.

According to the agricultural office, the annual rainfall of Himbirti is about 335mm. which is much lower than the average rainfall central highland climatic zone of Zoba Maekel. The f Himbirti opine that there has been a severe decline in annual rainfall during the last 10 years. Apart from the declining trend, rainfall has also been erratic in distribution, which has devastating effect on crops and livestock production. It creates a situation of high level of uncertainty.

The total population of Himbirti is estimated to be 7715 with 1650 families. The people of Himbirti speak Tigriniya, a major language of Eritrea, predominantly spoken in the highlands. They belong to both Muslim and Christian communities. The livelihood of the population of Himbirti is based on monsoon agriculture. The farming system is traditional which entails the use of oxen for ploughing and produces for subsistence. The main crops produced are Barley, wheat, sorghum, millet, maize, beans and peas. The herding of livestock, which is traditional in nature, is also part of the life of the village dwellers. Animals such as cows, oxen, sheep, goats and donkeys are reared. As farming is the main source of income in Himbirti, about 80 per cent of its population depends on it (Table 2).

Himbirti comes under the Gala Nefhi Sub-Zone administration of Zoba Maekel. It has social service such as health service, education, transportation, water supply and electricity. Education is provided to every citizen free of cost. In Himbirti there is one Kindergarten, one elementary school, one junior secondary school. A Secondary school is available 5 km away from Himbirti.

Table 2
Population of Himbirti Village

Age	*Population Size*	*Percentage*
0-17	1993	26.00
18 and above	5722	74.00
Total	7715	100

Sampling Plan: The research aims at studying the socio-economic consequences of drought. Thus, for this purpose both quantitative and qualitative research methodologies were used. Both the interview schedule and face to face interviews were conducted in order to collect the required information for the research. The interview schedule was intended to find out the demographic composition of the village community, to assess the socio-economic problems caused by drought and to observe the coping mechanisms adopted by the community.

In order to have an overview of the socio-economic condition of the population and the possible effect of drought in Eritrea, various concerned agencies such as Ministry of Agriculture, Eritrean Relief and Rehabilitation Commission, and local government administration were contacted. In the second stage an intensive study of the Himbirti village was done to have a first hand assessment of the situation. The household was considered as the basic unit of study. There were 140 households which were randomly selected and information was gathered from the heads of each household. Information was also gathered from health personnel, school directors and village administrators. For this purpose structured and semi-structured interviews were conducted. A local educated guide was taken along for the purpose of translation of Tigriniya to English. In addition, extensive review of secondary data was also made.

Demographic Structure of the Study: In order to determine the relationship between the occurrence of drought and its effect on the village community, it is important to discuss the socio-demographic structure of the sample households:

Age: The majority of the household respondents belong to the age group of 54 years and above. They constituted about 57 per cent of the total respondents and the lowest percentage belongs to the age group of 42-47 years. The remaining respondents belong to the age group of 24-29 and 48-53. Their corresponding percentage is 8.60 and 20.00 per cent respectively. The reason why the young people are not adequately represented in the sample is their compulsory participation in their national service. However, the elderly population has been exposed to recurrent drought situation and is better able to share their experiences (Table 3).

Size of the households: The size of household is an indicator of growth of population in a society. It also indicates the size of the dependent population in the community. Out of the total population taken for this study, 40 (28 per cent) had 8-9 members followed by 36 (26 per cent) households having 6-7 members. The rest 28 and 24 household had 2-3, and 4-5 members respectively. This reflects upon the fact that in Himbirti, the family size is large and hence the dependency ratio is high (Table 4).

Table 3
Respondents Age Distribution

Age group	*Number of Respondents*	*Percentage*
18-23	-	-
24-29	12	8.60
30-35	-	-
36-41	12	8.6
42-47	8	6.0
48-53	28	20.0
54 and above	80	57.0
Total	140	100

Table 4
Size of the Household

Size of Household	*Number of Respondents*	*Percentage*
1	4	3.00
2-3	28	20.00
4-5	24	17.00
6-7	36	26.00
8-9	40	28.00
10 and above	8	6.00
Total	140	100

Gender Distribution of Respondents: In the village out of the total population 80 (57 per cent) of the household were found top be male headed whereas 60 (43 per cent) were female headed. Many of the female heads are in fact the war widows and they seem to be more disadvantaged than others (Table 5).

Table 5
Gender Distribution

Gender	*Number of Respondents*	*Percentage*
Male	80	57.00
Female	60	43.00
Total	140	100

Marital Status: For the purpose of this study most elderly members of the households were selected to represent the data. A large majority of 83 per cent of the respondents were reported to be married. A considerable number of 11 per cent of the respondents were the war widows and unmarried and divorced were 3 per cent each (Table 6).

Educational Level: A large majority of the villagers consisting of 63 per cent of the respondents were illiterate. A significant number of 37 per cent had lower level of education and only 6 per cent of the respondents were having secondary level of education. Thus, in Himbirti majority of the people were either illiterate or had lower level of education only (Table 7).

Table 6
Respondents Marital Status

Marital Status	*Number of Respondents*	*Percentage*
Married	116	83.00
Unmarried	4	3.00
Divorced	4	3.00
Widow	16	11.00
Total	140	100

Occupational Distribution: Eritrea predominantly an agrarian society and about 80 per cent of population is dependent on agriculture. The reflections of Eritrean economic structure can be clearly observed in Himbirti. A large majority

Table 7
Respondents Educational Level

Educational Level	*Male*	*Percentage*	*Female*	*Percentage*	*Total Number*	*Percentage*
Illiterate	44	29.00	44	29.00	88	63.00
Elementary	24	17.00	4	3.00	28	20.00
Middle	20	14.00	4	3.00	24	17.00
Secondary	4	3.00	4	3.00	8	6.00
Total	88	62.00	52	38.00	140	100

of 77 per cent of the respondents were found involved in farming activities. The rest 23 per cent were employed in different off-farm activities such as trading (6 per cent), government jobs (3 per cent), daily laborers (8 per cent) and soldiers (6 per cent). Thus, most of the villagers depend largely on farming activities. The agricultural production found to vary considerably from year to year depending on climatic factors such as monsoon and drought (Table 8).

Table 8
Respondents Occupation

Occupation	*Number of Respondents*	*Percentage*
Farming	108	77.00
Trading	8	6.00
Government Employees	4	3.00
Daily Laborers	12	8.00
Soldiers	8	6.00
Total	140	100

Socio-economic Effects of Drought: Drought sets off a vicious cycle of socio-economic impacts beginning crop yield failure, unemployment, erosion of assets, decrease in income, worsening of living conditions, poor nutrition and subsequently, decreased risk absorptive capacity, and thus, increasing vulnerability of the poor to another drought and other shocks.

The effects of drought are manifested in many ways. The main effects are observed on supply of food and water, health of the people and on domestic animals. On the basis of the degree or severity of impact of drought on the people, shortage of food supply was given the highest ranking. The loss of livestock was ranked second. Then health problem was mentioned as another area affected by drought (Table 9).

Table 9
The Effects of Drought

Problem faced	*Rank*
Shortage of Food and Water	1
Loss of Livestock	2
Health Problem	3
Others	4

Drought greatly influence the supply of food items and consequently food intake. The people were found to change their feeding schedule by taking recourse to austerity measures. Unlike the normal practice, where people usually eat thrice a day, they were now eating twice or once a day. As a result, malnutrition and ill health follow. Only few better off people could follow the normal food schedule.

Daily Food Intake: The frequency of daily food intake is not by itself a complete approach of measuring the level of malnutrition and disease. However, as a matter of fact, people do not get adequate nutritious food as a result of drought. It can be discerned from the table that 8 per cent of the households in Himbirti face serious shortage of food supply and hence take food only once in a day. A large number of household (46 per cent) take food twice a day and a similar percentage (46 per cent) of households are better off and normal feeding habit thrice a day (Table 10).

Table 10
Daily Food Intake by Households

Feeding Frequency	*Households*	*Percentage*
Once a day	12	8.00
Twice a day	64	46.00
Thrice a day	64	46.00
Total	140	100

Frequency of Visits to the Clinic: Although most of the respondents could not specifically indicate the scope and type of diseases experienced by them because of drought situation, they expressed that many people lost weight and become anaemic as a result of inadequate food. Hence, their frequency of visit to clinics increases (Table 11).

Table 11
Frequency of Visit to Clinics

Frequency of Visit	*Number of Respondents*	*Percentage*
Once a week	24	17.00
Once a month	52	37.00
Once a year	24	17.00
others	40	29.00
Total	140	100

Loss of Livestock: Drought causes tremendous loss of livestock in rural areas. This loss is caused because of lack of availability of fodder and drinking water for livestock. Livestock are also lost by people as they take resort to selling them for their own survival. In Himbirti village loss of livestock can be assessed by looking into livestock ownership of people in pre-drought and post-drought situations (Table 12 & 13).

Table 12
Livestock Ownership in Pre-drought Situation

Types of Livestock	*Livestock Quantum*	*Number of Inhabitants*	*Percentage*	*Percentage*
OxenandCow	Nil	14	40%	40%
	1-2	9	26%	60%
	3-4	4	11%	
	5 and above	8	23%	
Donkey	Nil	21	60%	60%
	1	4	11%	40%
	2	8	23%	
	3-4	2	6%	
Sheep	Nil	28	80%	80%
	5-10	3	9%	20%
	11 and above	4	11%	
Goat	Nil	29	82%	82%
	1-3	2	6%	
	4-6	1	3%	
	7 and above	3	9%	18%

The loss of livestock i.e., cattle, sheep, goats and donkeys can be seen clearly through the above tables. Accordingly, all goats are lost after the occurrence of drought, while ownership of other livestock has decreased significantly due to drought. Hence, drought causes a long term and all round effect on the lives of people.

The socio-economic effect of drought is a major concern for the people. The rural people in general and the women and children in particular were the most vulnerable social groups to the effects of drought. Many villagers lost their livestock under drought situations. The families which used to produce 5-10 quintals of grain could produce less than one quintal of grain under the drought conditions. As a result, 6792 villagers became dependent on food aid (WFP). The food aid available was however, less than adequate. Thus, people took other initiatives as other supportive mechanisms. Many including women worked in the school construction project near Mai-Nefhi as daily laborers. Others worked as casual laborers in different government projects. Many earned their livelihood by selling tea or by selling hand made baskets in the local markets.

Table 13
Livestock Ownership in Post-drought Situation

Types of Livestock	*Livestock Quantum*	*Number of Inhabitants*	*Percentage*
OxenandCow	Nil	25	71.00
	1-2	7	20.00
	3-4	3	9.00
	5 and above	-	-
Donkey	Nil	30	86.00
	1	5	14.00
	2	-	-
	3-4	-	-
Sheep	Nil	35	100
	5-10	-	-
	11 and above	-	-
Goat	Nil	-	-
	1-3	-	-
	4-6	-	-
	7 and above	-	-

Shortage of potable water is another area of problem, caused by drought. A barrel of clean water is available at Eritrea 6 Nakfa (1USD = 15 Nakfa), which the poor can not afford. As a result, the majority of the villagers walk long distances to fetch water from the micro dam or from hand driven water pumps. The unavailability of fire wood is another problem for most of the households.

Information obtains from the health clinic located at Himbirti village; provide information on impact of drought on health conditions of the villagers. It reported an increase frequency and intensity of anaemia and other related diseases caused by mal-nutrition. The information reflected that the children and women were the worst affected by drought in Himbirti.

Coping Mechanisms: Drought onset is periodic, slow and insidious. Therefore, communities in drought prone areas must be constantly prepeared to insulate themselves from the probability of drought and finally, when overwhelmed, to ensure survival. But, community's response to drought varies depending upon its social and economic structures.

In agrarian societies, there are traditional ways of coping drought. These include:

1. Heavier reliance upon agricultural diversification to mitigate the effect of drought as different crops have different water requirements and they also vary in terms of their tolerance to drought.
2. Water conservation practices are also used when the need arose. Widening of the spacing of plants and/or planting fast maturing crops in case the drought persists.
3. Borrowing from relatives and/or community chiefs.
4. Working off farm and/or shifting to craft activity.
5. Using wild fruits and roots.

The mitigation of the impact of drought has been a key area of focus of Eritrea since independence as evident from programs such as 'the national action program to combat desertification and mitigate the effects of drought, draft for interim poverty reduction strategy etc'. However, the human and the social costs of droughts remain devastating. The present study provided insights into how farmers at Himbirti changed their behavior patterns to cope with drought situations. According to the interviewees a number of adaptive approaches were undertaken by the villagers, the giverment of Eritrea and by other agencies to cope with drought situation. Neverthless, the degree of intervention taken at the family and the community levels are more effective in terms of their consistency and sustainability.

The victims of drought were found to have taken recourse to multiple coping mechanisms to mitigate the effects of drought. They used various alternatives for generating income. Few decreased the cultivable area because of lack of water planted vegetables as a source of income. Others had the support of the community (from Kins living outside the village).

Many people sold livestock at depressed prices owing to lack of fodder or agricultural work for the livestock and on many occasions for buying food. There were members and families who migrated to other places or Zobas (regions) in search of livelihood. The coping mechanisms were ranked by the villagers as follows (Table 14).

Table 14
Traditional Coping Mechanisms at the Family Level

Coping Mechanisms	*Rank*
Reduced number of Livestock by Selling	1
Off-farm Employment	2
Community Co-operation	3
Internal Migration	4
Others	5

Major Findings

Drought is a recurring phenomena in Eritrea. With 80 peercent of the population dependent on agriculture, the livelihood of Eritreans remains vulnerable due to severe crop failure, loss of livestock and asset depletion. Eritrea was overwhelmingly affected by drought in 2002-2003. In Himbirti village, the effect of drought were clearly been observed. The socio-demographic features of Himbirti village and the effects of drought upon its people can be summarized as follows:

1. The dependency ratio of the people in the village was very hifgh because of large size of families. A large number (28 per cent) of the families were found to have 8-9 members and only 3 per cent families were single member families.
2. A large majority (57 per cent) of the families were headed by male, whereas 43 per cent of the families were female headed. Most of the female heads were war widows. The impact of drought on female headed families was more severe.
3. A large majority (83 per cent) of the respondents were reported to married. Widowed, divorced and unmarried together represent 17 per cent of the total respondents.
4. A large number (63 per cent) of the villagers were reported to be illiterate, and 37 per cent were found to have attended elementary and junior levels of schooling.
5. An overwhelming majority (77 per cent) of the villagers were farmers. The rest 23 per cent worked as daily laborers, government servants and traders. Thus, majority of the villagers depended on agriculture as a source of earning livelihood.
6. As coping mechanisms as a result of drought, people had to bring change in their feeding frequency. Daily food intake of the families which was in normal situations, thrice a day had to be reduced to twice a day or even once a day by almost 57 per cent of the population. Thus, people reduce expenditures on basic needs, leading to mal-nutrition and in extreme cases starvation.
7. The income level of people deteriorated drastically because of crop failure as a consequences of drought. This was reported by 80 per cent of the respondents.

8. Members or even families migrate to other places for livelihood and involve in off farm activities such as constructions labors. They also send children to work as laborers and work at minimum wages to generate some income.
9. The number of livestock greatly decreased as people sale livestock at lower prices owing to lack of fodder or agricultural work and sometimes to get little money.
10. Production of food grain decreased tremendously as a consequence of drought as cultivable area decreased because of lack of water. Hence, the families which in average used to produce 5 to 10 quintals of grain in normal circumstances could produce less than 1 quintal of grain during drought situations.
11. Except the few well off people, consisting of 12 per cent of the population, the rest 88 per cent of the population had to depend on international food aid.
12. The female headed families were the most disadvantaged and most of them made a living by selling tea and or by selling hand made baskets in the local market.
13. Availability of drinking water and firewood are serious problems in the village. A considerable number of the population was found to carry water from distant places. To fulfill the need of firewood villagers indulge in indiscriminate deforestation which in turn lead to recurrence of drought.
14. Most of the respondents mentioned selling of livestock as a first coping mechanism to drought followed by off farm employment, community cooperation and internal migration as other coping mechanisms.

Conclusion

Drought sets off a vicious cycle of socio-economic impacts beginning crop yield failure, unemployment, erosion of assets, decreasing in income, worsening of living conditions, poor nutrition, and subsequently decreased risk absorptive capacity, and thus increasing vulnerability of the poor to another drought and other shocks. The disastrous effect of drought has been particularly acute in the State of Eritrea. Eritrea lies in the Sahelian rainfall zone of Sub-Saharan Africa. Here the land is arid and semi-arid and is characterized by erratic rainfall. Due to its geographical locations in the arid and semi-arid regions of the African Sahel Belt, Eritrea lacks adequate rainfall. Thus, drought in Eritrea is a recurrent phenomenon. The Eritrean society is highly vulnerable to drought as more than 80 per cent of its population depend on agriculture for their livelihood. The magnitude of socio-economic stress experienced by the victims of drought is very severe. In Eritrea, people could mitigate the impact of drought to a larger extent by taking recourse to several coping mechanisms. They could succeed to insulate themselves from the disastrous consequences of drought and hence could ensure survival through these indigenous coping mechanisms. But, as drought is a recurrent phenomenon in this Sub-Saharan country, it continues to have a negative impact on Eritrean economy and on the lives of millions of rural poor. However, the impact of drought on the overall development indicators may decrease if proper measures are taken to mitigate them.

Recommendations

It is very apparent that drought is causing serious problems to the rural people. Thus, the Eritrean government must take effective measures to deal with this recurrent phenomenon. The following measures may be adopted to counter the adverse effects of drought:

1. Develop a multi-tiered strategy combining statewide economic and sect oral policies with well targeted efforts at the micro level.
2. Continue to accelerate the ongoing changes in the economic structure at the macro level.
3. Encouraging alternative employment options in the secondary and tertiary sectors.

4. Facilitating growth of the tertiary sector as Eritrea has tremendous potential to develop its tourism industry.
5. Supporting the development of livestock sector, particularly poultry and dairy, as an important buffer to absorb the drought impacts on rural economy.
6. Encouraging the shift in cropping pattern from more water intensive to less water intensive crops would decrease vulnerability to drought impacts. For instance, horticulture development may be encouraged.
7. Encourage investment in sectors with significant employment potential for the labors displaced from the agriculture sector, such as certain services, construction, mining and quarrying and fishing.
8. Construction of micro dams and digging of water wells as sources of water conservation.
9. Enhancing afforestation programs.
10. The last but not the least, creating a supporting institutional and policy framework.

References

Oram, P.A. (1989), *Sensitivity of Agriculture Production to Climate Change and Food Security,* International Rice Research Institute, London.

Alexander, D. (1993), Natural Disasters, Grilford and Kimmi's Biddler Ltd., London.

Eritrea Profile (2003), Drought and the Race Against Time to Save Lives in Eritrea, Eritrean Profile, March 1, 2003, pp. 3.

MOA (2002), *The National Action Programme for Eritrea to Combat Desertification and Mitigate the Effects of Drought,* Prepared by the Ministry of Agriculture, Asmara, Eritrea.

UN (2004), *Eritrea 2004: Consolidated Appeals Process,* Prepared by United Nations, Geneva, Switzerland.

Bryant, E.A. (1997), *Natural Hazards,* Cambridge University Press, UK.

CIDA (2002), *Combating Desertification: Building Bridges,* Published by Canadian International Development Agency, Canada.

GTZ (1996), Resource Conservation: Combating Desertification, Published by German Development Cooperation, Eschborn, German.

Norton, G.W. and Alwang, J. (1993), *Introduction to Economic and Agricultural Development*, McGraw-Hill, Inc., USA.

EEA (1995), *A Draft Paper of National Action Programme to Address Desertification*, Prepared by Eritrean Environmental Agency, Asmara, Eritrea.

GOE (2003), *Draft for Interim Poverty Rreduction Strategy*, Prepared by Government of the State of Eritrea, Asmara, Eritrea.

Mohammed Salih, (1994), *Inducing Food Insecurity: Perspectives in Food Policies in Eastern and Southern Africa*, Stockholm, Sweden.

22

ERITREAN TRADE WITH ITALY IN POST-INDEPENDENCE PERIOD–AN ANALYTICAL STUDY

Ravinder Rena

Introduction

The Cabinet of Ministers in its October 2005 meeting underlined that there is a need to focus on trade and investment partnerships rather than on looking for external assistance. An imaginative economic strategy towards the neighbours could do to boost foreign trade. Asmara is now ready to use the clout of its market to alter its bilateral relations with the neighbours. Peace process stalemate, drought reduces pace of growth in the last few years.

The government of Eritrea has been taking measures to promote economic integration in the region. These include incentives and facilities to promote border trade between Eritrea and its neighbours, reduction of tariffs for goods from the rest of Sub-saharan Africa and removal of restrictions on investment. Surely, the Eritrean Chamber of Commerce, Ministry of Trade and Industry see access to the Eritrean market as a leverage that must be used to obtain mutual benefit (Rena, 2005: 7).

If Eritrea looks at the strategic significance over the long term of economic integration with her neighbours, it should be more than eager to bilaterally force the pace of creating a single market in Africa and end the economic partition of the continent.

Unlike in the past, all the countries in African continent are seeking to globalize their economies. Besides, African countries are trying to have a single currency for Africa by 2020. It can be stated that all the countries are under compulsion to take full advantage of the natural imperatives for market integration with each other. There are some countries in the region, which remain reluctant to seek shared economic prosperity, there are some other countries in Africa that are beginning to see the implications of the logic of globalization and the consequent need to become part of the African union. Libya, Pakistan, United Arab Emirates, Bahrain etc., are seeking deeper linkages with Eritrea. Djibouti, Yemen, Sudan want duty free access for their goods to the Eritrean market. Qatar, France and Italy, which have already agreed to cooperate in promoting Eritrea's economy, are seeking a modernization of this relationship and removal of many distortions that have crept into the trading regime between them and Eritrea. For instance, Eritrea and Italy signed recently a memorandum of understanding regarding bilateral aviation ties (Rena, 2005: 7).

North East African states can hope to draw large amounts of foreign investments only on the basis of having an access to the America, Europe and some other countries within Africa, which become an engine of Africa's regional growth. The economic success of the neighbouring countries is linked with that of the trade and fiscal policies of every country in the region. The question is no longer whether the region will integrate. The unanswered questions are about how effectively and quickly the country will take advantage of this altered reality in the African continent over the last decade.

By facilitating regional integration through bilateral or multilateral measures, Eritrea is trying its best to build congenial and harmonious relations with its neighbours and rest of the World. However, it also helps itself. Eritrea cannot hope to prosper amidst collapsing economies and failed states in its neighbourhood. Nor can it hope that a bilateral-oriented approach will resolve economic problems.

The Government of Eritrea has increasingly come to see the importance of putting trade and commerce at the centre of Eritrea's regional diplomacy. The government is trying to put across Eritrea's renewed commitment to push the region towards an African Economic union. But these words have little meaning unless matched by deeds in recasting the Eritrean trade policy towards the neighbours.

That Eritrea stands to gain from trading with its neighbours is appreciable. Since economic pragmatism has been so rare, the Government of Eritrea, reported to have declared to have close trade links with its neighbours. The President Issayes Afwerki visited Italy recently to develop the trade between the two countries. He expressed the hope that "the Italian entrepreneurs are readily interested to invest in Eritrean tourism, construction, manufacturing sectors etc., however, the transit trade with its neighbours would significantly expand Eritrea's strategic options. But the new debate in Eritrea on trade with its neighbours is a welcome one. It is a big intellectual leap for the Eritrea's establishment to debate the "role of the Government" in coping with the "global economic challenges" to the nation.

Italy has colonized Eritrea for over 50 years. The key legacy of Italian colony was the development of skilled manpower, construction of infrastructure developing mechanized agriculture etc. The manpower developed includes factory workers, electricians, technicians and mechanics etc. During the period there was apprenticeship given by Italians in areas of middle professional development. Potentially it has developed a work force in Eritrea, which is geared toward Italian need. This has to continue now as the potential is still there (Rena, 2006: 35-40; Mesghinna, 1988, 65-69).

Why Italo-Eritrean Trade is Important?

The trade ties between Italy and Eritrea is important for both countries because: Over half of Eritrean exports to Europe are to Italy. At the same time Italian investment in Eritrea was also important for African economy in general Eritrean economy in particular. However, it can also be a bridge to develop trade link with Africa. If Italy invest in Eritrea it will have an access and control of the sea, henceforth, an access and control of the sea to the whole Europe. Therefore, Eritrean control the access to the Red Sea ports means maintaining the European trade link with Asia and oil producing Arab countries. One typical example of Italo-Eritrean trade could be Agro-Industry: Italy should invest on Agro-Industry which serve the Italian market in the fast delivery like banana, mango orange, water melon, fish etc. In addition, cotton (which was the traditional ownership of Italy), is only a matter of developing. Which may produce and process raw materials semi finished materials can be either exported or else. Most of the population also speaks Italian language. There are two important ports, which might be of importance to facilitate all the trade relations.

General Introduction

Eritrea got its independence on 24 May 1991 from Ethiopia and is located in the Horn of Africa, bordered in the north and west by Sudan, in the south by Ethiopia and Djibouti, and in the east by the Red Sea. It has an estimated population of about 4 million and a total land area of some 12.2 million hectares. Its annual population growth is estimated at 2.9 per cent. Eritrea has nine ethnic groups and six administrative *zobas* (provinces/regions). The country has six agricultural zones defined by climate, altitude, soils, and population density. They are: (1) The Central High Land Zone; (2) The Western Escarpment Zone; (3) The South Western Lowland Zone; (4) The Green Belt of the Eastern Escarpment of the Highland Zone; (5) The Coastal Plains Zone and, (6) The North-western Lowland zone.

Eritrea is a small country with a population size (4 million) of one region of Italy (Toscana). It is only 5.8 per cent of Italian population, where as, with a relatively large geographical land area with small population of 4 million (density is 28 per square k.m). The land is nearly 40 per cent of that of Italy. (Italy is only 2.4 times greater than Eritrea in geographical size where as the population is nearly 20 times than that of Eritrea). When it comes to economic well being the gap is greater. (The ratio in per capita income is 74 times greater than that of Eritrea).

Italy at present is an influential member of the world states in general and European Economic Union in particular. Eritrea is a small country who can be just another player, but on another level. It has got primary resources, which might benefit Italy. It has the resources where Italy can make business. (e.g., Salt and fish).

Given in to account Eritrea as a strategic place in the Red Sea region. Italy as a colonial power in the Horn of Africa has a colonial historical ties in the area. (Somali, Libya, Eritrea). Eritrea as a former Italian colony has historical, colonial trade relationship with Italy. Therefore, on the basis of this historical relationship it may be justifiable to try to strengthen and develop a sustained trade links between the two countries. It is also important to note that we are in an exciting period of a new millennium. This millennium with new technology, new thinking, new skill new rules and new form of international economic order and a period of globalization where the world is trying to be close together.

Due to lack of recent data an attempt is made to analyze the date up to 1998 and there are some gaps in the data presentation due to several factors. The methodology used preparing this paper is both qualitative and quantitative methods where the data is been collected from different reports, books news papers etc. The organization of the paper is as follows: the first part discusses the introduction, colonial legacy of Italy and profile of the country. Second part provides the trends of Itlo-Eritrean trade. Third part deals with the factors that influence the trade between these two nations and the final part provides concluding remarks of the study.

Italo-eritrean Trade

When one talks about trade, the first thing that comes to mind is the external market of this import/export, i.e. the destination. The main influencing factor of export is market. With out market an export is no export at all. Hence it would be more crucial to talk about the direction and destination of the market (Tekeste, 1987; Rena, 2006). However when it comes to Italo-Eritrean import/export activities then one can say it is at its preliminary stage *(For further details see the general trends of Italo-Eritrean trade exchange).*

President Isaias Afwerki visited Italy on 24th November 2003 and held talks with the president of Umbria Province of Italy, Signora Lorenzeti, and the governor of Peruja-Signor Loki, on bilateral and trade relation between the two countries.

Table 1
Import-export between Italy and Eritrea (1993-1997)
(value in millions of lire)

	1993	*1994*	*1995*	*1996*	*1997*	*1998*
Export	23,509	46,140	76,749	129,508	101,664	–
Percentage	96.26%	66.34%	68.74%	–21.50	–100%	–
Import	843	271	2,749	5,673	5,059	–
Percentage	–67.81%	913.29%	106,35%	–10,83%	–100%	–
Balance	22,667	45,869	74,000	123,835	96.606	–

Source: ICE Instituto commercio estro, 1998.

We can also observe from Eritrean trade point of view from 1995 up until 1998 trade was not progressing, as it should be. In fact in the case of 1996 it went dawn when compared with trade that 1995. Export, however it started to pick up in 1998. For further details see the Table 1.

The following Table 3 provides the structure of Italian regional export as from 1994 up until 1998. As indicated below some regions are well connected with Eritrean demands. For example in 1994, three regions from north Italy, Lombardia, Emilia Romagna and Piamonte has exported over 70 per cent of Eritrean demands (E. Romagna 32.9 per cent Lombardia 31 per cent, and Piamonte 11.6 per cent). The structure of Italian regional export (in the series of years from 1994 to 1998) in the northern part of the country has changed slightly. In fact Lombardia has drastically reduced its export from 31.1 to 21.3 per cent (ICE, 1998). These reduction of export implies less growth for export towards Eritrea from the region. Although unexpected high increase (200 per cent) of export has been detected from the region in 1997, however a year later (i.e. in 1998) again slided dawn by 100 per cent. Details are explained in the following Table 3.

Table 2
Trade trends in Italy and Eritrea During the Period 1992-1998

	Eritrea (Value in millions of Naka)			*Italy (Value in billions of lire)*		
Year	*Total exports*	*Total imports*	*The trade balance*	*Exports*	*Imports*	*The trade balance*
1992	(6.1) 46.1	(48.9) 367.1	(42.8) –321.1 (87.4%)	(110) 219.436	(116.1) 232.111	2.8
1993	(27.2) 203.97	(149.2) 1119.13	(122.2) –915.48 (82%)	(133.1) 266.214	(116.5) 232.991	0.4
1994	(52.1) 397.19	(265.7) 1993.15	(212.6) –1595.96 (80%)	(154.2) 308.046	(136.7) 272.382	16.9
1995	(70.5) 528.83	(338.0) 2535.53	(267.4) -2006.70 (79%)	(191.3) 381.172	(167.8) 335.661	23.2
1996	(69.3) 520.43	(408.2) 3062.85	(338.0) -2542.42 (83%)	(195.2) 388885	(160.1) 321.286	-4.3
1997	(50.0) 374.99	(408.1) 3060.33	(358.2) -2687.34 (88%)	(204.1) 409.128	(178.7) 357.587	11.3
1998	-	-	-	(210.1) 420.303	(187.1) 374.213	4.6

Source: Eritrean Figures from the ministry of trade and industry, 1998 and Italian figures are collected from ISTAT, 1998.

Note: 1 US$ is equivalent to 7.50 Eritrean nakfa. 1 USD is Equivalent to 2000 Italian Lire. The figures in bracket are converted currencies in US$.

Italy is one of he main European partners of Eritrea. In fact Eritrean Exports to Italy is nearly 38 per cent of the European share. The above trade exchange between Italy and Eritrea concerns all the regions and provinces. As can be observed in the above table that the highest trade exchange was between 1994 and 1996. Italy has exported to Eritrea items valued 129,508 billion lire. This export is doubled by 101 per cent from the previous year (1995). As far as import is concerned Italy has imported 843,271 billion lire worth of items in 1993, which was the highest in eight years period.

Table 3
Percentage share of Itlo-Eritrean
Regional Export Structure During the Period 1994–1998

	Region	*1994*	*1995*	*1996*	*1997*	*1998*
1.	N. West	45.4	38.7	42.1	74.6	48.2
	Piamonte	11.6	16.9	16.4	9.4	20.2
	Lombardia	31.1	21.3	22.8	64.7	27.0
	Liguria	2.6	0.6	2.9	0.5	1.0
2.	North.East	45.0	36.3	32.9	13.5	31.2
	Trento Alto	1.2	0.0	0.1	0.2	0.3
	Veneto	7.0	6.3	6.9	5.3	10.6
	Friuli Venez.	3.8	0.2	0.6	0.6	3.7
	E. Romagan	32.9	29.7	25.3	7.5	16.6
3.	Central	6.4	18.8	19.4	8.0	13.9
	Toscana	2.0	8.3	13.1	5.6	8.6
	Umbria	1.9	3.6	1.1	0.9	0.6
	Marche	0.6	1.5	0.8	0.3	0.9
	Lazio	2.1	5.3	4.5	1.2	3.8
	Total N. centre	96.9	93.8	94.4	96.1	93.3
4.	Middland	3.1	5.9	5.4	3.4	6.3
	Abruzo	0.2	1.7	0.1	0.3	0.3
	Molize	–	–	0.1	0.1	0.2
	Campania	1.6	3.0	2.6	1.9	3.3
	Puglia	1.3	1.0	2.2	1.0	2.5
	Basilicata	–	0.0	0.2	0.0	0.0
	Calabria	–	0.2	0.2	0.1	0.0
5.	Isles of Italy	0.0	0.3	0.2	0.5	0.4
	Cicilia	0.0	0.2	0.2	0.4	0.4
	Sardegna	–	0.0	0.0	0.0	0.0
	Non specifie	0.0	–	0.0	0.0	0.0
	Total South Italy	3.1	6.2	5.6	3.9	6.7
	Italy	100.0	100.0	100.0	100.0	100.0

Source: ISTAT, Roma Italia, 1999.

Note: The direction of Italo-Eritrean exports can be seen in to two categories: 1. The direction of Erirean trade towards (a) Ethiopian market and (b) the rest of the world. 2. Italian trade towards (a) European market and (b) and the rest of the World. (with all most insignificant trade share to Africa).

Table 4
Exports to Eritrea as from Italian Regions

Sl. No.	*Region*	*Export to Eritrea*	*Percentage change from 1997*
1.	Nord centre	94.858	-23.8
2.	Northwest Italy	49.016	-49.3
3.	Piamonte	20.557	-69.3
4.	Lombardia	27.478	-67.2
5.	Liguria	981	53.8
6.	Northeast Italy	31.737	80.9
7.	Trentino alto edige	305	52.4
8.	Veneto	10.789	57.2
9.	Fruili venezia guilia	3.798	390.3
10.	Emilia romagna	16.845	73.6
11.	Central Italy	14.106	36.8
	Toscana	8.713	21.1
12.	Umbria	642	-44.9
13.	Marche	895	136.0
14.	Lazio	3.855	145.0
15.	Mezogiorno	6.806	34.7
16.	Middland Italy	6.442	44.4
	Abruzzo	328	-9.0
17.	Molise	173	56.0
18.	Campagna	3.381	34.2
19.	Puglia	2.538	88.9
20.	Basilicata	17	-
21.	Calabria	6	-95.7
22.	Isles of Italy	364	-38.4
23.	Sicilia	360	-34.5
24.	Sardegna	4	-89.9
25.	Other unspecified.	-	-
26.	Italy	101.664	-21.5

Source: ICE, 1999.

In the year 1995, trade situation with Italy has improved drastically. For example in 1995, Eritrea exported to Italy goods valued 618,85 million lire in electronics. But after 1995, the picture of trade has changed. By 1998, trade gap narrowed drastically. These happened especially for items like: leather products, textiles and communication and electronics. Italo-Eritrean trade has been going on for ages. But the extent of trade exchange changes from time to time. The type of items of export is much more similar nearly all times. For further details see the following Table 7.

Table 5
Trade by Commodity Section (values in millions of birr)

Item Code	*1995*	*1995*	*1996*	*1996*	*1997*	*1997**
	Export	*Import*	*Export*	*Import*	*Export*	*Import*
0	141.25	426.73	92.42	542.86	46.48	327.85
1	19.75	10.65	26.19	23.51	7.39	10.11
2	156.12	65.91	123.00	116.49	61.27	34.30
3	0.11	48.22	0.25	39.51	0.05	28.22
4	2.16	28.82	2.61	55.01	1.09	35.92
5	12.03	144.20	13.35	209.74	3.89	90.91
6	100.32	478.10	88.29	733.82	37.22	334.08
7	20.19	1,165,95	27.71	1091.14	6.31	560.21
8	76.88	166.94	146.61	250.78	39.80	109.78
Total	528.83	2535.53	520.43	3062.85	203.52	1531.45

Source: Ministry of Trade and Industry various Reports.
Note: *Data for 1997 include only for the first half.
0- food and live animals, 1-beverage and tabaco. 2-crude materials except fuel. 3-Mineral fuel lubricant, related material. 4-animal and vegetable oil. 5-chemicals and related materials. 6-manufactured goods classified chiefly material 7-machinery and transport. 8-miscellaneous manufactured articles.

The two countries have a reasonable trade development in the year 1998 when compared with 1995. In the year 1995, Eritrea barely exported. But 4 years later, Eritrean export performance has improved. If we see the processed and unprocessed leather products (3,670 million lire) and textile products and fish are some of the imported materials to Italy. However, we have also seen Italian exports flourishing to Eritrea especially machinery foodstuff, electrical equipment and communication materials has been some of the main export items to Eritrea (ICE, 1998).

Factors that Influence Italo-eritrean Trade

Eritrea is a war-devastated country, it has a long way to go to achieve to improve the standard of living of its people and establish sustained and strong economy. The economic policy is based on free trade and liberalized policy. It is strategically an important country of East African nations with high potential of natural resources. It became independent in 1991. Therefore, as a new country, it needs to trade with various nations. Italy is placed in a best position to fulfill this gap. When we are talking about trade relationships between the two different countries we are talking about two different economies: the developed economy (Italy) and the non-developed economy (Eritrea). There are certain factors to persuade the Italian export to Eritrea. These factors include: Colonial ties, Commercial relationship between the two countries, Import substitution effect (take over

Table 6
Trade Exchange on Main Products between Italy and Eritrea in 1995
(value in millions of lire)

Item no.	*Export*	*% change*	*Import*	*Balance*
1.	5.559	69.70	0	5.559
2	4.208	421,72	0	4.208
3	3.152	416,00	0	3.152
4.	2.631	238,33	0	2,631
5.	2.306	-42,15	0	2.306
6.	1.872	82.80	0	1.872
7.	1.718	113.40	0	1.718
8.	1.436	493.97	0 –100	1.436
9.	1.304	83,28	0	1.304
10.	1,149	218,28	0	1.149
11.	1,124	64,51	0	1.124
12.	1.073	408,28	0	1.073
13.	1.024	-1.143	0	1.024
14.	976	716,59	0	976
15.	957	99,15	0	957
16.	952	513,57	0	952
17.	938	618,85	15	923
18.	917	569,01	0	917
19.	873	250,40	0	873
20.	800	275,06	0	800

Source: ICE, 1998.

Note: 1-agricultural machineries. 2-cars and motor cycles 3-car spare parts.4-semi processed articles
5-vegetable products. 6-various types of machinerie.7-utensils and other metallic articles.
8-articles of plastic materials. 9-corrugated steel 10-steel construction. 11-machines for construction and mining and metal works. 12-Fiber textile products. 13-tube and steel.
14-Conserved fruit juice and legumes. 15-electrical wires. 16-pram and wheelchairs for children and disabled 17-electronis and Telecom materials.18-petrochemical Products. 19-various electrical materials. 20-Machinery for wood work papers and washing machine.

from Ethiopia), Moral responsibility of Italy towards Eritrea, Primary resources available for trade, The International ports (Assab and Massawa), Geo-economic strategy. For further detail let as see each one of the following factors for trade.

Table 7
Italy-Eritrean Trade-Main Products

Products	*Import*	*Value change*	*Export*	*Value change*	*Balance*
1.	3.679	-29.07	5	-89.22	-3.695
2.	509	165.53	532	-72.70	23
3.	300	244.61	149	-99.73	-151
4.	124	119.28	22	-92.60	104
5.	87	-	-	-	-87
6.	80	-	-	-	-80
7.	73	416.31	1.172	-42.73	1.099
8.	45	-	612	493.73	568
9.	30	-	1.403	-21,88	1.372
10.	19	-	509	-27.72	490
11.	18	-	3.185-	20.96	3.167
12.	17	-	0	-100,00	-17
13.	9	-	583	574	-
14.	9	-	2.101	174.16	2.092
15.	9	-	3.537	52.41	3.528
16.	8	-	0	-	-8
17.	5	-	943	612.75	937
18.	5	32.08	10.616	81.29	10.611
19.	3	-	6.233	48.13	6.229
20.	3	-	11	-81.17	8

Source: ICE, 1999.

Note: Value in millions of lire for the year 1998 and comparison of the previous years.
1. leather and leather products 2-cloth products 3-airspace materials 4-communication and electronics 5-fish products 6-processed leather products 7-Semi processed products 8-office machinery, 9-plastic materials 10-industrial machinery 11-Utensil machinery's 12-wood and wood products. 13-construction materials 14-radio-TV and other electronic equipment 15-finished metal utensils 16-watches 17-electrical materials lamps and electrical apparatus for electricity 18-machinery 19-electrical equipment 20-different articles of wood.

Colonial Trade Ties

Italy has colonized Eritrea for over 50 years. During this period the Italian economic involvement was relatively big in the horn of Africa. The Italian Government embarked Eritrea for control of other colonial powers and to relief its own economic problems. For this reason Italy has invested in Eritrea a considerable amount of money for buildings, infrastructure and institutions. The structure of the Italian colonial economy in Eritrea had two main components one of, which had a lot to do with trade relations in the region. Primarily, usage of the natural resources of the colony, secondly, to develop Eritrea so as to make it an entry pot for transit trade and as a staging post for the economic and political penetration in the horn of Africa.

In the year 1882, Italy seized Eritrea through the Red Sea ports of Assab in 1886 and Massawa in 1889. The plan of Italian government was to transferee Eritrea into a permanent settled colony. By 1941, when Italian colonial occupation ended 70,000 Italians had indeed settled there in Eritrea. Most of them were farmers. History claims between 1893 and 1895 approximately 400,000 hectares was given to the Italians mainly to cash crops destined for European markets. The second phase of the Italians settlers was from 1897 to 1907 in this period further 70,000 hectares was added to the Italian settlers, which made it to be nearly 482,000. Another objective of the Italian settlers was to exploit mineral resources. By the years 1906 1.2 million lire has been spent in mining surveys ((Tekeste, 1987; Mesghena, 1988; Rena, 2006).

Commercial Ties During the Colonial Period

Italians had a laissez fair type of trade doctrine to make Eritrea a center of attraction. And it was successful in doing so. In this respect between 1902 and 1906 the value of imports from Eritrea tripled. This way the extent of trade between Eritrea and Italy had considerably expanded. For further details can be seen in the following Table 8.

Table 8
Trade Relationship between Italy and Eritrea During the Period 1902-1907 (Value in Italian Lire)

Year	*Imports*	*Exports*
1902	1,805,445	2,373,205
1903	1,609,527	2,607,581
1904	4,618,560	3,942,183
1905	4,813,459	4,490,461
1906	5,931,797	9,022,486
1907	3,943,243	5,009,905

*Source:*Mesghena, Yemane (1988) *Op. cit.*, p. 200.

Table 9
Some of the Former Italian Owned Factories

Italian factory	*New Names*	*No. of Employees*
Grazianin Fabrica	Cement Factory	124
Baratolo Fabrica	Textile Factory	1956
Guerra Fabrica	Tiles and Marble Factory	220
Naffi Fabbrica	Printing Press	125
Monopolio Fabrica	Tobacco Factory	63
Malaria Fabrica	Wear Factory	115
Fenili Vino Fabrica	Wine and Liquor Beverage	77

Source: Eritrean Chamber of Commerce, Asmara Eritrea, 1984.

Eritrea has become an Italian trade associate especially in terms of cotton cement and other commodities exported to Italy. For this Italy consolidated its position in Eritrea by building infrastructure and other essential investments in the country. Some of the positive consequence of Italian rule are; the construction of serviceable transportation network and other infrastructures. There is 119 km. Railway road connecting Asmara-Massawa with a considerable engineering complexity. In 1911 a road construction of Asmara - Agordet line with the cost (in 1928) cost of 48,000.000 Lire. Road construction in total Italians built was 3,600 km. Therefore, the changes, which the Italian rulers brought to Eritrea, had a drastic impact. For example, once all most rural population they developed an urban sector (Mesghena, 1988; Rena, 2006). During those years there were many factors owned and run by Italian nationals residing in Eritrea. Therefore, this historical economic cooperation has to continue for the mutual benefit.

The above table refers the new names given by the Eritrean government to those factories. They have also developed factories where the raw materials may be processed for the market in Europe. These factories include textile factory (Baratolo factory) Tobacco factory (Monopolio factory), Tiles and construction factory (Guera factory) Printing factory (Naffi factory) are some of the examples, which were owned by the Italians in Eritrea. Henceforth, the continuity of these factories is crucial to the government of Eritrea, because the machinery and other spare parts to formulate the production process is imported from Italy and mainly operated by the Italians.

Import Substitution (taking over Ethiopian market)

Eritrean exports seemed to have somehow secured and privileged market in Ethiopia until 1997. It was a market being exploited due to more non-economic factors than economic factors. In a sense it is a market which is not so different from domestic market given its proximity, (for example, zero tariff privilege, and the same currency). From 1992 to 1997, the direction of Eritrean exports can be seen from two broad categories (Rena, 2004). These of Ethiopian market and the rest of the world. The Ethiopian market is the market, which involved through time due to a number of factors among which proximity, regional location, social and cultural ties are the major factors. In otherwords, firstly: it is the outcome of the past colonisation and the close social and cultural ties of the people reflected in similar tastes and preferences.

Table 10
Trade Balance Between Eritrea and Ethiopia from 1993 up to half of 1997

Year	*Import from Ethiopia*	*Export to Ethiopia*	*Balance*
1993	63,938,197	123,579,747	+
1994	90,786,808	181,491,011	+
1995	146,820,200	354,298,842	+
1996	261,781,354	342517,024	+
1997 1st half	157,788,261	134,403,694	+

Source: Ministry of Trade and Industry, 1998.

Secondly: the fact that the country is less distant transportation cost, which reduces the overall production cost and thus lower prices of products. Furthermore, Eritrea's trade balances with Ethiopia seen to be positive up to 1997 (see the table above). But after the introduction of Eritrean currency Nakfa on 8th November 1997 the trade between two countries has been deteriorated. At present there is no more trade relations between the two countries. Hence, Italian government has an opportunity to take over the imports and exports opportunities that were held by Ethiopia.

Italy-Eritrea's Biggest European Trading Partner

Large share of imports to Eritrea comes from Italy i.e. 14.1 per cent of the 38 per cent of all products imported from Europe. And 42.1 per cent of all products exported to Europe (i.e. 6.7 per cent) are from Italy. The main export commodities of Eritrea are textiles, footwear, leather goods salt and fish. The main imports of Eritrea are food items machinery and equipment, a petroleum product, and industrial inputs.

Table 11
Eritrean Exports to Italy (Value in nacfa, 1998)

Commodity	*1995*	*1996*	*1997*	*1998*
1	681,760.00	32,493.00	114,427.00	207,014.00
2	288,000,000	1,198,625,00	741,600,00	115,200,00
3	-	-	-	2,440,00
4	12,966,366,00	20,409,429,00	17,303,465,00	10,037,690,00
5	-	600,00	-	-
6	110,00	325,270,00	59,265,00	6,650,00
Total	13,936,236,00	21,966,417,00	18,218,757,00	10,368,994,00

Source: Ministry of Trade and Industry, 1999.
Note: 1. food and live animals. 2-crude materials, inedible except fuel. 3-chemicals and related products. 4-manufactured goods classified chiefly by material. 5-machinery and transport equipment. 6-Miscellaneous manufactured articles.

As from Eritrean figures of trade, the exports to Italy sided from 1.4 billion in 1995 to 1.0 billion. Lack of demand for import machineries and transport equipment may be the main cause for the reduction of exports to Eritrea. These may be is due to the shortage of hard currency in the country.

Table 12
Eritrean Imports from Italy During the Period 1995-1998

Code Number of the Item	*1995*	*1996*	*1997*	*1998*
0	982,009.00	9,587,647,00	14,855,480.00	50,779,721,00
1	520.88520	526,260,00	887,947,00	1,167,510,00
2	5,027,220.00	5,371,985,00	5,681,595,00	4,992,155,00
3	9,505.020.00	1,896,825,00	4,971,735,00	1,116,280,00
4	12,694,163,00	1,338,470,00	1,044,028,00	1,357,160,00
5	17,623,257,00	31,743,738,00	13,482.203,00	11,585,266,00
6	57,671,587,00	68,506,729,00	68,960,455,00	89,826,621,00
7	296,546,040,37	246,868,911,00	269,888,892,00	256,759,850,00
8	26,701,882,00	28,626393,00	35,279,087,00	44,639,794,00
Total	437,272,063.57	394,466,958,00	415,051,422,00	462,224,357,00

Source: Ministry of Trade and Industry (1999) Official Statistics., Asmara, Eritrea.

Note: 0–food and live animals. 1-Beverage and tabacco. 2-crude materials inedible except fuel.
3-mineral fuels lubricants and related materials. 4-animal and vegetable oils fats and waxes. 5-chemicals and related products, N.E.S 6-manufactured goods classified by material.
7-machinery and transport equipment. 8-miscellaneous manufactured materials. 9-total.

Unlike Eritrean exports, trade imports from Italy have been progressing rapidly. For example in 1995, the extent of import was Nacfa 437 million. Although there was a slight diminish in 1996 by Nacfa 394 million in 1997 the figure returned at Nacfa 415 million. The highest import was recorded in 1998 and that was Nacfa 462 million.

However, we have not seen much trade exchange especially in exports to Italy from Eritrea. For example if we see the above table trade exchange between the two countries are limited. Almost 99 per cent was being sent by Italy as can be seen in the table -12. The direction of export by Eritrea was mostly confined to Ethiopia (Ethiopia export to Eritrea 65.8 in 1997). It can be said trade of Eritrea was only confined to limited areas. The table below shows that 80.08 per cent of the exports was limited to African continent. The second biggest exporting partner is North America the third is Europe. In Europe the highest trading partner (6.72 per cent) exports and 38.0 per cent of imports in which 14.4 per cent is from Italy.

Table 13
Direction of Trade with the
Rest of the World-Origin of Exports in 1996

Area	*Percentage value of imports*	*Percentage value of exports*
Africa	16.6	80.08
Europe	38 (14.4% to Italy)	6.72 (42.2% Italy)
North America	2.71	7.66
Asia and Middle East	41	5.52
Ociana	0.08	0.01
Others	1.09	-

Source: Ministry of Trade and Industry (1995), Asmara, Eritrea.

Where as on the other side of the coin if we see the over all total export of Eritrea to Europe is limited. Italy occupies a tiny portion of the total. The reason is; Eritrean export was only confined to Ethiopia (Africa), which holds 80.08 per cent of the total export of Eritrea.

Moral Responsibility

The colonial army was also a common destination for Italy. Thousands of Eritreans were sent to Libya and Somalia to fight along side Italy. In 1938, around 70.000 Eritreans conscripted for Italy against colonial war with Ethiopia. In those years from 1935 to 1936 alone Eritreans simultaneously launched a war to help Italy against Ethiopian forces. In this war hundreds of thousands Eritreans has been killed. The war lasted for 5 years from 1935 to 1941. Therefore, the Italian colony needs to feel moral responsibility on Eritrea and should act accordingly for the benefit of the two nations.

Availability of Primary Resources

The potential exports and imports of Eritrea are varies: The agricultural sector in Eritrea can produce large quantity of products by using modern cultivation and fertilization plant production and harvesting techniques. During the Italian colony, there were many successful large commercial plantations, particularly in the lowlands and eastern side of the country, which produce a wide variety of cash crops like cotton, fruits and vegetables and banana. The main area for potential exports includes cash crops, cotton, salt, sesame, fish tobacco, and fruits and vegetables, flowers, livestock and livestock products. The horticulture project in Gahtelay and Adi Nefas used to run by individual Italian nationals residing in Eritrea is an indication for possible ways of diversifying agricultural export. As far as livestock is concerned, there is variety of them. The highest producing regions are Sahel, Gash Setit and Barka. Nearly 50 per cent of the total goats found in Barka and Sahel. There are around 7 to 8 million herds of sheep, goats and cattle however; there is a need for a modern production method, for higher and competitive standard. If this is done there is no doubt that the total export quantity will increase. Besides, in 1997 a large quantity of sodium chloride, salt foot wear was exported to Italy.

The Ports of Massawa and Assab

As early as 1869 an Italian missionary named Guiseppe Sappeto purchased a small land in the port of Assab. The reason was to house a Rubbiano company. But later by 1882 Italians occupied the whole of Assab and by 1885, the Italians occupied the port of Massawa. By January 1890 Eritrea was declared the colony of Italy (Rena, 2006:40-45).

At present, the ports of Massawa and Assab are the two international ports, which may be found in the Horn of Africa. They are spread along the line of Red Sea coast of nearly 1200 kilometers. The two ports contribute higher income to the national economy. Nearly 96 per cent of the whole country goods come through these two ports. The port of Masssawa serves nearly 90 per cent of incoming goods. Where as the port of Assab used to serve 60 to 70 per cent of Ethiopian goods (before Ethio-Eritrean conflict). These two ports generate 26 per cent of the national income from port revenue. In addition Eritrea has great potential to develop fishery sector. In the past Eritrea, has been selling a high quality and good quantity fish, potential out side the country. Many experts said that the country owns a high quality fish potential. It is found that there are various types and quantities of fisheries in Eritrea.

Geo-economic Strategic Area

It is said long ago the meeting factor of these two countries (Italy and Eritrea) was the strategic position of Eritrea to be able to reach the other parts of the world. Due to its geographical position the nation has served for around 100 years as a trade corridor between the Ethiopian highlands and the commercial center of the Red Sea, the Mediterranean and the Indian Ocean; this contributed to the development and strength of trade relationship in the region. Thus, regional commerce in animal, forest product timber, hides butter, bees, wax, ivory, gold and other precious mineral formed the basis of the regional trade and external trade until the colonial era. It is located on an important Sea route between Europe and Asia. Even before the Suez Canal opened in the mid 19th century, increasing its strategic significance Eritrea attracted the European power. Italy, France and Britain become interested in territories and borders of the Red Sea.

Conclusion

Eritrea has become an Italian trade associate especially in terms of cotton cement and other commodities. Unlike Eritrean exports, trade imports from Italy have been progressing rapidly. Lack of demand for import machineries and transport equipment may be the main cause for the reduction of exports to Eritrea. The agricultural sector in Eritrea can produce large quantity of products by using modern cultivation and fertilization plant production and harvesting techniques.

The port of Masssawa serves nearly 90 per cent of incoming goods. Where as the port of Assab used to serve 60 to 70 per cent of Ethiopian goods. These two ports generate 26 per cent of the national income from port revenue. Due to its geographical position the nation has served for around 100 years as a trade corridor between the Ethiopian highlands and the commercial center of the Red Sea, the Mediterranean and the Indian Ocean; this contributed to the development and strength of trade relationship in the region.

Acknowledgments

The author would like to thank Eritrean Ministry of Trade and Industry and the Institute of Foreign Commerce (ICE) for providing the relevant statistical data.

References

Attilio Celant (1999), *Per Una Geografia del commercio Estro Italiano,* Roma: In Societa Geografica Italiana.

Ethiopian Mapping Authority (1988), National Atlas of Ethiopia, Addis Ababa: Ethiopian Mapping Authority.

Federica Guizzani (1999), *La regione di un confine colloniale. Eritrea", 1898 –1908".* L'Harmattan Italia. "Il politico e la memoria editrice L'harmattan,. Via bava, torino Italia.

Government of Eritrea, Ministry of Trade and Industry various Reports.

ICE (1998), *"Instituto Dell Comercio Estro,"* (Various Statistical Documents).

ISTAT (1998), *"Year Book on Various Statistical Information-1998"* (Various Statistical Documents).

Ministry of Trade and Industry (1998), Various Documents, Asmara: The State of Eritrea.

Rena, Ravinder (2006), A Hand Book on the Eritrean Economy: Problems and Prospects for Development Dar Es Selaam (Tanzania): New Africa Press.

Rena, Ravinder (2005), A Comprehensive History of Eritrea, Asmara (Eritrea): Millennium Publishers.

Rena, Ravinder (2005 22nd October), Some Observations about Eritrea's Trade Linkages, Asmara: Eritrea Profile (A Weekly Bulletin of News and Views) Ministry of Information and Culture, Vol. 12 (65), p. 7.

Tekeste, Negash (1987), Italian Colonialism in Eritrea–1882-1941 Policies, Praxis and Impact, Sweden: Uppsala University.

Trevaskis, G.K.N. (1960), Eritrea: A Colony in Transition, London: Oxford University Press.

UNDP(1996). Human Development Report, UNDP.

UNDP(1997). Human Development Report, UNDP.

UNDP(1999). Human Development Report, UNDP.

UNICEF(1994). Children and Women in Eritrea.

Yemane Mesghinna (1988), Italian Colonialism: A Case Study of Eritrea 1869-1934, Motive, Praxis and Result, Lund (Sweden): Skifter Utgivna av Ekonomisk-historika foreningen i Lund, Vol. LVII.

23

IMPACT OF MICRO-CREDIT AMONG POOR WOMEN IN ERITREA: AN EMPIRICAL STUDY

Shankar Chatterjee

Poverty Ratio in Eritrea

Poverty is a great problem in the developing countries of the world. Eritrea, as a young nation is also not free from high poverty ratio. For determining poverty ratio about its population income criterion has been adopted in Eritrea also. Based on income two categories of poverty for its population has been determined- poor and extreme poor. If income of any person is 240 Nakfa per month that is 240 Nakfa per capita/ month then the person is treated as Below Poverty Line (BPL category) and extreme poverty line, the same is 150 Nakfa. For determination of poverty in Eritrea, National Statistics and Evaluation Office (NSEO) of Government of Eritrea conducted household Living Standards Measurement Survey (LSMS, hence LSMS will be used) in 2003. According to LSMS, 66 per cent of their total population was unable to get sufficient food (calorie terms) vis-à-vis other essential goods and services to lead healthy life. Of the 66 per cent population, 37 per cent were in the category of extreme poor that is they live below the food poverty threshold. It is pertinent to mention here that the Report used the words-"Poor" and "Extreme Poor".

Concentrations of poor are more in urban areas than the rural areas— 64.64 per cent poor in rural areas against 70.32 per cent in urban areas. This may be attributed to the fact that poor have been migrating to urban areas for search of livelihood. Asmara, the capital city of Eritrea is also not free from high poverty ratio as poverty ratio in Asmara is approximately 56 per cent. One noteworthy point of the Report is that, "the proportion of the population that is poor and dependent on food assistance has increased because of the adverse effects of the recent border war and severe drought". Some important findings with respect to women issues are (Source: LSMS and Dimensions of Poverty, NSEO, Eritrea, 2003).

(a) Of the total households of Eritrea, the women headed 30 per cent households. Of the 30 per cent of Women-headed household 18 per cent were widows.

(b) On an average female worker earns less than half of the men.

(c) A majority of the poor rural women earn their income through manual labor particularly through construction works and agriculture.

(d) Women-headed households have comparatively less hold assets including livestock than non-women headed household.

In the present age everyone believes that without the development of women, a nation cannot develop. Participation of women in all the sphere of life enhances their role in development process. Mention may be made here that Fourth World Conference of Women held in Beijing, China in the year 1995, declared that "develop the fullest potential of girls and women of all ages, ensure their full and equal participation in building a better world for all and enhance their role in the development process". It further stated that, "promote women's economic independence, including employment and eradicate the persistent and increasing burden of poverty on women..." The women are as dynamics as men. In many respects their works in numerical term cannot be measured as all the household works they carry are without payment. It is estimated that in addition to work within the household women provide 60 to 80 per cent of agricultural labor in Africa and Asia and around 40 per cent in Latin America (Todaro, 2000).

Table 1
Some Basic Particulars about Eritrea

Sl. No.	*Particulars*	*Data*
1.	Life Expectancy at Birth (2002)	52.7 years
2.	Adult Literacy rate (% ages 15 & above) (2002)	56.7
3.	Combined gross enrolment ratio for primary, secondary & tertiary schools (%) (2001-02)	33
4.	Education Index	0.49
5.	GDP Index	0.36
6.	Population without sustainable access to an improved water source (%) (2000)	54
7.	Children underweight for age (% under 5 years) (1995-2002)	44
8.	Population below income poverty line (%) (1990-2001)	53
9.	Annual population (%) growth rate (1975-2002)	2.4
10.	Urban population (% of total) (2002)	19.5
11.	Per capita GDP (US $) (2003)	190
12.	GDP (% growth–2002-03)	3.0
13.	Per capita GDP (% growth 2002-03)	0.8

Source: Human Development Report 2004, UNDP and World Development Indicators, World Bank, 2005.

The Government of Eritrea is serious to eradicate poverty from the country. Altogether four surveys have been conducted at the initiation of Government of Eritrea in recent years. The objectives of these surveys were to get a through idea about the nature, causes and extent of poverty in Eritrea. Apart from household Living Standards Measurement Survey (LSMS) by National Statistics & Evaluation Office in 2003 (as mentioned already), another survey was conducted in 2003 that is known as Rural Livelihood Security Assessment. The other two are– Participatory Poverty Assessment (PPA) & Second Demographic and Health Survey (EDHS).

After the independence of Eritrea in 1991, the government has initiated from, Savings and Micro Credit Program popularly known as SMCP (hence SMCP will be used). It is the first largest Eritrean micro finance institution under government-owned in terms of both members and amount of credit for eradication of poverty. Economists believe that micro-finance is essentially a process to activate and involve people in the theme of self-help and mutual-help, so that they can manage their livelihoods on sustainable basis. SMCP extends credit to those persons who are basically poor and without access to formal financial services. In fact, in the language of SMCP, the statement is "Bank to the village". That is villagers get their credit in the village itself without any hassle, which this author also has found true during the course of field study.

SMCP extends credit to its beneficiaries (client in SMCP's language, however as a common word beneficiary is used hence forth) under Two tiers– First-tier and Second-tier. First-tier credit is given to the beneficiaries forming groups. The groups, which are formed under First-tier, are known as Solidarity Groups. All the groups are under one umbrella that is known as Village Bank (VB). Under one Village Bank minimum members should be 35 and maximum should be 105.If members exceed more than 105 then another Village Bank (VB-2) has to open in the same village, thus third one will be VB-3 etc. Again from all the members Solidarity Groups are formed. Thus under the umbrella of one Village Bank many Solidarity Groups are formed. Under First-tier a beneficiary can borrow money up to ten cycles that is ten times. After repayment of first loan, second loan may be sanctioned and so on. But all the group members have to repay. In other words no one can be defaulter. In case of First-tier if members of the group repay timely loan then after five cycles individually credit may be sanctioned to each member. Here also all the group members have to repay the loan. This is termed as First-tier B. Both First-tier A & B members are under the control of Village Bank. Three members group-one chairperson (a Government official known as Village Administrator), one secretary and one treasurer (both are selected from the beneficiaries) control Village Bank. The secretary and treasurer get lump sum honorarium. The repayment is made in the village. The treasurer of the Village Bank immediately gives the receipt. On the other hand, Second-tier beneficiaries include individual person. The beneficiaries are under the direct control of SMCP, not under Village Bank. The beneficiaries are given loan only no subsidy is involved here. The Second-tier beneficiaries can borrow up to six times/ six cycles.

Regarding interest payment, it may be mentioned that rate of interest under First-tier is 16 per cent per annum with simple rate of interest. Rate of interest is calculated on the basis of declining method. For example if a person borrows 5000Nakfa (Interest rate is 16% for first installment) and repays 4000 Nakfa then rate of interest will be calculated on 4000 Nakfa, etc. In case of Second-tier beneficiaries albeit rate of interest is 16 per cent but if it is repaid within stipulated time then 2 per cent is refunded to the beneficiary. Thus finally Second-tier beneficiary has to repay 14 per cent interest. The reason is that Second-tier beneficiary is extended much more higher loan amount then the First-tier beneficiary. The cases of beneficiaries studied are presented later on of this article. The Annual Report of SMCP reveals that maximum amount of loan is extended under First-tier (90.8 %) and Second tier accounts only 9.2 per cent. This is a noteworthy point as group lending dominates than individual lending. The Annual Report of SMCP 2005 shows that for last several years' repayment rate was declining but in the year 2005 it went up to around 83 per cent, against 79 per cent. The noteworthy point is that from 1996 onwards more and more women beneficiaries are extended assistance from SMCP. For example, in 1996 under first tier 30 per cent of women beneficiaries (clients) were extended credit, which went up to 40.60 per cent in 2005. Under Second tier although in 1996 no one was extended credit, but in 1997 percentage of women beneficiaries assisted was 14.29 which went up to 37.52 per cent in 2004. That is within a span of eight years, it went up to several times. Percentage of women beneficiaries (clients) covered from 1996 to 2005 may be seen in Table 2

The table reveals that less than a decade women beneficiaries have been greatly benefited by SMCP credit. During 1998 and 1999, due to war normal situation was disturbed so coverage was not high..

Table 2
Percentage of Women Beneficiaries Covered under SMCP Credit

Year	Percentage of Women beneficiaries	
	I-Tier	II-Tier
1996	30.00	-
1997	30.26	14.29
1998	27.62	6.45
1999	29.60	14.29
2000	30.18	29.00
2001	37.00	36.00
2002	40.00	36.00
2003	40.00	39.00
2004	42.60	42.04
2005	*40.60*	*37.52*

Source: SMCP 2005 Annual Report, Asmara, Eritrea.

To get an idea about the impact of SMCP credit, a study was conducted at Anseba zoba (province), headquarters of Anseba namely Keren is located at about 90 kilometers away from Asmara. SMCP has been functioning in this region since its inception. Number of beneficiaries in 2004 was 2697, which was increased to 3839 in 2005.An increase of 42 per cent was observed over a period of one year. With regard to disbursement of credit, a sum of 6.44 Million Nakfa was disbursed in 2004 that was increased to almost 100 per cent in 2005. Thus, it is evident that more and more poor persons have been benefited from SMCP credit. Regarding delivery of credit it may be mentioned that a team of officials consisting of banker, SMCP official and village administrator come to the village and deliver credit in presence of villagers. Thus villagers need not go to the bank or SMCP office to check up their case. This process also prevents corruption (as SMCP officials informed), because everything happens in presence of villagers. For repayment of loan, beneficiaries need not go to bank. Locally a person is recruited to collect the money and immediately receipt is given to the beneficiary.

Economic Activity wise SMCP's Credit

Analysis of economic activity wise credit reveals that out of total loan disbursed (1 July 1996 to 31 December 2004) under

First tier trade and service got top priority as out total disbursement 56.16 per cent share of trade and service was 56.16 per cent, followed by agriculture 42.95 per cent and manufacturing 0.88 per cent. On the other hand, under Second tier share of trade and service was more than 70 per cent (72.74%) of total loan disbursed. Next to it was agriculture (20.47%) and manufacturing (6.79%). This data at the prima facie mean that poor persons are more interested in trade and service than any other activities. Inclination towards the tertiary activity is an indicator of development. Interestingly last eight and half years cost of loan amount has come down. The cost per Nakfa loaned were 21,5, 4.7, 4.5,6, 5.4, 5.2, 8 and 9.6 Nakfa starting from 1996 to 2004. This clearly indicates cost effectiveness and efficiency of the program. To get an in-depth idea about the impact of micro-credit among poor women beneficiaries the study was carried out.

Methodology: The study was conducted in the month of May 2006. As mentioned already study was conducted in Anseba province of Eritrea. For the purpose of the study one village namely Hagaz and one town Keren were visited. Hagaz village is located 25 kilometers further away from Keren. In other words Hagaz is located at about 115 kilometers away from Asmara. Keren is headquarters of Anseba region. So the study is spread over to both in town vis-à-vis in rural areas as a sequel. Altogether 6 women beneficiaries were randomly studied, for which Participatory Rural Appraisal (PRA) method was adopted.

Results: The study has been carried out with the objective of assessing impact of micro-credit among poor women. Beneficiaries were randomly selected and in-depth study was made. The results of the study reveal that poor women with the help of micro credit could change their economic plight. Before the project they had to face economic hardship as a sequel children suffered. After the project the situation completely changed as poor women are not only earning income, but also economically they are self-sufficient, which has given them moral boost. The direct impact of the result is that children have been benefited. The women have proved that they are successful entrepreneurs also. The women are managing a computer center to petty business. It was observed that psychologically they are prepared to face any eventuality. A detailed discussion is made in the following.

Discussions

Both the study area i.e. Hagaz and Keren are having minimum social facilities like electricity, drinking water, health center, high schools etc. Six cases of women beneficiaries are presented covering both the places.

Case-1

Mrs. Tsion of Hagaz village is a beneficiary of SMCP under Second tier. She is around 33 years old person having three children. Thus her total member of family is five. In the year 2005, she was extended an amount of 25,000 Nakfa with this she expanded her grocery business. The activity fetched her good income so within a year she repaid entire loan amount. She was enthusiastic to expand her business. On the day study she informed that she had applied an amount of 40,000 Nakfa as second cycle loan to expand her business. To a query about earning of profit, she revealed that on an average a sum of 5, 000 Nakfa was earned by her.

Case-2

Mrs. Amna of Hagaz village is around 39 years old is a member of self-help group. The group member consists of three women. All are the beneficiaries of First tier. Amna is having only one child. Her husband is a freedom fighter. Along with the group members she was sanctioned an amount of 3000 Nakfa in the year 2005. With this amount she started sheep and goat rearing business. She informed that within a couple of months she would be able to sell some sheep and goats. Thus she was expecting good return from her primary activity. She expressed her happiness for getting the loan fro SMCP.

Case-3

Mrs. Syeeda, a widow of 30 years old of Hagaz village is having 2 children. Her husband died in war. She is the beneficiary of First tier-A. She gets 500 Nakfa per month as pension. With this meager amount she was facing problem to manage her family. She along with another two persons of the village (3 – member group) was extended SMCP credit in the year 2005. She got a loan amount of 3000 Nakfa with which she started grocery business. The business brought joy in her family as she could able to earn 500 Nakfa per month. She happily informed that after repaying the amount the group members would apply for second cycle.

Case-4

Mrs. Rumana of Keren is 26 years old educated woman. She is having two children, besides her husband. She is the beneficiary of Second tier. She had a desire to set up computer typing works etc. as she had undergone training on computer. In 2003 she was extended an amount of 20000 Nakfa as loan from SMCP. With the amount she purchased computer and established her computer shop in Keren town. Motivated with the earning she applied for second cycle loan. She got an amount of 40,000 Nakfa in the year 2005. She expanded her business. On the day of interview she informed that she had two computers and one worker. After making all payments etc, she could able to earn 5000 Nakfa per month. She spends the amount for the welfare of the family.

Case-5

Mrs. Zamila Nagash of Keren is 35 years old woman. She is having only one child so with her husband a small family of three. In the year 2005, she got a loan of 15000 Nakfa as Second-tier beneficiary and with the amount she started hairdressing shop exclusively for ladies in Keren town. She hired a room at a cost of 600 Nakfa per month. She her self manages the shop. With all her effort she could able to earn an amount of 1500 Nakfa per month even after repaying of loan. She is happy with her business and planning to expand it by borrowing second cycle loan immediately after repayment of first loan.

Case-6

Mrs. Luchcha of Keren is a 35 years old woman with husband and eight children. She is a beneficiary of First-tier B, on the day of survey. As a special case she was considered directly as First-tier B category beneficiary. In the year 2003, she was extended a loan amount of 5000 Nakfa. She expanded her grocery shop with this amount. After repayment of first loan, she got an amount of 7000 Nakfa as second cycle loan in the year 2004, which she refunded within the stipulated time. In the year 2005, she was given a sum of 10000 Nakfa. Since she repaid the amount within the time so she got a loan of 13000 Nakfa in 2006. With these entire amounts she expanded her grocery business. Since her family members are more so after using minimum grocery items for her family, she could able to earn a sum of 1000 Nakfa per month.

It is evident from all the cases that all the women except one who were extended SMCP loan were earning income from their respective activities. Many of the beneficiaries even borrowed several times. Only in one case a beneficiary is expected earning from sheep selling. It is hearting to mention that no one have any grievances against officials or members of Village Bank.

A few of the beneficiaries mentioned that rate of interest is comparatively high; otherwise they did not have any other problem.

Conclusion

The study reveals that SMCP credit has brought change in the quality of life of the beneficiaries. Not only economically they are now socially and culturally also advance. They are self-confidence to manage the enterprise. They talk to the people freely even to the outsiders. Whatever extra they are earning spending for the welfare of the family members particularly for the welfare of the children. The greatest security for the family is now "food security". Thus family members feel that they are not having any "no-moon days, all the days are full-moon days." In other words their dark days are over. To quote Rabindranath Tagore, (First Noble Laureate from India in literature) " where the mind is without fear head is held high"

Reference

Eritrea Basic Education Statistics (2001/02), Ministry Education, Eritrea.

Living Standards Measurement Survey (2003), Eritrea.

Savings & Micro Credit Program (2005), Annual Report, Asmara, Eritrea.

Todaro P. Michael, (2000), Economic Development, Addison–Wesley, USA.

24

HUMAN RIGHTS: GENDER DISCRIMINATION AGAINST FEMALE CHILDREN IN NIGERIA

Hakeem Ijaiya

Introduction

Section 42 of the Constitution of the Federal Republic of Nigeria, 1999[1] provides for freedom from discrimination on the grounds of ethnic group, origin, gender, religion, circumstances of birth, disability, or political opinion[2]. Female children in Nigeria are subjected to all forms of gender discrimination such as early marriages, female genital mutilation and other forms of discrimination. Discrimination also affects other groups of children like male children, orphans, street children, disabled children or children born out of wedlock. The paper will discuss gender discrimination against female children in Nigeria and make recommendations on how to solve the problem.

Gender Discrimination

Section 42 (1) (2) of the Constitution of Nigeria makes provision for gender equality among male and female children. But as a result of culture and religious beliefs in the country, female children are often deprived of their fundamental rights to basic education, good nutrition, essential health care and all other basic needs, as well as protection against abuses, neglect, exploitation and slavery. Traditional practices such as early marriages and female genital mutilation are responsible for the discrimination against female children in Nigeria. These traditional practices have negative impact on the reproductive and health rights of the female children in Nigeria. Most of these practices have their roots in long-standing customs of particular communities in the country and they are often formulated ostensibly to achieve particular goals. While some of these practices may have noble goals and premised on sound moral principles[3], they nevertheless have adverse effects not only on the health of female children but their overall status in society[4]. They also have defective medical grounds and validity, understandably because at the time they are formulated and adopted, these communities either did not have access at all to orthodox medical services or these were too remote for them[5].

Early Marriages

One of the traditional practices common to many parts of Nigeria is early or child marriage. It is common in Nigeria to find girls under the age of 12 years been betrothed to adult males. Many pre-pubescent and adolescent girls are given away in marriage without their consent. Although it is a practice in vogue in several parts of the country, it is more prevalent among the Moslems of Northern Nigeria[6]. While the problem associated with child marriage are enormours[7], the existing legal rules have not provided any reasonable assistance in the matter. This is because there is no definite age specified in the relevant enactments as the marriageable age for girls in Nigeria.

The age of marriage is a highly controversial issue and varies from place to place. For instance, in the North West and North Central parts of Nigeria, 14 years is the age of marriage. While in the Northern and Central parts of Nigeria, the age of marriage is between the 2nd and 3rd menstruation, whereas in the Southern part of the country, the marriage age varies from between 16 to 18 years. Section 18 of the Marriage Act[8] allows persons under the age of 21 years to get married, provided that parental consent is given. The Matrimonial Causes Act[9] provides that one of the grounds upon which a marriage shall be void is when "either of the parents is not of marriageable age"[10] it does not go further to define the marriageable age. However, the Child Rights Act[11] attempts to infer the prescription of a marriageable age[12], Section 277 of the Act defines a child as a person under the age of 18 years.

The inconsistencies in the marriage age in Nigeria have negatively affected the rights of the female children. It limits the opportunities for them to accede to education, putting them in a disadvantaged position[13]. 36 million Nigerian female children are not educated.

Early marriage can be detrimental to physical, mental and emotional health. Apart from the fact that it deprives the female children from their rights to have control over their body and reproduction health, it puts them in position of complete dependency from their husband.

In the Northern part of Nigeria, where the majority of female children face the prospect of early marriage, there are reported cases of vesico-vaginal fistula, a condition caused by giving birth when the cervix is not well developed, because the pelvic bones have had insufficient time to develop to cope with child-birth[14]. Corrective operations often require the consent of the spouse, and more often then not the female children are abandoned or divorced by their husbands and ostracized by their communities[15]. 22 per cent of the teenage female children in Nigeria had at least one unwanted pregnancy. This situation is disastrous to the female children because it leads to severe discrimination within their own community or family. They are often punished for being pregnant or are excluded from school. Sociologically, early marriage creates enormous problems for the society. This is because upon the attainments of majority, such girl-wives may realize that they never really married their husbands on the basis of love and this could lead to breakdown of the marriage with the attendant social problems.[16]

Female Genital Mutilation

Female Genital Mutilation (FGM) refers to the surgical operation carried out traditionally on the female genitalia. It is often incorrectly referred to as female circumcision[17]. As Thomas[18] described it,

> Female Genital Mutilation is now a universally accepted term used to describe any interference with natural appearance of the female external genitalia using a blade, knife or any sharp instrument in order to bring about either a reduction in size of the clitoris or a complete removal of the vulva.

The World Health Organization (WHO) adopts a fairly more general definition by stating that:

> Female Genital Mutilation comprises all procedures that involve partial or total removal of the female external genitalia and/or injury to the female genital organs for cultural or any other non-therapeutic[19].

Female Genital Mutilation is practiced in the Southern and Eastern parts of Nigeria. The age of mutilation varies from 3 months to 17 years or just above the first pregnancy. Many female children faces health risks through mutilation, this include, HIV infection due to unhygienic methods that accompany the practice which in itself is a pubic health issue. One distressing feature of this practices is that crude instruments such as razor blades, knives, broken bottles and other sharp objects are mostly used for the operations which are often carried out by aged non-medical persons, intent on sustaining such practices in line with long-standing customs[20]. These instruments are invariably non-sterilized and the operations often carried out in unhygienic conditions with attendant health risks to the victim[21].

A number of reasons have been advanced for the practice of female genital mutilation in Nigeria. Prominent among these, is the belief that it helps to curb promiscuity among females[22]. This is predicated on the assumption that an uncircumcised woman is unduly sexually active which makes her sexual desires uncontrollable. However, not only is there no scientific validation of the assumption, there has not been any proper assessment of the comparative levels of promiscuity between circumcised and uncircumcised females. Indeed, the point must be made that female promiscuity is not necessarily dependent on the condition of the female genitalia but the result of a complex of social factors[23]. These include the social and family background of the female victim, her perception of the socialization process as well as other environmental conditions.

Furthermore, it is also said that the purpose of the exercise is to clean up the female genitalia which, in its naturally state is considered unsightly and dirty and so promote hygiene and provide aesthetic appeal[24]. However, such concern for purity and decency can only be legitimate if it is founded on sound medical reasons, which is manifestly lacking in this case.

In addition, the belief is rife among several communities that circumcision makes for easy and safe delivery of babies. The belief is that the presence of uncircumcised clitoris would greatly interfere with the child delivery process as it is capable of causing serious obstruction to the process. Again, medical evidence completely disproves this assertion as the clitoris is not known to be involved at all in the delivery process, since it has its own patently different function in the female body constitution[25].

The obnoxious practice of female genital mutilation and scarification which have the objective of suppressing female sexuality affect girls physically, psychologically and socially. Physically, the girl is in constant pain and torture, and there is excessive bleeding which sometimes leads to death after the genitals have been mutiliated[26]. At times, infection sets in, either due to the unsterilized instrument used or lack of care of the affected area. Socially, the practice rather than discouraging promiscuity has been the source of increased promiscuity as circumcised female are impelled by the spirit of adventure to have sexual relations with several men all in a bid to gain sexual pleasure[27].

Female genital mutilation has been outlawed in Edo[28], Delta and Cross River States[29] of Nigeria. Also as a result of public enlightenment and mobilization by the Federal Government and its agencies, FGM are diminishing in other states in Nigeria. But the practice of FGM remains widespread in the country and the proportion of the female population having undergone genital mutilation is high.

Other forms of Discrimination

The other forms of discrimination against female children in Nigeria are protection from abuse and access to education.

Protection from Abuse

There is clear disparity in the severity of sanctions for children abuse, depending on both, the age and the gender of the children victim.

In the Northern part of Nigeria for instance Section 216 of the Criminal Code Act[30] States that:

> Any persons who unlawfully and in decency deals with a boy under the age of fourteen years is guilty of a felony, and is liable to imprisonment for seven years

While Section 222 of the Criminal Code Act reads:

> Any person who unlawfully and indecently deals with a girl under the age of sixteen years is guilty of misdemeanor and is liable to imprisonment for two years, with or without caning. If the girl is under the age of thirteen years, he is guilty of a felony and is liable to imprisonment for three years, with or without caning.

Sections 216 and 222 of the Criminal Code Act are discriminatory against female children in Nigeria. The provisions insufficiently define acts of abuse against which female children should be protected.

Access to Education

The percentage of female children attending school in Nigeria compared with male children is very low. This is particularly the situation in the Northern part of Nigeria, where the highest rate of illiteracy (70%) was registered, and while female children attending schools are very few[31]. This is as a result of early child marriage.

Conclusion and Recommendations

Nigeria ratified the Convention on the Rights of the Child (CRC) in 1991 and other international instruments that affects the rights of the children such as the Convention on the Elimination of all Forms of Discrimination against Women (CEDAW), the Convention against Torture and Other Cruel Inhuman or Degrading Treatment or Punishment and the Convention on the Elimination of All Forms of Racial Discrimination. It is also part of the International Convention on Civil and Political Rights and to the International Convention on Economic, Social and Cultural Rights. Further, it signed but did not ratify the Optional Protocol on children in armed conflict and the Optional Protocol on the sale of Children, child prostitution and child pornography and the African Charter on the Rights and Welfare of the Child. But the legislation to implement them, the Child Rights Act (CRA) was first drafted in 1993 and adopted in 2003. The CRA was enacted in only 10 states out of the 36 states of the federation.

Section 14(2) (b) of the Constitution of Nigeria States that "the security and welfare of the people shall be the primary purpose of a government...". It is obligatory on the government to fundamentally pursue the security and welfare of the children at all times. In order to protect the rights of the female children in Nigeria, based on the following recommendations:

(a) The CRC and other international conventions as enshrined in the Child Rights Act must be adopted and implemented in all the states of the federation.

(b) The government must ensure full compliance with the United Nation Convention on the Rights of the Child and the Child Rights Act 2003, which set the marriage age at 18 year.

(c) The government must enact law on Female Genital Mutilation and also carry out a nation wide campaign on the dangers of FGM.

(d) The government should implement policies to eradicate all forms of gender discrimination against female children, including a policy of integration in formal schools.

(e) The government should collaborate with CRC and other specialized international institutions as well as NGOs in establishing, monitoring and implementing a comprehensive programms that would promote the interest of the children.

(f) It is most obvious that the government alone cannot create awareness on the rights of the female children in Nigeria. The burden of creating awareness lies on human rights conscious individuals in various capacities be it academic, press, or organizations such as NGOs and the UN agencies.

(g) Finally, the world's attention should be on the modality for the protection of the rights of the children to help meet their basic needs, and to expand their opportunities to reach their full potentials. Therefore children need to know their rights, so that they can become human rights conscious. Parents needs to know the right of the children in order to control child violation. Government agencies need to know the rights of the children so as to enable them differentiate child rights from child privileges and charity. Legislators too need to know these rights in order to have a reorientation on the rights of the children.

Notes

1. Constitution of the Federal Republic of Nigeria (Promulgation) Decree 1999 No. 24.
2. The general framework within which human rights are protected in Nigeria are enshrined in the Constitution of the Federal Republic of Nigeria, 1999. Chapter IV contains an elaborated Bill of Rights. The rights guaranteed include the right to life (Section 33); the right to personal liberty (Section 35); the right to fair hearing (Section 36) and the right to freedom of movement (Section 41) Section 42 prohibit unjustifiable discrimination on basis of "ethnic group, place of origin, sex, religion or political opinion". As for penal infractions, codes, Nigeria has two seperate one applying to Southern Nigeria (Criminal Code) and one applying to Northern Nigeria (Penal Code). These provide for offences against persons, including homicide, assaults and different kinds of sexual and gender-specific violations such as rape.

3. In some areas, the off-springs of such a union are still ascribed to the late husband and not the biological father, a practice which is in itself repugnant to natural justice, equity and good conscience.
4. For further reading see Ezeilo J. Women and Children's Rights in Nigeria Women's Aid Collective, Enugu, 2001 pp.25-26, Omonubi – Mc Donnell, M. Gender Inequality in Nigeria, Spectrum Books Ltd, Ibadan, 2003 p.8
5. It is on this score that traditional herbal practitioners have held sway in these communities with the veneration of age-long dogmas and beliefs on reproductive and health matters.
6. This is often assumed to be predicated on religious injunction as contained in the Holly Koran.
7. Some of these are social and mental problems.
8. Cap. 218 Chapter 218 Volume XI, Laws of the Federation of Nigeria, 1990.
9. Cap. 220 vol. 8 Laws of the Federation of Nigeria, 1990.
10. Section 3(1) (e) of the Matrimonial cause Act.
11. No. 26 of 2003. This followed on the heels of the UN Convention on the Rights of the Child, 1989.
12. This would be the ordinary assumption since the constitution regards age as crucial to the exercise of the civic responsibility of participating in the political process.
13. According to a NDHS Survey, 19% of girls cited marriage as a reason for leaving school. NDHS, quoted in: Oxfam: Women and Poverty in Nigeria, CRC/C15/Add.61, 30/10/96. Also available under htt://www.unchr.ch/tbs/doc.nsf/(Symbol)/CRC.c.15. Add.61. En? Open Document.
14. UNICEF, quoted in Integrated Regional Information Network (IRIN), Nigeria: Focus on the challenge of enforcing children's rights, November, 2002. Available under htt://www.irinnews.org/print.asp?. Report ID = 30878
15. Oxfam: Women and Poverty in Nigeria, ibid.p.58. Available http://www.irinnews.org/print.asp?. Report ID= 30878.
16. The psychological trauma generated by this condition can better be imagined than seen as this could degenerate to psychiatric problems and other socially unacceptable conditions.

17. This is because the process is in no way comparable to the circumcision of the male organ, where simple circular cut is made to remove the well-defined foreskin alone. However, the various states laws and even some academic writers still refer to it as circumcision, see for example the Cross River State's Girl – Child Marriages and Female Circumcision Law, 2000, Female Circumcision and Genital Mutilations (Prohibition) Law of Edo Sate, 1999 and Rivers State Abolition of Female Genital Mutilations (Prohibition) Laws of Edo State, 1999 and Rivers State Abolition of Female Circumcision Law, No. 2 of 2001.
18. Thomas, I. M. "Female Genital Mutilation as a contradiction of Moral, Medical and Ethical Values being a keynote Address delivered at the National Symposium on Female Genital Mutilation organs by Women's Centre for Peace and Development, (WOPED) at Ikeja, Lagos on 25th May, 2000 extract in WOPED News. Vol. 2 Nos 1 & 2, July, 2000, p. 24
19. The World Health Organization (WHO) is an International Organization that cater for the health and welfare of the children.
20. This is an harmful traditional beliefs.
21. For further reading, see Obiora, L.A. Bridges and Barricades: Rethinking Polemics and Intransigence in Campaign Against Female Circumcision (1975) 47 Case Western Reserve Law Review p. 275.
22. This reason appears to be common in most of the communities and countries where the practice is vague, see Slack, A. T. "Female Circumcision: A Critical Appraisal "Human Rights Quarterly Review Vol. 12 No. 4 (1988) p. 437 at 445.
23. Indeed, some of these other factors can have profound influence on the productivity of females promiscuity; for instance, a girl from a broken home without proper parental care and guidance is more likely to be swayed to promiscuous conduct as she may treasure more, the companion outsiders.
24. Mainly to the men, Nahid Toubia describes such beliefs and practices as part of the global subordination of women, see Toubia, N. "Female Genital Mutilation" in Women Rights Human Rights: International Feminist Perspectives, Peter J.O. Wolper, A (eds) Routledge, Inc. 1995, p. 224 at 236.
25. For further reading see Thomas, I.M op. cit. p. 25.

26. For further reading see Akumadu, T.U. Repudiating Repugnant Customs: The Call to Ban Female Genital Mutilation in Nigeria, Women's Centre For Peace and Development WOPED, 2000 p. 11.
27. For further reading see Akumadu, T.U. Beast of Burden: A study of Women's Legal Status and Reproductive Health Rights in Nigeria, Civil Liberties Organization 1998 p. 39.
28. Edo State of Nigeria took a commendable lead in enacting law against female genital mutilation which is one of the dehumanizing practices in Nigeria, known as Female Circumcision and Genital Mutilations (Prohibition) Law, 1999. Section 4 (a) (b) of the law provides the categories of offenders. These include "any person who offers herself for circumcision or genital mutilation" and "any person who coerces, entices, or induces any person to undergo female circumcision or genital mutilation".
29. River State of Nigeria also enacted the Abolition of Female Circumcision law No. 2 of 2001. Section 2 (2) (a) of the Law makes it an offence for any person to deny any female her right or privilege simply because she refused to be circumcised.
30. Cap. 77 Chapter 77 Laws of the Federation of Nigeria, 1990.
31. Info taken from UNICEF, quoted in Integrated Regional Information Networks (IRIN), Nigeria: Focus on the challenge of enforcing children's rights, November, 2002.

INDEX

Q & R